T0178800

Early Detection and Early Intervention in Developmental Motor Disorders

Clinics in Developmental Medicine

Early Detection and Early Intervention in Developmental Motor Disorders: From Neuroscience to Participation

Edited by
Mijna Hadders-Algra
MD, PhD, University Medical Center Groningen, Developmental Neurology, Groningen, The Netherlands

2021
Mac Keith Press

© 2021 Mac Keith Press

Managing Director: Ann-Marie Halligan
Senior Publishing Manager: Sally Wilkinson
Publishing Co-ordinator: Lucy White

First published in this edition in 2021 by Mac Keith Press
2nd Floor, Rankin Building, 139–143 Bermondsey Street, London, SE1 3UW

British Library Cataloguing-in-Publication data
A catalogue record for this book is available from the British Library

Cover designer: Marten Sealby

ISBN: 978-1-911612-43-8

Typeset by Riverside Publishing Solutions Ltd
Printed by Hobbs the Printers Ltd, Totton, Hampshire, UK

Contents

Author Appointments

Schirin Akhbari Ziegler   PT, PhD, Head of Master Programme for Paediatric Physiotherapy, Zurich University of Applied Sciences ZHAW, School of Health Professions, Institute of Physiotherapy, Winterthur, Switzerland

Margret Buchholz   OT, PhD, Senior lecturer, Senior Occupational Therapist, Specialist in Occupational Therapy, Institute of Neuroscience and Physiology, Sahlgrenska Academy at University of Gothenburg; DART Centre for AAC and AT, Sahlgrenska University Hospital, Gothenburg, Sweden

Debra Field   OT, PhD, Occupational Therapist Sunny Hill Health Centre, Clinical Assistant Professor, University of British Columbia, Vancouver, BC, Canada

Mijna Hadders-Algra   MD, PhD, Professor of Developmental Neurology, University Medical Center Groningen, Beatrix Children's Hospital, Developmental Neurology, Groningen, The Netherlands

Leena Haataja   MD, PhD, Professor of Paediatric Neurology, Helsinki University Hospital and University of Helsinki, Helsinki, Finland

Hayley C Leonard   PhD, Department of Psychological Sciences, School of Psychology, Faculty of Health and Medical Sciences, University of Surrey, Guildford, UK

Roslyn Livingstone   MSc(RS), Occupational Therapist Sunny Hill Health Centre, Investigator BC Children's Hospital Research Institute, Clinical Instructor University of British Columbia, Vancouver, BC, Canada

Annette Majnemer   OT, PhD, Vice Dean, Education, Faculty of Medicine and Health Sciences; Professor, School of Physical & Occupational Therapy, McGill University; Senior Scientist, Research Institute – McGill University Health Centre and the Centre for Interdisciplinary Research in Rehabilitation, Montreal, QC, Canada

Monika Novak-Pavlic   PhD Candidate, PT, MSc, CanChild Centre for Childhood Disability Research, School of Rehabilitation Science, McMaster University, Hamilton ON, Canada

Lindsay Pennington   PhD, Reader in Communication Disorders, Population Health Sciences Institute, Faculty of Medical Sciences, Newcastle University, Newcastle upon Tyne, UK

Peter Rosenbaum   MD, FRCP(C), DSc(HC), Professor of Paediatrics, McMaster University; Canada Research Chair in Childhood Disability 2001–2014; Co-Founder, CanChild Centre for Childhood Disability Research, Hamilton, ON, Canada

Barbara Sargent   PhD, PT, PCS, Assistant Professor of Clinical Physical Therapy, University of Southern California, Division of Biokinesiology and Physical Therapy, Los Angeles, CA, USA

Laurie Snider   OT, PhD, Director and Associate Dean, Faculty of Medicine and Health Sciences; Associate Professor, School of Physical & Occupational Therapy, McGill University; Research Institute-McGill University Health and the Centre for Interdisciplinary Research in Rehabilitation, Montreal, QC, Canada

Alicia Jane Spittle   BPhysio, MPhysio, PhD, Professor of Paediatric Physiotherapy, Department of Physiotherapy, School of Health Sciences University of Melbourne; Victorian Infant Brain Studies, Murdoch Children's Research Institute, Melbourne, Australia

Gunilla Thunberg   Assistant Professor Senior University Hospital Speech Language Pathologist, Lecturer Institute of Neuroscience and Physiology, Sahlgrenska Academy at University of Gothenburg; Dart Centre for AAC and AT, Sahlgrenska University Hospital, Gothenburg, Sweden

Foreword

Developmental motor disorders such as cerebral palsy and developmental coordination disorder are common conditions with consequences for motor function in everyday life, along with comorbidities in many cases. Whilst these conditions occur due to disruption of brain development occurring in early life, historically there have been significant delays in diagnosis and little focus on evidence-based intervention. Thankfully, this situation is changing and so it is the perfect time for this book to emerge.

It has been an absolute pleasure to read and review this book, for two reasons. Firstly, the topic is dear to my heart and until recently was very much neglected, perhaps due to previous rather negative views on the effects of early intervention for developmental motor disorders, and therefore a lack of urgency around early detection. Those who read this book will understand the importance of a shift in viewpoint, as well as the need for and challenges of research in this field. Secondly, my personal education around early detection and early intervention is inextricably linked to Professor Hadders-Algra, through happy times spent at conferences and educational courses in Groningen. Professor Hadders-Algra is a great and supportive teacher as well as the author of many key original research articles in early detection and early intervention. I will never forget sitting in one of her teaching sessions as every single attendee was asked in turn to voice their opinion on a video of an infant's movements, before the correct answer was revealed. There was a quiet and growing confidence in the room as we kept going through this process, that I hope readers can also gain through this book. Links to videos of infant movement are also included here for the reader, and are a real strength, saying much more than even well-chosen words can say alone.

The introductory section of the book already gives a glimpse of the enormity of the challenges faced in early detection and early intervention in the clinic as well as their importance. It also includes a profound personal reflection by the author on disability: 'Why do we characterize persons with a disability by their disability? ... What prevents us from being open to the idea that everybody has different abilities, everybody has strengths and weaknesses?'

The next sections cover neurodevelopment from a neuroanatomical and neurophysiological viewpoint, starting antenatally and continuing through the first two years of life. This is used as the basis for insights into behavioural changes during normal development and how damage to the developing brain restricts and reshapes development. The main focus is on the motor system as the infant progresses from general movements through to increasingly sophisticated voluntary control. However, a whole chapter is devoted to sensory, language, cognitive, and socio-emotional development with an acknowledgement of the rich interconnection between all these domains. This understanding is in my opinion critical to providing high quality early intervention.

The book then covers the general principles of assessment but also specifically the details of the psychomotor properties of assessments and some very practical information about 'how to become an assessor' for each. The last section of the book is devoted to early intervention. It starts by situating intervention within the context of the family, considering the impact on caregivers and how to support them in looking after themselves as well as in nurturing their infant's development. Early intervention in the neonatal period, and in the remaining months of the first two years, are both covered, with discussion of the evidence base and acknowledgement of what is still not known. Intervention is rightly defined broadly and includes the use of environmental modifications such as augmentative and alternative communication and powered mobility. The figures really bring this chapter to life, showing how young children can participate with much enjoyment if appropriate support is provided.

There are some thoughtful concluding remarks, including the following quote about intervention which really resonates with me: 'Each intervention session carries the implicit message that "something is wrong".'

I strongly believe that to support infants with developmental motor disorders and their families, we have to supplement our knowledge with an understanding that there is no right way to be and that we are all in this together, just trying to find the best way through.

So, who should read this book? It chimed personally with both my clinical interest in neurodevelopmental disorders as a consultant paediatric neurologist and my specific research and teaching interests in early detection and intervention as a clinical senior lecturer. I would therefore strongly recommend it to all practitioners working with high-risk infants, including those in the neonatal intensive care unit and paediatric inpatient and community settings. The combination of theoretical and practical information with more philosophical insights would provide value for paediatricians, neonatologists, neurologists, those working in neurodisability, and therapists, and provides a vital standpoint to build on for those wanting to teach and expand the evidence base in this area for the future.

Anna Basu
Clinical Senior Lecturer and Honorary Consultant Paediatric Neurologist,
Population Health Sciences Institute, Newcastle upon Tyne, UK
Director, EI SMART

Preface

This book aims to guide the reader through recent advances in early detection and early intervention in developmental motor disorders. Its subtitle (*From Neuroscience to Participation*) emphasizes that the book's specific goal is to create a knowledge bridge between neurodevelopmental theory and clinical practice. The focus of the book is on early life, that is, on the prenatal period and the first two years after term age. The first 1000 days are characterized by a wealth of dynamic changes in the child's brain and behaviour. These changes are the basis of opportunities for and challenges in early detection and early intervention.

The book's theoretical framework for functioning in daily life is the International Classification of Functioning, Disability and Health, Children & Youth version (ICF-CY). The ICF-CY underscores the fact that quality of life does not only depend upon the presence or absence of impairments. Many factors play a role, including personal and environmental factors. In early life, the major environment is the family. Hence, the book pays ample attention to the family, in particular in the chapter discussing early intervention (Part VI).

Part I consists of two introductory chapters. Part II describes the neurodevelopmental mechanisms in early life. Part III and IV discuss typical and atypical development respectively. Focus is on motor development, but also specific attention is paid to sensory, cognitive, and language development. It is gradually acknowledged that the various developmental areas are tightly linked, with consequences for early intervention. These sections of the book are illustrated by multiple video recordings. Part V is dedicated to early detection of developmental motor disorders. It starts with a chapter that succinctly and clearly explains psychometric properties, whereas the following chapters systematically describe the most commonly used tests (including summarizing tables). Part VI critically discusses the methods of early intervention that are mostly applied and the evidence of their effectiveness. A specific chapter addresses the family and another one assistive devices.

I am grateful that I was allowed to edit and contribute to this multi-author book. It is my way to serve the infants with and at risk of developmental disorders and their families. The collaboration with the other authors was simply a joy – a first-hand privilege to be able to read and discuss their contributions.

I gratefully acknowledge the critical and constructive remarks of colleagues and friends who read the first drafts of the chapters that I wrote: Schirin Akhbari Ziegler; Eva Brogren Carlberg; Bjørg Fallang; Roelof Hadders; Darlene Huisenga; Heike Philippi; Joachim Pietz, Uta Tacke and Ying-Chin Wu. I also thank the parents who allowed me to use images (figures and/or video-recordings) of their infants to illustrate this book. Last, but not least, special thanks to Anneke Kracht for her skillful assistance in the creation of the figures and video-recordings.

Mijna Hadders-Algra
Groningen
December 2020

Video Captions

VIDEOS ACCESS

The videos cited in the book are free to view via the Mac Keith Press website. Contact admin@mackeith.co.uk for more information.

Video 3.1   Primary variability during progression in prone at 11 months CA: variation without adaptation. An 11-month-old boy is able to crawl on hands and knees. He uses a repertoire of combinations of movements in the neck, trunk, shoulders, elbows, wrists, hips, knees, and ankles (variation). His crawling movements do not consist of an automatic selection of efficient movements: he tries out which movements may be performed and when he tries to crawl onto the mattress he almost topples over. The trying out and the toppling event reflect that his crawling movements are not adaptive.

Video 3.2   Secondary variability during progression in prone at 13 months CA: variation with adaptation. A 13-month-old boy is able to crawl on hands and knees. Like the boy in Video 3.1, he also uses a repertoire of combinations of movements in the neck, trunk, shoulders, elbows, wrists, hips, knees, and ankles (variation). However, in contrast to the boy of Video 3.1, this boy immediately selects from his movement repertoire those crawling steps and body movements that suit the situation best. His crawling movements are efficiently adapted to the situation, that is, to the crawling over the mattress and to changes in the direction of crawling. Thus, his crawling movements are varied and adaptive.

Video 3.3   Impaired variation during progression in prone at 9 months CA. A 9-month-old girl uses abdominal crawling for prone locomotion. In her crawling she almost consistently uses the same movement pattern of the left leg, which shows only a few crawling initiatives and is mostly dragged along in a rather extended posture. The rest of the body shows a typical amount of variation.

Video 5.1   Typical preterm GMs in two infants of 34 weeks PMA. A pair of twins of 34 weeks show the typical waxing and waning of GM activity. They also show continuously changing combinations of movement patterns of joints all over the body. The continuous changes refer to the aspect of variation, the changing combinations of patterns in all participating joints refer to the aspect of movement complexity. It is clear that movement complexity and movement variation are tightly intertwined. The trunk is clearly involved in GM activity, as reflected for instance by the relatively high tilts of the pelvis. The movements of infant I are more fluent than those of infant II; nevertheless, the quality of GMs of both infants is entirely within the typical range.

Video 5.2   Typical writing GMs at term age. A 3-week-old term born boy shows writhing GMs. Like the GMs of the infant in Video 5.1, his GMs are characterized by movement complexity and movement variation. The movements illustrate the relatively forceful aspect of writhing. The trunk participates less abundantly in the GMs than during the foetal/preterm phase (see Video 5.1).

Video 5.3   Typical fidgety GMs at 3 months CA. A 3-month-old girl shows typical fidgety GMs. Like the GMs of the infants of Videos 5.1 and 5.2, also her GMs are characterized by movement complexity and movement variation. On top of that, as a modulation of basic GM activity, she shows fidgety movements: tiny, elegant, dancing movements that occur irregularly all over the body.

Video 5.4   Typical head balance at 3 month CA. A 3-month-old girl shows age adequate head balance: she is able to keep the head upright and to rotate the head in any desired direction. Nonetheless, her head balance is not perfect, as still some wobbling movements are present. But this is typical at this age.

Video 5.5   Prereaching at 3 months CA. A 3-month-old boy shows prereaching movements. The expressions of his face clearly indicate that he is interested in the toy. He fixates the toy and in response his arms begin to move, the prereaching movements. These arm movements are not directed to the toy. If the arms would have been directed to the toy his arm movements would have been classified as 'reaching movements'. This boy shows 'flapping movements' as prereaching. See for another example of prereaching movements Video 6.5.

Video 6.1   Sitting behaviour: variation without adaptation. An 8-month-old infant approaches the ability to sit independently. In order to maintain balance, he tries out many combinations of movements of his legs, trunk, and head (variation). He loses balance easily, illustrating that he often is not able to select a pattern that assists balance maintenance (no adaptation).

Video 6.2   Sitting behaviour: variation with adaptation. A 10-month-old infant demonstrates that he – similar to the infant of Video 6.1 – also has a varied repertoire of sitting postures and movements consisting of many combinations of movements of the legs, trunk, and head (variation). His sitting behaviour is adaptive: he easily and efficiently is able to adapt his sitting posture to the playing situation and he does not lose balance.

Video 6.3   Variation with little adaptation during walking. A 14-month-old infant has 4 weeks of walking experience. He shows a typical repertoire of variants of walking, that is, various combinations of ankle, knee, hip, trunk, head, and arm movements (variation). Yet, most of the time he has difficulties selecting the most efficient walking and balancing strategy (little adaptation), which is illustrated by his falls, his irregular steps, and his inability to step on the mattress.

Video 6.4   Variation and adaptation during walking. A 17-month-old girl shows – like the infant of Video 6.3 – a typical varied walking repertoire. But this infant's walking is adaptive: her walking is easy and efficient and the girl promptly adjusts her walking movements to the tasks at hand (changing direction, stepping across the mattress).

Video 6.5   Prereaching movements. A 3-month-old girl looks at the object and moves her arms in response. However, the arms do not move to the object, but to the midline to end in mutual touching of the hands: prereaching. If the arms had moved to the object, the arm movements would have been classified as 'reaching movements'. See Video 5.5 for another variant of prereaching movements.

Video 6.6   Emergence of reaching movements. A 3-month-old girl shows a mix of prereaching movements (flapping arm movements not directed to the object and arm movements that end with mutual touching of the hands, but not of the object) and an occasional reach (i.e. an arm movement directed to and touching the object).

Video 6.7   Variation with little adaptation during reaching. A 6-month-old girl shows a varied repertoire of reaching movements (variation). She is able to get hold of two objects – in each hand one – but she is not able to master the milestone 'is able to grasp and hold three objects'. Most of her reaching movements do not consist of efficient movements that immediately reach the object. In general, the reaching hand does not directly land near or at the object, requesting additional correction movements to get the object: hence little adaptation.

Video 6.8   Variation with adaptation during reaching and grasping. A 15-month-old girl shows a varied repertoire of arm movements during reaching and a varied repertoire of hand and finger movements during grasping. Both the movements of her arms (reaching) and those of her hands (grasping) are efficient and adaptive: the arm movements are efficiently directed to any toy location and the hands are easily adjusted to the type of toy and task. The adaptive quality of her hand movements is also illustrated by the way in which she gently picks the third object with her right index finger while holding two other objects in her hands.

Video 6.9   Shaping of the varied vocal repertoire. An infant aged 3.5 months is in dialogue with her mother. The infant tries to select from her varied infant vowel repertoire the vowels that have adult-like frequency characteristics. The selection is guided by auditory and visual feedback.

Video 7.1   Atypical GMs without fidgety movements at 3 months CA. A 3-month-old boy shows movements with virtually absent movement complexity and variation (definitely abnormal GMs) and without a sign of the typical dance of fidgety movements (absent fidgety movements). He also shows cramped-synchronized movements (i.e. movements in which all body parts move in an *en bloc* synchrony). His GMs and his neuroimaging (periventricular leukomalacia) indicate that he is at very high risk of being diagnosed with CP.

Video 7.2   Mildly abnormal GMs at 3 months CA. A 3-month-old girl shows GMs with moderately reduced movement complexity and variation (mildly abnormal GMs). The reduction in movement complexity and variation is most pronounced in the upper part of the body. The girl shows fidgety movements, but their quality is abnormal. The fidgety movements are not small and elegant, but rather gross and jerky (exaggerated fidgety movements).

Video 7.3   Atypical GMs with fidgety movements at 3 months CA. A 3-month-old girl shows GMs with a marked reduction of movement complexity and variation (poor repertoire GMs, definitely abnormal GMs (see Table 7.1). Nonetheless, she does show fidgety movements all over the body. This means that she is at high risk of a developmental disorder, such as CP or cognitive impairment. Her risk is, however, lower than that of the infant of Video 7.1.

PART I

Introduction

Introduction

Mijna Hadders-Algra

This book provides an overview of early detection and early intervention in developmental motor disorders. Developmental motor disorders are defined as disorders characterized by limitations in mobility due to an altered organization of the brain that had its origin in early life. This definition has two main components. The first component consists of the limitations in mobility. Mobility is the term of the International Classification of Functioning, Disability and Health, Children & Youth version (ICF-CY) to describe activities and participation with a motor component (World Health Organization 2007; Fig. 1.1). Examples are changing and maintaining body position; moving around and walking; and carrying, moving, and handling objects. The second component is the altered organization of the brain originating in early life. The altered organization may consist of a congenital malformation, a prenatal, perinatal, or neonatal lesion of the brain, or a more subtle disruption of the developmental processes occurring in the brain during the prenatal, perinatal, and neonatal period (Hadders-Algra 2018).

So far, so good. However, at an early age it is generally not easy to determine which infant will be diagnosed later with a developmental motor disorder. In clinical practice, the diagnostic trajectory often starts with a careful monitoring of infants who are at high risk for developmental disorders, for instance infants who had been critically ill in the newborn period, such as infants born preterm, or infants with intrauterine growth retardation, hypoxic-ischaemic encephalopathy, a complex congenital heart disease, or a lesion of the brain. It is well known that these infants are at high risk of developmental disorders, including motor disorders (Mercuri and Barnett 2003; De Kieviet et al. 2009; Miller et al. 2016; Van Iersel et al. 2016; Huisenga et al. 2020). But not all high risk infants have an impaired outcome (e.g. about half of the preterm infants have a favourable outcome). In addition, a substantial proportion of children with a developmental disorder has an uneventful prenatal, perinatal, and neonatal history. Part V of this book addresses how we best can detect the infants at high risk for developmental motor disorders.

In older children, two groups fulfil the criteria of developmental motor disorder. First, children with cerebral palsy (CP), who have limited mobility due to a congenital malformation or an early lesion of the brain (see Text Box 1.1). Second, children with developmental coordination disorder (DCD; see Text Box 1.2). Children with DCD also have a limited mobility, but mostly the limitations are less marked than those in children with CP. In the majority of children with DCD, no evident lesion of the brain can be demonstrated. However, neuroimaging studies suggest that the brains of these children exhibit minor alterations in organization (Peters et al. 2013; Wilson et al. 2017; Brown-Lum et al. 2020).

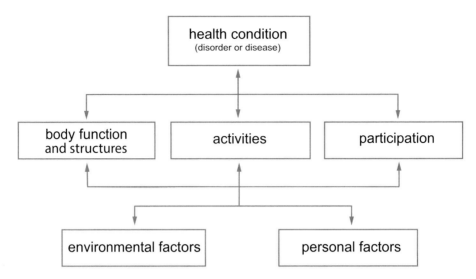

Figure 1.1   Diagram of the ICF-CY. The diagram illustrates the dynamic interactions between the various entities determining a child's health condition and his activities and participation.

Text Box 1.1 Cerebral Palsy

Cerebral palsy has been defined as 'a group of permanent disorders of the development of movement and posture, causing activity limitation, that are attributed to non-progressive disturbances that occurred in the developing foetal or infant brain. The motor disorders of cerebral palsy are often accompanied by disturbances of sensation, perception, cognition, communication, and behaviour, by epilepsy and by secondary musculo-skeletal problems' (Rosenbaum et al. 2007, p. 9).

Rosenbaum (2014) highlighted that:

- The focus of the definition is on limitations in activities and participation and not on impairments in body structure and function.
- CP is a developmental disorder, implying that the permanent disorder originating in early life is characterized by changes in clinical manifestation over the lifetime.
- CP is characterized by heterogeneity in clinical manifestation (i.e. by variation in signs, severity, and co-morbidity).

To cope with the heterogeneity in the manifestation of CP, functional classification systems have been developed to characterize the individual's gross motor function (Gross Motor Function Classification System; GMFCS; Palisano et al. 1997), manual ability (Manual Ability Classification System, MACS; Eliasson et al. 2006), communication (Communication Function Classification System, CFCS; Hidecker et al. 2011), feeding and eating (Eating and Drinking Ability Classification System, EDACS; Sellers et al. 2014), and visual function (Visual Function Classification System, VFCS; Baranello et al. 2020). In addition, the clinical manifestation of CP can be described using the distribution of neurological impairments: spastic CP (unilateral or bilateral), ataxic CP, or dyskinetic CP (Rosenbaum 2014).

Text Box 1.2 Developmental Coordination Disorder

The diagnostic criteria of developmental coordination disorder (DCD) described in the *Diagnostic and Statistical Manual of Mental Disorders*, fifth edition (DSM-5, American Psychiatric Association 2013) are:

A. The acquisition and execution of coordinated motor skills is substantially below that expected given the individual's chronological age and opportunity for skill learning and use. Difficulties are manifested as clumsiness (e.g. dropping or bumping into objects) as well as slowness and inaccuracy of performance of motor skills (e.g. catching an object, using scissors or cutlery, handwriting, riding a bike, or participating in sports).

B. The motor skills deficit in Criterion A significantly and persistently interferes with activities of daily living appropriate to chronological age (e.g. self-care and self-maintenance) and impacts academic/school productivity, prevocational and vocational activities, leisure, and play.

C. Onset of symptoms is in the early developmental period.

D. The motor skills deficits are not better explained by intellectual disability (intellectual development disorder) or visual impairment and are not attributable to a neurological condition affecting movement (e.g. CP, muscular dystrophy, degenerative disorder).

At an early age, children with CP and DCD do not fulfil the diagnostic criteria of their disorders. Due to the substantial developmental changes occurring in the brain during the first postnatal years (see Chapter 3), it takes developmental time before the disorders become fully expressed. Generally, CP is first diagnosed from about the end of the first postnatal year onwards, whereas in some children it may take several years before the clinical picture is established (Smithers-Sheedy et al. 2014; Granild-Jensen et al. 2015). DCD is typically not diagnosed before the age of 5 years (Blank et al. 2019). However, the last version of the *Diagnostic and Statistical Manual of Mental Disorders* (i.e. its fifth edition [DSM-5]) introduced for the diagnosis of DCD the new criterion that the symptoms start in the early developmental period (criterion C, Text Box 1.2). Yet, the evidence supporting this criterion is limited.

Developmental motor disorders are the main theme of the book. It should be realized, however, that developmental disorders usually are not restricted to limitations in one domain. For instance, limitations in mobility are often accompanied by limitations in learning and communication. Two major factors explain the high rate of limitations in multiple domains: (1) adversities that interfere with early brain development generally do not affect single functional systems; (2) the high degree of interrelation between development in the various domains. For instance, limited mobility hampers the infant's discovery of the world, which, in turn, negatively impacts cognitive development and, vice versa, limitations in learning (e.g. in exploratory drive) interfere with motor development.

The book zooms in on the prenatal period and the first 2 years post-term – the first 1000 days of life. It uses the ICF-CY as framework of reference. The ICF-CY emphasizes that activities and participation in daily life do not only depend on body function and structure, but also environmental and personal factors (Fig. 1.1). What the latter may imply is recounted in the reflections on disability presented in Text Box 1.3. The book starts with the clinical picture of early detection and early intervention. Next, in Part II, the neurodevelopmental mechanisms occurring in early life are discussed, including vulnerability and plasticity. Part III comprises chapters on typical development. It not only discusses motor development but also sensory and cognitive development. It is increasingly recognized that motor development is strongly interrelated with developmental changes in other brain functions (Diamond 2000). The strong interrelation explains why children with developmental motor disorders often have comorbid disorders, such as learning disorder, autism spectrum disorder, and attention deficit and hyperactivity disorder (Novak et al.

Text Box 1.3 Reflections About Disability – A Personal Point of View

- *Disability or different abilities?* Why do we characterize persons with a disability by their disability? Is it because the disability is frequently quite visible? Are we scared by this view as the disability confronts us with the vulnerability of human existence? What prevents us from being open to the idea that everybody has different abilities, everybody has strengths and weaknesses? Isn't being able to share a smile when the sun warms the skin and the wind strokes the hair equally valuable as being able to write a chapter?
- *Walking or wheeling?* Families and professionals often choose as a major goal of early intervention the achievement of the ability to walk (independently). Of course, I won't deny that it is convenient to be able to walk without help. However, when the walking costs an enormous effort, it is perhaps better to skip this activity and save the energy for communication, other forms of social interaction, learning and applying knowledge. I learnt this well from personal experience. I acquired a partial spinal cord lesion at the age of 16 years. The physicians doubted whether I would be able to walk again. However, being somewhat on the hyperactive side of the spectrum, I massively practised and regained the ability to walk. Over time, the walking deteriorated and I realized how much upright stance and walking interfered with communication and cognitive function. When I started to use the wheelchair, I 'regained my brain'.
- *Interdependency.* Disability is associated with dependency (i.e. a condition that is the opposite of autonomy and independency that are advocated as ultimate goals for individuals in Western industrialized societies). Actually, I think, that the Western societies can learn from other societies, such as the Asian and African societies that focus more on interdependency (Nisbett and Miyamoto, 2005). These societies acknowledge more than the Western that humans are social beings, with a brain that is totally tuned to interaction with others (Chen et al. 2018). The interdependency implies that all humans depend on other human beings. In general, we consider it as typical that we depend on the pilot of an aircraft when we fly, or on the employees of a supermarket when we go shopping, but we feel embarrassed by the idea that we might need assistance when visiting the bathroom. Again, from personal experience, dependency in this situation does not differ from that in the other ones. You just get confirmation that the large majority of fellow humans are friendly and respectful, and that humans indeed are social beings.
- *Assistive devices.* Families and professionals may have a negative view on assistive devices, as they underline that the infant has specific impairments or limitations. But we perhaps should try to root out this view, as assistive devices are meant to do what their name tells: to assist, to make life easier. It is interesting to consider the change over the last five decades in the perception of the visual assistive device 'glasses'. Fifty years ago, wearing glasses was regarded as negative; children with glasses were called names and bullied. However, nowadays glasses have an entirely positive aura; they are part of fashion and used to express a person's identity.

2012; Blank et al. 2019). Part IV discusses atypical motor development. After the preparatory chapters of Parts I to IV, the heart of the matter follows: Part V provides an overview of the methods available for early detection, and Part VI summarizes early intervention methods, including their evidence on effectiveness. Special attention is paid to the family (Chapter 12) and environmental adaptations (Chapter 15).

Finally, two practical remarks. First, the infant ages used in this manual always refer to ages corrected for preterm birth, unless otherwise indicated (e.g. foetal ages and gestational ages of preterm infants). This is not further indicated in the text. Second, writing about individuals who may be male or female gives an author the awkward choice of consistent referral to all gender typologies by using expressions such as he/she, or the selection of a specific gender. The latter results in a text that is easier to read, but this option has the disadvantage that an impression of 'neglect' of other gender identities occurs. We opted for a single gender option to facilitate readability, and choose the female gender when referring to the professional and the male gender when referring to the child. However, we would like to stress our gender-neutral intentions.

REFERENCES

American Psychiatric Association (2013) *Diagnostic and Statistical Manual of Mental Disorders*, 5th edn. Washington DC: American Psychiatric Association.

Baranello G, Signorini S, Tinelli F, et al. (2020) Visual Function Classification System for children with cerebral palsy. *Dev Med Child Neurol* **62**: 104–110. doi: 10.1111/dmcn.14270.

Blank R, Barnett AL, Cairney J, et al. (2019) International clinical practice recommendations on the definition, diagnosis, assessment, intervention, and psychosocial aspects of developmental coordination disorder. *Dev Med Child Neurol* **61**: 242–285. doi: 10.1111/dmcn.14132.

Brown-Lum M, Izadi-Najafabadi S, Oberlander TF, Rauscher A, Zwicker JG (2020) Differences in white matter microstructure among children with developmental coordination disorder. *JAMA Netw Open* **3**: e201184. doi: 10.1001/jamanetworkopen.2020.1184.

Chen C, Martínez RM, Cheng Y (2018) The developmental origins of the social brain: empathy, morality and justice. *Front Psychol* **9**: 2584. doi: 10.3389/fpsyg.2018.02584.

De Kieviet JF, Piek JP, Aarnoudse-Moens CS, Oosterlaan J (2009) Motor development in very preterm and very low-birth-weight children from birth to adolescence: a meta-analysis. *JAMA* **302**: 2235–2242. doi: 10.1001/jama.2009.1708.

Diamond A (2000) Close interrelation of motor development and cognitive development and of the cerebellum and prefrontal cortex. *Child Dev* **71**: 44–56.

Eliasson AC, Krumlinde-Sundholm L, Rösblad B, et al. (2006) The Manual Ability Classification System (MACS) for children with cerebral palsy: scale development and evidence of validity and reliability. *Dev Med Child Neurol* **48**: 549–554.

Granild-Jensen JB, Rackauskaite G, Flachs EM, Uldall P (2015) Predictors for early diagnosis of cerebral palsy from national registry data. *Dev Med Child Neurol* **57**: 931–935. doi: 10.1111/dmcn.12760.

Hadders-Algra M (2018) Early human brain development: starring the subplate. *Neurosci Biobehav Res* **92**: 276–290. doi: 10.1016/j.neubiorev.2018.06.017.

Hidecker MJ, Paneth N, Rosenbaum PL, et al. (2011) Developing and validating the Communication Function Classification System for individuals with cerebral palsy. *Dev Med Child Neurol* **53**: 704–710. doi: 10.1111/j.1469-8749.2011.03996.x.

Huisenga D, La Bastide-Van Gemert S, Van Bergen A, Sweeney J, Hadders-Algra M (2020) Developmental outcomes after early surgery for complex congenital heart disease: a systematic review and meta-analysis. *Dev Med Child Neurol*, Epub ahead of print. doi: 10.1111/dmcn.14512.

Mercuri E, Barnett AL (2003) Neonatal brain MRI and motor outcome at school age in children with neonatal encephalopathy: a review of personal experience. *Neural Plast* **10**: 51–57.

Miller SL, Huppi PS, Mallard C (2016) The consequences of fetal growth restriction on brain structure and neurodevelopmental outcome. *J Physiol* **594**: 807–823. doi: 10.1113/JP271402.

Nisbett RE, Miyamoto Y (2005) The influence of culture: holistic versus analytic perception. *Trends Cogn Sci* **5**: 467–473.

Novak I, Hines M, Goldsmith S, Barclay R (2012) Clinical prognostic messages from a systematic review on cerebral palsy. *Pediatrics* **130**: e1285–1312. doi: 10.1542/peds.2012-0924.

Palisano R, Rosenbaum P, Walter S, Russell D, Wood E, Galuppi B (1997) Development and reliability of a system to classify gross motor function in children with cerebral palsy. *Dev Med Child Neurol* **39**: 214–223.

Peters LH, Maathuis CG, Hadders-Algra M (2013) Neural correlates of developmental coordination disorder. *Dev Med Child Neurol* **55** (Suppl 4): 59–64. doi: 10.1111/dmcn.12309.

Rosenbaum P (2014) Definition and clinical classification. In: Dan B, Mayston M, Paneth N, Rosenbloom L, editors, *Cerebral Palsy: Science and Clinical Practice.* London: Mac Keith Press, pp. 17–26.

Rosenbaum P, Paneth N, Leviton A, et al. (2007) A report: the definition and classification of cerebral palsy, April 2006. *Dev Med Child Neurol* **49** (Suppl 2) 8–14.

Sellers D, Mandy A, Pennington L, Hankins M, Morris C (2014) Development and reliability of a system to classify the eating and drinking ability of people with cerebral palsy. *Dev Med Child Neurol* **56**: 245–251. doi: 10.1111/dmcn.12352.

Smithers-Sheedy H, Badawi N, Blair E (2014) What constitutes cerebral palsy in the twenty-first century? *Dev Med Child Neurol* **56**: 323–328. doi: 10.1111/dmcn.12262.

Van Iersel PA, Algra AM, Bakker SC, Jonker AJ, Hadders-Algra M (2016) Limitations in the activity of mobility at age 6 years after difficult birth at term: prospective cohort study. *Phys Ther* **96**: 1225–1233. doi: 10.2522/ptj.20150201.

Wilson PH, Smits-Engelsman B, Caeyenberghs K, et al. (2017) Cognitive and neuroimaging findings in developmental coordination disorder: new insights from a systematic review of recent research. *Dev Med Child Neurol* **59**: 1117–1129. doi: 10.1111/dmcn.13530.

World Health Organization (2007) *International Classification of Functioning, Disability and Health, Children & Youth Version (ICF-CY)*. Geneva: WHO Press.

SUGGESTIONS FOR FURTHER READING

Dan B, Mayston M, Paneth N, Rosenbloom L (2014) Cerebral Palsy: Science and Clinical Practice. London: Mac Keith Press.

Graham HK, Rosenbaum P, Paneth N, et al. (2016) Cerebral palsy. Nat Rev Dis Primers **2**: 15082. doi: 10.1038/nrdp.2015.82.

Early Diagnosis and Early Intervention in the Clinic

Leena Haataja

SUMMARY POINTS

- The age at which typically developing infants attain various milestones varies widely. This makes early diagnostics of developmental disorders into a challenging task.
- The use of formal developmental screening tools and validated neuromotor and neurological examination tools improves early identification of motor disorders.
- Early clinical signs of cerebral palsy (CP) are not unequivocally specific for CP. Instead, these signs are manifestations of any injury, disorder, or dysfunction of the central nervous system.
- Early detection of CP is based on a combination of detailed patient history, validated neurological examination, or neuromotor assessment and brain imaging.
- Consider the possibility of an alternative condition mimicking CP if the clinical presentation and/or history is unusual and/or neuroimaging is negative.
- Early intervention in infants with or at high risk of CP is associated with short term better outcomes in child and family. No evidence is available on the long term effects of early intervention in children with CP.

Early detection and intervention are clinically relevant for infants who are at high risk of a developmental disorder. There is no internationally agreed consensus definition of the 'high-risk' of infants but expert recommendations are available (https://newborn-health-standards.org/). It is agreed that preterm children born <32 weeks of gestation have a higher risk of developmental disorders than infants born at later gestation. Also, infants who are born at or after 32^{+0} gestation and have one or more significant risk factors are regarded as being at high risk of long-term disability. Examples of significant risk factors are brain injuries verified with neuroimaging, such as grade III intraventricular haemorrhage and venous infarction, hypoxic ischaemic encephalopathy grade II/III, neonatal sepsis or meningitis, foetal growth restriction or being born small for gestational age, and severe social or other serious family problems exposing child to the risk of deprivation and violence.

Early detection of developmental problems relies on a combination of detailed patient history, developmental assessment, structured and validated neurological examination or neuromotor assessment, brain imaging, and further aetiological investigations (e.g. neurophysiological or genetic investigations) when appropriate for differential diagnostics. Delay in early motor development is often the decisive feature leading to further investigations, but the delay itself doesn't provide direct aetiological support for neurological diagnostics (e.g. for CP). Therefore, a neurological examination is needed. This examination aims to delineate objective neurological findings that correlate with the neuroanatomy of the possible lesion of the central nervous system. Accordingly, the neurological assessment furnishes relevant information for differential diagnostics and future prediction in the clinical context.

Irrespective of the applied methods of neurological and neurodevelopmental examination, specific features of the rapidly developing young nervous system must be recognized as an integral part of the diagnostic process. Accordingly, in most situations longitudinal follow-up examinations are required to comprehend the evolution of the neurological, cognitive, and behavioural findings in an infant.

The major developmental motor disorders in childhood are CP and developmental coordination disorder (DCD). CP has prevalence of two cases per 1000 livebirths in high-income countries (Himmelmann and Uvebrant 2014), though the prevalence is presumably higher in low-income countries. DCD is the most common non-CP motor disorder in childhood with prevalence estimates of 5–6% (Blank et al. 2019). Both in CP and DCD, motor problems interfere with independent age-appropriate activities of daily living and participation. A male predominance is a constant finding across studies both in CP and DCD, and the risk of developing CP or DCD is higher the lower the gestational age at birth is (Sellier et al. 2015; Blank et al. 2019). In contrast to CP, the formal diagnosis of DCD under the age of 5 years is recommended only in cases of severe impairment since young children with motor delay may show spontaneous catch-up. Also the young child's collaboration and motivation to perform functional tests may cause problems in interpretation and reliability of the diagnostics (Blank et al. 2019).

The current chapter focuses on CP since the clinics of CP during the first two postnatal years well illustrate the possibilities and challenges of early diagnostics and early intervention. First, the definition, clinical spectrum, and classification of CP is discussed. The second section addresses clinical practice with the use of evidence-based examinations aiming at early identification of high risk of CP and diagnostics. In the third section, the role of brain imaging as a part of clinical workup of early diagnostics is discussed. The last section addresses the accumulating research evidence on early intervention and its application to clinical settings at present. However, before we move to these sections, we first meet Mesi. Mesi's history illustrates the challenges and possibilities in early detection and early intervention. In Mesi's history the family plays a large role. However, more recently, the role of the family has increased even more, emphasizing the role of family autonomy (see Chapters 12–14).

CASE HISTORY: MESI

'She is three years of age and she is such a joyful little girl!' said Mesi's mum today on the phone. Things were very different when Mesi was born from a twin pregnancy at 26+1 weeks of gestation, 4 weeks after premature rupture of membranes ending with chorioamnionitis. Her size was appropriate for gestational age (birth weight 760g), but she was born in a very poor condition with Apgar scores of 1/1/1 (at 1, 5, and 10 minutes). Immediately after birth, she developed severe hypoventilation problems, so severe that her survival was questioned. The first cranial ultrasound did not show any definite abnormalities, but at 2 weeks of age intraventricular haemorrhage grade I was seen on the right side and a venous infarction on the left side. She did not develop hydrocephalus and she did not have any seizures. Due to severe bronchopulmonary dysplasia (BPD), it was impossible to take a brain magnetic resonance imaging (MRI). Mesi developed stage I retinopathy of prematurity that did not require treatment. At the age of 3 months corrected age (CA), she was discharged from the hospital with an oxygen concentrator that she continued to need during the following 3 months.

During her stay in the neonatal ward, Mesi received physiotherapy once a week that aimed to enhance her tolerance to sensory stimuli and to balance her increased extensor tone and tendencies to asymmetry. The parents and responsible nurses took part in the therapy sessions, so that the intervention strategies could be integrated in the daily care-giving activities. When Mesi was discharged from the hospital, the parents received additional advice on how to take care of their daughter in the light of her increased extensor tone.

Mesi was seen by the paediatric neurologist for the first time at 6 weeks of CA. She performed the Hammersmith Neonatal Neurological Examination (HNNE). It revealed that Mesi had poor asymmetric visual orientation and that her spontaneous movements showed little variation and were jerky. She also had axial hypotonia and asymmetry in limb tone between left and right.

At 3 months of CA, Mesi had improved in her social eye contact and her extensor tone had decreased. Her Hammersmith Infant Neurological Examination (HINE) showed a global score of 33/78 indicating a high risk of CP. However, it was obvious that her extreme BPD affected her performance and, accordingly, the HINE scores attained. The General Movement Assessment revealed movements with little variation and no fidgety movements. In line with guidelines of the University Hospital of Helsinki, Mesi was recommended a weekly physiotherapy session at home with at least one of the parents present during the session. Physiotherapy was paid for by the hospital. As a part of regional practice, parents were given instructions on how to perform individualized exercise and stimulation with Mesi between therapy sessions. At 5 months of CA, Mesi obtained the official diagnosis of CP (ICD-10 G80.9). Her right limbs were clearly spastic, but also the tone in her left leg was atypical; it showed varying muscle tone. The trunk was very hypotonic; posture control and goal directed movements were impaired. In addition to physiotherapy sessions, now provided twice a week at home, she received adaptive seating to enhance eye–hand coordination and feeding.

At 8 months CA, Mesi had learnt to turn around and at 12 months CA she had reached the developmental stages of crawling, stable sitting, and standing with support. The X-ray of the hips indicated typical development. She was walking independently at 15 months CA.

At 3 years, an asymmetry in walking is seen, mainly manifested by a less active dorsiflexion of the right ankle. During 'running' the unilateral problem becomes more evident; it is more challenging to maintain balance and stereotyped posturing and tone in the right limbs increases. Her diagnosis is set as a spastic hemiplegia (G80.2) and her GMFCS level is II. She is keen on practising and participating in age-appropriate physical activities (e.g. riding a push-bike is one of her present favourites). She uses her left hand age-appropriately, but she manages many daily tasks, like eating independently, also with the right hand or bimanually. Her communication skills are in the typical range for her age. At 2 years she started in day care (inclusive policy) and the physiotherapy, which is paid by the National Social Insurance Institution, continues once a week either in the day care or at home. At present, the most difficult problems are the presence of sensory over-reactivity in the right upper limb and fatigue in busy social situations. The clinical follow-up continues in the multidisciplinary paediatric rehabilitation unit in the children's hospital.

Mesi's parents are overtly happy with their active, persistent, and cheerful daughter. Mesi's development has been much more favourable than anyone had expected. It is impossible to know which factors contributed most to her outcome. However, we know for sure that her parents took care that Mesi practised every day and that her parents have a remarkable sensitivity, which they used to let Mesi discover her own activities and her own world. This, most likely, has already made her an actor in her own life.

CEREBRAL PALSY

Definition

CP is defined as a group of disorders of the development of movement and posture, causing activity limitation, that are attributed to non-progressive disturbances that occurred in the developing foetal or infant brain (Rosenbaum et al. 2007). In addition, CP is often accompanied by comorbidities like disturbances of sensation, hearing and visual deficits, communication and learning problems, intellectual disability, epilepsy, and behavioural and skeletal problems. The description of CP highlights its true clinical challenge: its large heterogeneity in phenotype. In addition to the fact that every child is a unique individual, every child with CP is different.

To date, various risk factors – in isolation or in additive or interactive combination – have been reported for CP (see Chapter 3). Nonetheless, the mechanisms leading to CP are currently not well understood. The clinical impression is that the aetiology of CP acts more as a vicious circle of multifactorial negative incidents than as a single incident.

Classification

The classical way to describe CP is based on its topographic features (i.e. the parts of the body involved in CP). Accordingly, hemiplegia refers to functional impairment dominating in one side of body and diplegia refers to the predominance of functional limitation in both legs. When all four limbs are affected equally, the condition is called either quadriplegia or tetraplegia. In clinical practice, topographical description is challenging since there is no definite objective measure to define, for instance, at what point diplegia changes into quadriplegia. The Surveillance of Cerebral Palsy in Europe (SCPE) has provided an alternative way to classify CP: it classifies CP into unilateral (one side of body) or bilateral (both sides of body) CP. According to the Australian Cerebral Palsy Register Report, unilateral CP covers 38% of all children with CP, whereas bilateral CP, including diplegia and quadriplegia, covers 37% and 24%, respectively (ACPR Group 2013).

In addition to the topographic definition of CP, the predominant features of the motor impairment are classified. The SCPE expert group has recommended using the following CP sub-types: spastic CP, dyskinetic CP (including both dystonic and choreo-athetotic types), ataxic CP, and non-classifiable CP (Cans 2000). The majority of children with CP have the predominantly spastic types (86%; ACPR Group 2013). In the dyskinetic and ataxic sub-types, signs of spasticity may also be present. If there is a combination of clinical findings of both spasticity and dyskinesia or ataxia, SCPE recommends classifying the type of CP according to the dominant clinical feature. In young children (i.e. children younger than 2 years of age), it may be difficult to define the type of CP. Therefore, best practice is to communicate this difficulty with the family and leave the type first as 'non-classified' until the type becomes clear with increasing age. The definitions of different subtypes (Table 2.1) and the hierarchical classification tree of CP subtypes shown in Figure 2.1 are good clinical guides (Cans 2000). The advantage of using the SCPE classification is that it allows for harmonization of diagnostic criteria both at local and national level. Such harmonization is the base for benchmarking the quality of diagnostic processes, national or international CP registers, and intervention trials.

In clinical practice, the use of classifications is hampered by two problems. The first problem is that the phenotype of CP evolves over time due to physical growth, overall development, and interventions. The changing phenotype interferes with the classification of the sub-types of CP. The second problem is that the topographic classification of CP, not the SCPE classification, form the defining criteria in the

Table 2.1 Definitions of sub-types of cerebral palsy (modified from the Surveillance of Cerebral Palsy in Europe; Cans 2000)

Spastic CP (minimum two criteria)

    – abnormal pattern of posture and/or movement pattern

    – increased tone

    – brisk/clonic tendon reflexes and/or positive Babinski response

Dyskinetic CP

    – abnormal pattern of posture and/or movement pattern

    – abnormal repetitive involuntary movements

       Dystonic CP comprises two different stages:

       *hypokinesia (e.g. stiff, passive motion)

       *hypertonia, rigid posturing

       Choreoathetoid CP comprises two different stages:

       *hyperkinesia (excessive rapid, jerky movements)

       *hypotonia

Ataxic CP

    – **both** abnormal posture and/or movement pattern

    – **and** abnormal movement co-ordination (strength, accuracy)

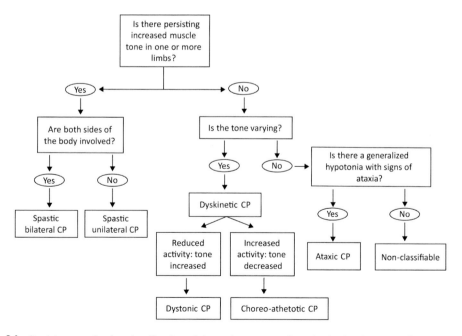

Figure 2.1 Decision tree for the classification of the various types of cerebral palsy (based on Cans 2000).

International Classification of Diseases (WHO ICD-10). It is this ICD-10 classification that many hospitals are obliged to use as a source for codes of diagnosis in official patient records, therewith hampering the widespread use of the SCPE classification.

The type of CP is not equal to the functional performance of a child with CP even though this is often used as an approximate of the child's performance. In addition to disclosing the type of CP, it is also important to tell parents that the majority of children with CP will walk either independently or with aids. The communication on the child's gross motor potentials is facilitated by the use of two tools: the Gross Motor Function Measure (GMFM) and the Gross Motor Function Classification System (GMFCS). The GMFM is used to evaluate change in the gross motor function over time in children with CP (available at www.canchild.ca). The GMFCS addresses the severity of mobility limitations (Palisano et al. 1997). It describes performance of children with CP in five distinct levels. The evolution of gross motor function by age has been integrated into the classification criteria by age bands (criteria before 2nd birthday, between 2nd and 4th birthday, between 4th and 6th birthday, between 6th and 12th birthday and between 12th and 18th birthday) (available at www.canchild.ca). In children older than 2 years, the GMFCS has shown to be relatively stable over time. Yet, in children younger than 2 years who have been classified according to the GMFCS, about 40% of the children change classification level when they grow older, with the majority moving to a less functional level (Gorter et al. 2009).

The GMFCS has been the foundation model for other functional classification systems, of which the most widely used are the Manual Ability Classification System (MACS), the Communication Function Classification System (CFCS), the Eating and Drinking Ability Classification System (EDACS), and Visual Function Classification System (VFCS) (see Chapter 8).

EARLY IDENTIFICATION OF CEREBRAL PALSY

Early Clinical Signs of CP

In the neonatal period and in early infancy, the clinical signs of developmental motor disorders are often very unspecific. In addition, the behavioural state and the somatic stability of the infant should be taken into account when performing a neonatal or infant neurological examination, especially during the first year of life. If the infant is unstable, hungry, in pain, or crying constantly, reliability of neurological findings is questionable and findings should be interpreted with caution.

Early clinical signs of CP are not specific to CP; instead, they are general signs that signal any possible injury or disorder of the central nervous system. It is debated if CP can be diagnosed before 2 years of age as the clinical phenotype changes in parallel to the rapidly developing central nervous system. The pathway of how early unspecific neurological findings change into specific signs of CP is always individual. The timing, size, and aetiology of the spectrum of brain injuries related to CP vary, and neuroplastic changes modifying the injured neural network together with ongoing individual motor development despite CP as well as the infant's unique environment all play a role in the clinical presentation. In a minority of infants, the diagnosis of CP can be confirmed during the first months of life. Nonetheless, it is possible with the available evidence-based assessment methods to detect at early age the infants with the highest risk of developing CP (Novak et al. 2017). The common early signs and findings of CP are listed in Table 2.2.

The practical management to use systematically evidence-based assessment tools (see below) is limited by the finding that 25–50% of children with CP lack signs of neurological abnormality and do not have typical risk factors suggestive of CP in neonatal period (Bax et al. 2006). Accordingly, these infants are

Table 2.2   Examples of common early signs and neurological findings in infants developing CP

- Invariable or poor attention and vigilance
- Seizures
- Head growth failure
- Persisting infantile reactions
  - grasping reflex in hands
  - Moro reflex
  - asymmetric tonic neck reflex (ATNR)
- Cranial nerve dysfunction
  - asymmetrical or poor facial movements
  - poor or inconsistent visual attention and tracking
  - strabismus or other abnormal eye movements
  - feeding problems
- Abnormal quantity or quality of spontaneous movements
  - passive or excessive movements
  - monotonous or asymmetric movement pattern
  - stiff, cramped, dystonic, or other abnormal movements
  - frequent or constant tremor
  - asymmetric use of hands
- Tone abnormalities
  - poor head control
  - increased extensor tone
  - distal spasticity in limbs
  - constant fisting of hands
  - truncal hypotonia
- Abnormal tendon reflexes
  - exaggerated reflexes
  - clonus
- Delayed motor development

not regarded to be at risk of neurological abnormalities and therefore they are not referred to follow-up clinics run by specialists. This may cause a significant delay in the diagnosis of CP.

Differential Diagnosis of Cerebral Palsy

Common conditions causing motor delay without specific signs of CP are dissociative motor development (benign typical variant; gross motor development only transiently lags behind other aspects of development), bottom-shuffling, constitutional ligament laxity, idiopathic toe-walking, or DCD. In children with CP of unknown aetiology, brain imaging is recommended (Ashwal et al. 2004). If neuroimaging is negative or unspecific or if there are atypical features in the history (e.g. family history of CP), genetic disorders (e.g. hereditary spastic paraplegia, spinocerebellar ataxia, microdeletions or microduplications, or other chromosomal aberrations) and metabolic disorders (e.g. mitochondrial disorders, biotinidase deficiency) need to be considered. In addition, neurophysiological investigations may be performed to rule out (e.g. an obstetric brachial plexus palsy) or to understand the aetiology of hypotonia with weak reflexes.

Evidence-based Assessment Tools in the Clinics

'Is my baby able to walk?' is one of the most common questions at the Neonatal Intensive Care Unit (NICU) follow-up consultations (see also Chapter 14). It is important to explain to parents of high-risk infants that developmental disorders including CP are defined by clinical criteria, and therefore these children are followed with sequential assessments. Parents need to be asked if they have any concerns about their child's vision, hearing, contact, hand function or motor development, asymmetries, or behaviour. One can also use standardized questionnaires (e.g. the Developmental Assessment of Young Infants [DAYC]) for parental reporting (Maitre et al. 2013).

A recent systematic review (Novak et al. 2017) reported that the best three tools to detect high risk of CP before 5 months CA are (1) neonatal MRI (86–89% sensitivity, 89% specificity); (2) General Movement Assessment (92–100% sensitivity, 82–100% specificity), and (3) the HINE (90% sensitivity, 90% specificity; but see also Chapter 10). Furthermore, after 5 months CA, the best tools to detect high risk of CP are brain MRI, the HINE, and the DAYC (Novak et al. 2017). The brain imaging in relation to CP is discussed below in this chapter and the assessment of general movements (GMs) is described in detail in Chapters 5 and 10. The HINE method is a simple, and quantifiable neurologic examination for infants between 2 and 24 months of age (Haataja et al. 1999, www.hammersmith-neuro-exam.com). It is discussed in Chapter 11.

CLINICAL NEUROIMAGING

CP is defined by clinical criteria, and therefore, by definition, brain imaging is not obligatory for the diagnosis if it cannot be done safely or the practical arrangement is not feasible due to technical or financial resources. From a clinical point of view, brain imaging is most useful for understanding the possible pathogenic mechanisms related to the development of CP and the clinical phenotype. Furthermore, brain imaging is advisable for the differential diagnostics, especially in cases where the clinical phenotype is ataxic CP, or when the clinical history lacks risk factors for CP or when the condition is progressive – which pleads against CP as it is a non-progressive disorder.

Brain MRI is preferred over other imaging modalities (Novak et al. 2017), and computed tomography (CT) is advised to be used only in emergency situations. Cranial ultrasound (cUS) is a practical bedside tool for brain imaging, particularly in preterm infants (De Vries et al. 2004, 2011). Major cUS abnormalities, such as grade III intraventricular haemorrhage, venous infarction, cystic periventricular leukomalacia, and focal infarctions, have been reported to show 95% and 99% specificity, and 76% and 86% sensitivity, respectively, for CP, in two different cohorts (≤32 weeks of gestation and 33–36 weeks of gestation) of high-risk preterm infants (De Vries et al. 2004). It is essential to understand that in order to achieve this accuracy by cUS, one must perform sequential cUS during the first 4–6 weeks after birth and have an additional one between 36 and 40 weeks postmenstrual age due to the variable time course for cysts, for example, to develop (De Vries et al. 2004).

Brain MRI is superior to reveal subtle white matter lesions, myelination of the posterior limb of internal capsule (PLIC), and cerebellar lesions (De Vries et al. 2011). Brain MRI is reported to reveal

> **Text Box 2.1** Advanced Neuroimaging
>
> It has been argued that the conventional MRI techniques lack sensitivity that could be achieved with more advanced neuroimaging techniques. Diffusion-weighted imaging (DWI) provides visual appearance related to restricted diffusion due to acute cellular swelling and cell damage in acute ischemia. This is seen in hypoxic-ischemic encephalopathy or in stroke (Rutherford et al. 2004), and, accordingly, DWI has become routinely included to the neonatal imaging protocols. Diffusion tensor imaging (DTI) is considered to reflect pathology in the microstructure of white matter. DTI metrics are reported to correlate with later motor development of preterm infants. Furthermore, low diffusion anisotropy in the PLIC is reported to correlate significantly with CP (Rose et al. 2007). DTI is not yet used in clinical routine; future studies are needed to delineate the role of DTI in clinical estimation of motor prognosis. Another available technique is proton magnetic resonance spectroscopy. It has been demonstrated that the deep grey matter lactate/N-acetyl aspartate (Lac/NAA) is the most accurate quantitative MR biomarker in the neonatal period for prediction of neurodevelopmental outcome after neonatal encephalopathy (Thayyil et al. 2010). Furthermore, the use of magnetic resonance spectroscopy is advised when an alternative diagnosis of CP is suspected.

abnormal findings in about 85–86% of children with CP (Krägeloh-Mann and Horber 2007; Reid et al. 2014). The type and frequency of different lesions vary according to the subtype of CP (Novak et al. 2017). Lesions are least often seen in children with ataxia (24–57%) (Reid et al. 2014). In general, white matter injury has been shown to be the most common injury type (19–45%). Grey matter injury has been reported to be the predominant type in 21%, focal vascular insults in 10%, malformations in 11%, and miscellaneous findings in 11% of all findings (Reid et al. 2014). The typical lesions seen in ataxic CP are mostly cerebellar malformations like cerebellar hypoplasia. The myelination of PLIC is a good predictor for motor outcome, for example in term-born infants with middle cerebral artery infarction outcome of hemiplegia is associated with the involvement of the parenchymal white matter, basal ganglia, and thalamus and the PLIC (Mercuri et al. 2004).

About 15% of children with CP is reported to have no detectable abnormality in conventional brain MRI. Multiple explanations may be offered for this apparent discrepancy. One possible explanation is that signs of a preterm brain lesion may be masked in the brain MRI at the conventional time at term age due to the substantial brain plasticity in early life. On the other hand, brain MRI in preterm infants at earlier ages (e.g. at discharge) may miss the developing myelination in the PLIC. Similarly, the initial injury may reorganize itself structurally to the extent that one is not able to confirm the possible primary lesion if the suspicion of CP is raised late in infancy. In clinical practice of extremely and very low birth weight infants, sequential cUS and brain MRI at term age are often combined in order to maximize the predictive imaging data available.

EARLY INTERVENTION

The term 'early intervention' is frequently used but a closer look reveals that it is used with variable meanings by different stakeholders. The ideas of changing or normalizing the child with, for example, CP through intervention should be history, but lack of verified knowledge of developmental disorders and diverse concepts of rehabilitation are still a huge challenge globally. At worst, the parents' despair is exploited by, for example, offering inefficient therapies with unrealistic promises to cure their child.

At present, intervention for children with developmental disorders could be described as a process of empowering the child and family to find their own meaningful goals. Meaningful goals are goals that matter to child and family in terms of the child's functional capabilities, activity, and participation in their own everyday environment. The possible comorbidities and child's general somatic well-being (e.g. nutrition status and growth) must be taken into account in order to create a holistic picture of the characteristics of the individual child and family. Realistic, measurable goals of intervention should be identified on an individual basis, and once agreed with the child and family, the International Classification of Functioning, Disability and Health (ICF) framework is recommended to be used as a common base to guide interventions (Mäenpää et al. 2017).

It is also disputed what 'early' means in the context of intervention (e.g. it is not uncommon to hear people arguing that interventions should not be started before the diagnosis of CP is established due to lack of evidence of their impact). The relevant question is if one can enhance the innate brain's plasticity with intervention as early as possible without concerns about possible negative effects by eliciting disturbing stimuli that could interfere with spontaneous neural repair mechanisms. The evidence from early intervention trials is scarce, and one of the difficulties in terms of increasing the power of systematic reviews is that the definitions of 'early' and designs of interventions lack consensus hampering systematic analysis. Furthermore, a large body of available literature consists of studies in which the majority of children were regarded as at high risk of CP but who did not develop CP (Herskind et al. 2015). Accordingly, it may be that the possible effect of intervention, if any, is masked due to an underpowered study (Hadders-Algra 2014). Based on available research evidence (Novak et al. 2017), one could justify setting the limit for early intervention before 6 months of age. Yet, concerning the available literature on possible effects of early intervention and the clinical experience of evolving clinical presentation of CP the approximate upper age limit for 'early' could be the first 2 years of life.

Evidence of Early Intervention in High-risk Infants

The debate of the role of early intervention has been going on for decades. It is of interest that already in 1990 Sharkey et al. reported a study showing significant developmental advantage at 18 months of age in infants with physical disability (majority later diagnosed as CP) if infants were referred before 9 months for intervention. The study result was not explained by patient characteristics or developmental level at onset of the study (Sharkey et al. 1990). The authors reasoned that parental factors may have played a strong role or may even have been the essential factor for the better response of early intervention rather than the direct infant treatment itself – even though it had not been possible to confirm this suggestion in the study setting. Later studies on systematic coaching of parents and how they can challenge daily activities in high-risk infants have reported positive effects on functional outcome (Dirks and Hadders-Algra 2011).

It is undisputed that brain plasticity is activity dependent. It has been concluded from meta-analysis that early interventions, including an enriched environment, which allow and encourage the infants themselves to be active and by doing so gain multiple and diverse sensory and motor stimuli via play, may be beneficial (Morgan et al. 2013). There is also some evidence that early intervention in the home environment is associated with better motor and cognitive improvement than early intervention in other environments (Rostami and Malamiri 2012). Despite scarce evidence of long-term effects of early intervention, a clear message to clinicians is that no evidence is available that indicates that early intervention is not beneficial (Herskind et al. 2015; Hadders-Algra et al. 2017).

Early Intervention in the Clinics

Early intervention in high-risk infants after discharge from the hospital can be organized at home and/or in clinics. In general, it is challenging to organize clinical services that cover both the clinical follow-up, including the demands of a multidisciplinary team in the case of comorbidities and individualized early intervention schemes.

From a clinical point of view, the first step in an early intervention policy is to systematize the assessment tools used in the NICU follow-up clinics and the outpatient clinics where children with developmental delays are referred. As indicated earlier in this chapter, the first signs of cerebral palsy are often unspecific, and early systematic detection of high-risk infant or early diagnosis of CP relies on evidence-based tools (Novak et al. 2017).

The next step is to develop a management policy of discussing with parents without delay if their child is regarded as a high-risk infant. It is of great importance to address parental concerns and well-being since bonding and the formation of the parent–infant relationship is based on their resources. It is advisable to have facilities that cover psychological and psychiatric support services for families facing stressful situations due to adaptation to suspected or diagnosed CP.

Based on available clinical evidence of positive effects of environmental enrichment and the home environment as a preferred intervention site, it is desirable that individually tailored intervention goals are integrated into daily activities (e.g. feeding, clothing, social communication, and play). Crucial in the intervention is that the infant is active and motivated to be active. Another key element for a successful implementation of intervention in everyday life practice is parental sensitivity to the infant's optimal vigilance and receptiveness (see Chapter 14).

Little evidence is available on the effectiveness of adaptive devices in early intervention (see Chapter 15). Based on clinical experience adaptive seating has an additive role to enhance feeding and eye–hand coordination in exploration of toys, and visual observation of environment in individual cases where for example, axial hypotonia and/or inability to control trunk posture delays independent sitting.

Since CP is often accompanied by comorbidities, clinical management has to cover collaboration between the paediatric neurology team and other disciplines (e.g. the ophthalmologist, audiologist, orthopaedist, and dietician). The comorbidities may also require early medical intervention, which is part of the holistic care of an infant with CP. For example, delayed treatment of strabismus may lead to amblyopia and unrecognized epilepsy may have major health consequences.

Clinical services covering systematic early intervention require administrative and financial decisions. It is advisable to arrange joined meetings with clinical staff involved and administration. If early intervention is truly taken as a management guideline, it should be offered equally to all high-risk patients in the region (https://newborn-health-standards.org/). The type and frequency of intervention should also be thoroughly discussed and harmonized since service providers need to have clear instructions and advice about what they are expected to provide to the child and family. Last, but not least, the families should be provided detailed information on regional early intervention policy and available clinical services.

CONCLUDING REMARKS

The wide biological variation in attaining motor milestones and mastering motor skills in early infancy turn early identification of developmental disorders into a challenge. Detection of infants with the highest risk of developing CP is possible before 6 months of life with the available evidence-based tools (General Movement Assessment, HINE, brain MRI). However, the diagnosis of CP can be confirmed in the first months of life only in a minority of children with CP. Evidence of the most effective early intervention in the clinics is still accumulating but methods that include both motor and sensory stimuli and that motivate children themselves in their natural home environment seem currently most promising.

REFERENCES

ACPR Group (2013) *Australian Cerebral Palsy Register Report, Sydney*, Cerebral Palsy Alliance, available at https://cpregister.com/wp-content/uploads/2018/05/ACPR-Report_Web_2013.pdf [Accessed 6 April 2019].

Ashwal S, Russman BS, Blasco PA, et al. (2004) Practice parameter: diagnostic assessment of the child with cerebral palsy: report of the Quality Standards Subcommittee of the American Academy of Neurology and the Practice Committee of the Child Neurology Society. *Neurology* **62**: 851–863.

Bax M, Tydeman C, Flodmark O (2006) Clinical and MRI correlates of cerebral palsy: the European Cerebral Palsy Study. *JAMA* **296**: 1602–1608.

Blank R, Barnett AL, Cairney J, et al. (2019) International clinical practice recommendations on the definition, diagnosis, assessment, intervention, and psychosocial aspects of developmental coordination disorder. *Dev Med Child Neurol* **61**: 242–285. doi: 10.111/dmcn.14132.

Cans C (2000) Surveillance of cerebral palsy in Europe: a collaboration of cerebral palsy surveys and registers. *Dev Med Child Neurol* **42**: 816–824.

De Vries LS, van Haastert IC, Benders MJ, Groenendaal F (2011) Myth: cerebral palsy cannot be predicted by neonatal brain imaging. *Semin Fetal neonatal Med* **16**: 279–287. doi: 10.1016/j.siny.2011.04.004.

De Vries LS, Van Haastert IL, Rademaker KJ, Koopman C, Groenendaal F (2004) Ultrasound abnormalities preceding cerebral palsy in high-risk preterm infants. *J Pediatr* **144**: 815–820.

Dirks T, Hadders-Algra M (2011) The role of the family in intervention of infants at high risk of cerebral palsy: a systematic analysis. *Dev Med Child Neurol* **53** (Suppl 4): 62–67. doi: 10.1111/j.1469-8749.2011.04067.x.

Gorter JW, Ketelaar M, Rosenbaum P, Helders PJ, Palisano R (2009) Use of the GMFCS in infants with CP: the need for reclassification at age 2 years or older. *Dev Med Child Neurol* **51**: 46-52. doi: 10.1111/j.1469-8749.

Haataja L, Mercuri E, Regev R, et al. (1999) Optimality score for the neurologic examination of the infant at 12 and 18 months of age. *J Pediatr* **135**: 153–161.

Hadders-Algra M (2014) Early diagnosis and early intervention in cerebral palsy. *Front Neurol* **24**: 185. doi: 10.3389/fneur.2014.00185.

Hadders-Algra M, Boxum AG, Hielkema T, Hamer EG (2017) Effect of early intervention in infants at very high risk of cerebral palsy: a systematic review. *Dev Med Child Neurol* **59**: 246–258. doi: 10.1111/dmcn.13331.

Herskind A, Greisen G, Nielsen J (2015) Early identification and intervention in cerebral palsy. *Dev Med Child Neurol* **57**: 29–36. doi: 10.1111/dmcn.12531.

Himmelmann K, Uvebrant P (2014) The panorama of cerebral palsy in Sweden. XI. Changing patterns in the birth-year period 2003–2006. *Acta Paediatr* **103**: 618–624. doi: 10.1111/apa.12614.

Krägeloh-Mann I, Horber V (2007) The role of magnetic resonance imaging in elucidating the pathogenesis of cerebral palsy: a systematic review. *Dev Med Child Neurol* **49**: 144–151.

Maitre NL, Slaughter JC, Aschner JL (2013) Early prediction of cerebral palsy after neonatal intensive care using motor development trajectories in infancy. *Early Hum Dev* **89**: 781–786. doi: 10.1016/j.earlhumdev.2013.06.004.

Morgan C, Novak I, Badawi N (2013) Enriched environments and motor outcomes in cerebral palsy: systematic review and meta-analysis. *Pediatrics* **132**: e735–746. doi: 10.1542/peds.2012-3985.

Mercuri E, Barnett A, Rutherford M, et al. (2004) Neonatal cerebral infarction and neuromotor outcome at school age. *Pediatrics* **113**: 95–100. doi: 10.1542/peds.113.1.95.

Mäenpää H, Forsten W, Haataja L (2017) Multiprofessional evaluation in clinical practice: establishing a core set of outcome measures for children with cerebral palsy. *Dev Med Child Neurol* **59**: 322–328. doi: 10.1111/dmcn.13289.

Novak I, Morgan C, Adde L, et al. (2017) Early, accurate diagnosis and early intervention in cerebral palsy: advances in diagnosis and treatment. *JAMA Pediatr* **171**: 897–907. doi: 10.1001/jamapediatrics.2017.1689.

Palisano R, Rosenbaum P, Walter S, Russell D, Wood E, Galuppi B (1997) Development and reliability of a system to classify gross motor function in children with cerebral palsy. *Dev Med Child Neurol* **39**: 214–223.

Reid SM, Dagia CD, Ditchfield MR, Carlin JB, Reddihough DS (2014) Population-based studies of brain imaging patterns in cerebral palsy. *Dev Med Child Neurol* **56**: 222–232. doi: 10.1111/dmcn.12228.

Rose J, Mirmiran M, Butler EE, et al. (2007) Neonatal microstructural development of the internal capsule on diffusion tensor imaging correlates with severity of gait and motor deficits. *Dev Med Child Neurol* **49**: 745–750.

Rosenbaum P, Paneth N, Leviton A, et al. (2007) A report: the definition and classification of cerebral palsy April 2006. *Dev Med Child Neurol Suppl* **109**: 8–14.

Rostami HR, Malamiri RA (2012) Effect of treatment environment on modified constraint-induced movement therapy results in children with spastic hemiplegic cerebral palsy: a randomized controlled trial. *Disabil Rehabil* **34**: 40–44. doi: 10.3109/09638288.2011.585214.

Rutherford M, Counsell S, Allsop J, et al. (2004) Diffusion-weighted magnetic resonance imaging in term perinatal brain injury: a comparison with site of lesion and time from birth. *Pediatrics* **114**: 1004–1014.

Sellier E, Platt MJ, Andersen GL, Krägeloh-Mann I, De La Cruz J, Cans C, on behalf of Surveillance of Cerebral Palsy Network (2015) Decreasing prevalence in cerebral palsy: a multi-site European population-based study, 1980 to 2003. *Dev Med Child Neurol* **58**: 85–92. doi: 10.1111/dmcn.12865.

Sharkey MA, Palitz ME, Reece LF, et al. (1990) The effect of early referral and intervention on the developmentally disabled infant: evaluation at 18 months of age. *J Am Board Fam Pract* **3**: 163–170.

Thayyil S, Chandrasekaran M, Taylor A, et al. (2010) Cerebral magnetic resonance biomarkers in neonatal encephalopathy: a meta-analysis. *Pediatrics* **125**: e382–395. doi: 10.1542/peds.2009-1046.

SUGGESTIONS FOR FURTHER READING

Dan B, Mayston M, Paneth N, Rosenbloom L, editors (2014) *Cerebral Palsy: Science and Clinical Practice*. London: Mac Keith Press.

Korzeniewski SJ, Slaughter J, Lenski M, Haak P, Paneth N (2018) The complex aetiology of cerebral palsy. *Nat Rev Neurol* **14**: 528–543. doi: 10.1038/s41582-018-0043-6.

www.hammersmith-neuro-exam.com

www.canchild.ca

https://newborn-health-standards.org/

SCPE Reference and Training Manual, http://www.scpenetwork.eu/en/r-and-t-manual/

PART II
Developmental Neurology

Neurodevelopmental Mechanism in Early Life

Mijna Hadders-Algra

SUMMARY POINTS

- Development of the human nervous system is a complex and long-lasting process.
- High developmental activity in the brain occurring prenatally and in the first postnatal year involves high plasticity.
- High plasticity of the young brain implies that brain lesions do not always result in a developmental disorder.
- High plasticity of the young brain interferes with early detection of developmental disorders; the young nervous system does not offer certainties.
- High plasticity of the young brain offers great opportunities for early intervention.

Developmental motor disorders have been defined as disorders characterized by limitations in mobility due to an altered organization of the brain that had its origin in early life. This implies a pivotal role of the developing nervous system. Therefore, this chapter first briefly summarizes the neurobiology of the developing human brain. The focus is on the developmental processes occurring before the age of 2 years. The second section addresses the windows of vulnerability and plasticity in the young brain. It also presents the major causes of atypical brain development that may underlie developmental motor disorders. The third section discusses the consequences of brain development for the clinical manifestation of developmental disorders. Finally, the fourth section reviews the prevailing theories on motor development, including their significance for early detection and early intervention in developmental motor disorders.

NEUROBIOLOGY OF THE DEVELOPING HUMAN BRAIN

The development of the human brain takes many years: it is around the age of 40 years that the nervous system obtains its full-blown adult configuration (Ouyang et al. 2017; Hadders-Algra 2018a). The developmental processes are the result of a continuous intricate interaction between genes and environment, activity, and experience. The processes occurring up until the age of 2 years are summarized in Figure 3.1 (Hadders-Algra 2018a).

Neural development starts in the fifth week postmenstrual age (PMA) with the development of the neural tube. Shortly after closure of the neural tube, specific areas near the ventricles start to generate

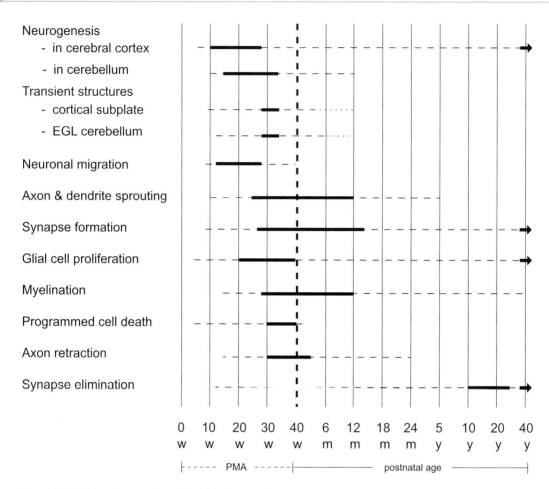

Figure 3.1 Schematic overview of the developmental processes occurring in the human brain. The bold lines indicate that the processes mentioned on the left are very active, the broken lines denote that the processes still continue, but less abundantly. The diagram is based on the review of Hadders-Algra (2018a). EGL = external granular layer; m = months; PMA = postmenstrual age; w = weeks; y = years.

neurons. The majority of neurons are formed between 5 and 25–28 weeks PMA. Cerebral cortex neurons are generated in the germinal layers near the ventricles. From these ventricular layers, they move radially or tangentially to their final place of destination in the more superficially located cortical plate. The process of migration peaks between 20 and 26 weeks PMA, with the peak occurring somewhat earlier in the occipital than in the frontal region. During migration, neurons start to differentiate (i.e. they start to produce axons, dendrites, synapses with neurotransmitters, the intracellular machinery, and the complex neuronal membranes). Interestingly, the first generation of neurons does not migrate to the cortical plate, but these neurons halt in the cortical subplate.

The cortical subplate is a temporary structure between the cortical plate and the future white matter (Fig. 3.2). It is the major site of neuronal differentiation and synaptogenesis in the cortex. It receives the first ingrowing cortical afferents (e.g. from the thalamus), and it is the main site of synaptic activity in the midfoetal brain (Kostović et al. 2015). In other words, the subplate is a major mediator of foetal (motor) behaviour. The subplate is thickest between 28 and 34 weeks PMA, when it is about four times

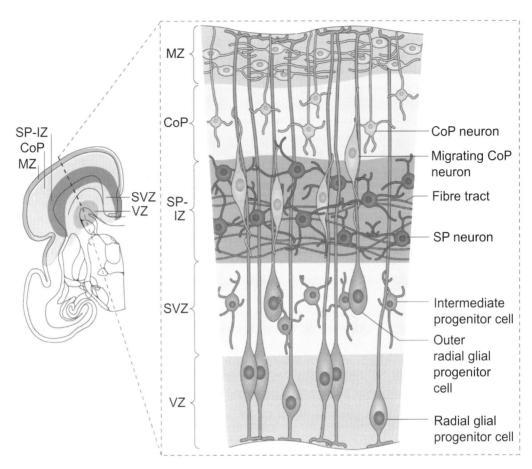

Figure 3.2 Schematic representation of the human cerebral cortex at 28 weeks PMA. On the left a coronal section is shown; the inset box on the right provides details of the developmental processes. The ventricular zone (VZ) and subventricular zone (SVZ) constitute the germinal matrices where cell division occurs. The first generations of cells are generated in the VZ, the later generations in the SVZ. The SVZ is a structure that expanded during phylogeny; it is especially large in primates. The radial glial cells span their shafts between the germinal layers and the outer layer of the cortex (marginal zone (MZ)). The first generation neurons have migrated to the subplate (SP) – they participate in the functional foetal cortex; later generations of neurons migrate to the cortical plate (CoP). Figure reproduced from Hoerder-Suabedissen and Molnár (2015) with permission from the authors and the Nature Publishing Group.

thicker than the cortical plate. From 25–26 weeks, the subplate gradually decreases in size as the subplate neurons undergo programmed cell death and later generated neurons start to populate the cortical plate. These developmental changes are accompanied by a relocation of the thalamocortical afferents that grow to their final target in the cortical plate.

As the cortical plate expands, the cortex increases in size and gyrification starts. It is estimated that cortical volume increases about twentyfold in the second half of gestation. In this phase the subplate decreases. This also implies that the human cortex during the third trimester of gestation is characterized by the co-existence of two separate but interconnected cortical circuitries: the transient foetal circuitries centred in the subplate and the immature, but progressively developing permanent circuitry centred in the cortical plate. The state of double circuitry ends when the subplate has dissolved. This situation is reached in the primary motor, sensory, and visual cortices around 3 months post-term, but first around the age of 1 year in the associative prefrontal cortex (Kostović et al. 2015).

Brain development also involves the creation of glial cells. The total final number of glial cells is – just like that of neurons – about 85 billion. Glial cell production occurs in particular in the second half of gestation. Part of the glial cells, the oligodendrocytes, take care of axonal myelination. Oligodendrocyte development peaks between 28 and 40 weeks PMA. Myelination is prominently present in the third trimester of gestation and the first 6 months postnatally. However, myelination is a long-lasting process that is first completed around the age of 40 years (Ouyang et al. 2017).

Brain development does not only imply the generation of neurons and connections, it also involves regressive phenomena. The process of neuronal death was already mentioned. It is estimated that in the mammalian central nervous system about half of the created neurons die off through apoptosis. The neurons die as the result of interaction between endogenously programmed processes and chemical and electrical signals induced by experience. Axon elimination in the human is best known from the corpus callosum and the corticospinal tract. Axon elimination in the corpus callosum occurs especially in the third trimester and the first 2 months post-term. Axon elimination in the corticospinal tract starts during the last trimester of gestation and continues during the first 2 postnatal years. As a result, the tract's initially bilateral corticospinal projections in the spinal cord are reorganized into a mainly contralateral fibre system. This reorganization is activity driven and use dependent. This is illustrated by the effect of an early unilateral lesion of the brain that induces asymmetrical activation of the spinal cord. This asymmetrical activity results in preferential strengthening of the activity from the ipsilateral projections from the contra-lesional hemisphere in comparison to the contralateral projections from the ipsi-lesional hemisphere (Williams et al. 2017). The elimination of synapses in the brain starts during the mid-foetal period. However, in the cerebral cortex synapse elimination is most pronounced between the onset of puberty and early adulthood.

From early age onwards neurotransmitters and their receptors are present in neural tissue. In the cortex catecholamines, serotonin, γ-aminobutyric acid (GABA) and excitatory amino acids including glutamate can be found from 8–10 weeks PMA. Interestingly, the noradrenergic α2-receptors in the brain's white matter and in many brain stem nuclei are transiently overexpressed in the peri-term period. In this period, also dopamine turnover is relatively high. The serotonergic axons penetrate at term age all cortical layers but rapidly decrease in density a few weeks thereafter. GABA function during early life differs from that in later life: during the major part of gestation it has an excitatory function. First during the third trimester GABA gets its inhibitory function. Evidence suggests that the glutamatergic n-methyl-D-aspartate (NMDA) receptors in the cortex have two transient periods of overexpression that occur between 13 and 21 weeks PMA and around term age. The data indicate that the peri-term period is characterized by a specific transient setting of various transmitter systems (i.e. by a temporary overexpression of the noradrenergic α2-receptors and glutamatergic NMDA-receptors), a relatively high serotonergic innervation, and a high dopaminergic turnover. It has been suggested that this specific neurotransmitter setting around term age induces an increased excitability, among others expressed by the motoneurons, and that this setting facilitates the transition from the foetal periodic breathing pattern to the continuous breathing needed for postnatal survival (Hadders-Algra 2018b).

The development of the cerebellum, that finally contains about 80% of the brain's neurons, deserves specific attention, as it has its own developmental timing. Cells in the cerebellum brings forth originate from two proliferative zones: (1) the ventricular zone which brings forth the deep cerebellar nuclei and the Purkinje cells, and (2) the external granular layer originating from the rhombic lip. Cell proliferation starts at 11 weeks PMA in the ventricular zone, and from 15 weeks onwards in the external granular layer. The external granular layer is a transient structure that produces the most numerous cells of the cerebellum, the granule cells. The external granular layer reaches its peak thickness between 28 and 34 weeks PMA. From this layer the granule cells migrate inward to their final destination, most often the internal granular layer. The latter layer grows in particular between mid-gestation and 3 months post-term. The external granular layer shrinks especially between 2 and 3 months post-term, but it takes until the second half of the first postnatal year to dissolve entirely.

In summary, during foetal life and the first 2 years post-term the brain shows high developmental activity. The most significant changes occur in the second half of gestation and the first 3 months post-term, in particular in the cortical subplate and cerebellum. As the transient subplate pairs a high rate of intricate developmental changes and interactions with clear functional activity, two phases of development have been distinguished: (1) the transient cortical subplate phase, ending at 3 months post-term when the permanent circuitries in the primary motor, somatosensory and visual cortices have replaced the subplate; and subsequently, (2) the phase in which the permanent circuitries dominate. In the latter phase, in particular during the remainder of the first post-term year, the brain's major developmental changes consist of axon reconfiguration, dendrite and synapse production, abundant myelination, and an integration of the permanent circuitries in the association areas (Hadders-Algra 2018a).

THE DEVELOPING HUMAN BRAIN: WINDOWS OF VULNERABILITY AND PLASTICITY

The preceding section sketched the ingenious development of the human brain with specific processes occurring during specific time windows. This implies that human brain development is characterized by specific windows of vulnerability and plasticity.

Windows of Vulnerability

The major groups of conditions that are associated with developmental motor disorders are summarized in Table 3.1. Whether or not a condition or risk factor, such as foetal growth restriction or preterm birth, will result in a developmental motor disorder depends on:

- The timing of the risk event (see below).
- The intensity of the risk event: a higher intensity is associated with a higher risk, e.g. serious hypoxia-ischaemia results more often in a developmental motor disorder than mild hypoxia-ischaemia.
- The duration of the risk event: a longer duration is associated with a higher risk, e.g. foetal growth retardation starting in the second trimester of gestation results more often in a developmental motor disorder than growth retardation starting in the third trimester of gestation.
- Whether the risk event occurs in isolation or as an experience in a chain of adversities. An example is the combination of maternal smoking during pregnancy, foetal growth restriction, chorioamnionitis, preterm birth, periventricular leukomalacia finally resulting in bilateral spastic cerebral palsy. The accumulation of unfavourable events is rather the rule than the exception (Stanley et al. 2000; see also Text Box 3.1).
- Resilience of infant and family. Knowledge on this important aspect of child development is limited. Resilience most likely is brought about by an interaction between nature – genes encoding specific forms of resistance – and nurture. This is reflected by the old finding of the cohort study of the Groningen Perinatal Project: infants with clear neonatal neurological dysfunction, who lived in families with rather well-educated parents, had four times less risk for later neurological dysfunction than infants with similar neonatal neurological impairment living in families with parents with limited

Table 3.1   Conditions associated with developmental motor disorders

Condition	Timing
• Malformation of the brain, e.g. lisencephaly or schizencephaly	prenatal: 1st half pregnancy
• Infections, e.g. CMV, chorioamnionitis, neonatal sepsis, meningitis	prenatal, perinatal, neonatal

• Exposure to toxic substances, e.g.
  • alcohol
  • mercury
  • corticosteroids
  • bilirubin
	
	prenatal
	prenatal and postnatal (breast feeding)
	postnatally in preterm infants
	neonatally in preterm and term infants

• Foetal growth restriction[a]	prenatal: 2nd trimester (early onset) and 3rd trimester (late onset)
• Preterm birth	between 22–24 and 37 weeks PMA
• Hypoxia-ischaemia	from midgestation onwards: prenatally, perinatally, neonatally in preterm and term infants

Based on Stanley et al. (2000), Mwaniki et al. (2012), Dan et al. (2014), Miller et al. (2016) CMV = cytomegalovirus.
[a]Birthweight <10th centile. [b]In 2014 the estimated global preterm birth rate was 10.6%, equating to almost 15 million live preterm births in 2014 (Chawanpaiboon et al. 2019).

education (Hadders-Algra et al. 1988). Another indication that family resilience may act as a protective factor is found in intervention studies in preterm infants. These studies suggest that programs facilitating responsive parenting (i.e. that promote the family's resilience) are associated with better cognitive outcome of the infant (Van Wassenaer-Leemhuis et al. 2016).

The effect of adverse factors impacting brain development strongly depends on the operational *timing* of the factor. An example is the exposure to ionizing irradiation: irradiation during the period of 8–15 weeks PMA reduces IQ with 21 points per 1Gy, irradiation during 16–25 weeks PMA with 13 IQ points per 1Gy, whereas later irradiation has not been associated with IQ reduction (Kal and Struikmans 2005). This differential effect illustrates that ionizing irradiation especially affects the

---

Text Box 3.1 Poverty and Child Development: Accumulating Effect of Adversities

Black et al. (2017) reported that about 250 million children younger than 5 years (i.e. 43% of children in low and middle income countries), are at risk of atypical development due to impaired living conditions. These conditions are associated with poverty and prenatal and postnatal growth stunting. Growth stunting is associated with less favourable cognitive and social development, in particular when it occurs before the age of 2 years. Poverty is associated with deficits in language and cognitive development. The effect of poverty is mainly mediated by low parental education, an unfavourable home environment (that may include family stress, child abuse and neglect, and non-optimal food), and prenatal and postnatal growth stunting. More often than not, the adversities coincide and accumulate, an accumulation that aggravates the negative effect of the single factors per se.

This also means that an environment that supports families in their provision of nurturing care and that promotes caregivers' nutrition and mental and physical health will facilitate infant growth and development.

Black et al. did not pay specific attention to motor development, but most likely the mechanisms of an accumulation of adversities and the beneficial effects of adequate infant care and nutrition, that are involved in cognitive and social development, hold also true for motor development.

process of neuronal proliferation. Another example of the effect of timing is the differential effect of hypoxic-ischaemic events in preterm and term infants. In preterm infants pathological findings after hypoxia-ischaemia are especially found in the periventricular and subplate areas and cerebellum, whereas in term infants the sites of predilection of pathology after hypoxaemia-ischaemia are the basal ganglia, thalamus, and the so-called watershed zones including the cortex and its underlying white matter (Volpe 2009; Rennie and Robertson 2014). These different vulnerabilities are based on the age dependent changes in neurodevelopmental activity and their accompanying changes in metabolic activity and vascularization.

Preterm infants are born at the time that developmental activity in the brain is maximal. Their untimely exposure to the stresses of extrauterine life in the peak period of brain development induces a high vulnerability for developmental disorders, such as cerebral palsy (CP), developmental coordination disorder (DCD), autism spectrum disorders (ASD), and learning disorders (Hadders-Algra 2018a).

Windows of Plasticity

Neuroplasticity refers to the brain's capacity to reorganize in response to external events and experience. The reorganization may occur at the level of neuron proliferation and at the level of network reorganization involving alterations in axons, dendrites, and synapses (Kolb et al. 2017). Neuroplasticity via neurogenesis is one of the aims of stem cell therapy in infants with neonatal hypoxic-ischaemic encephalopathy. This therapy is still in its infancy, but animal research and the first clinical trials showed that therapy with mesenchymal stem cells is promising and safe. The animal studies indicated that the trophic factors of the mesenchymal stem cells not only promote neurogenesis, but also the proliferation of oligodendrocytes and synaptogenesis (Wagenaar et al. 2017).

Axonal plasticity is especially known from reorganizational activity in the corticospinal system. In the section 'Neurobiology of the Developing Human Brain' the activity-driven reorganization of the initially bilateral projections into a contralateral projection was discussed. Animal research demonstrated that the asymmetrical activity in the spinal cord induced by an early unilateral brain lesion may be counteracted by provision of early stimulation of motor activity of the affected side. The latter promotes plasticity on the affected side, restoration of connections, and a more symmetrical outcome (Williams et al. 2017). These plastic changes are the putatively underlying mechanisms of constrained induced movement therapy (baby-CIMT) and intensive bilateral manual activities in infants (see Chapter 14). Based on the time window of the reorganizational processes in the corticospinal projections, it may be surmised that these interventions will be most effective when applied in the first year of life.

Neuroplasticity mostly occurs at the level of dendrite and synapse reorganization. Dendrites and synapses are very plastic; dendritic spines can rapidly modify their structure, and generate and delete synapses – presumably within minutes (Kolb et al. 2017). Animal experiments demonstrated that enriched environments and large sibling groups have a positive effect on brain weight, neuron soma size, the number of dendrites and synapses, and on cognitive development (Kolb et al. 2017). These effects are present over the lifetime but most pronounced at early age.

The dendritic and synapse reorganization may have restricted windows of plasticity. The phenomenon of the 'window of plasticity' is well known for amblyopia: if the infant's brain consistently lacks visual input from one eye, cortical cells lose their ability to respond to visual information. This visual deficit may be reversed, but success of treatment is larger before the age of 7 years than at older ages (Holmes and Levi 2018). Another example is the effect of intensive motor training in children after cerebral hemispherectomy for intractable epilepsy: the training effect on gross motor abilities is considerably larger in children of 5 years or younger than in older children (Fritz et al. 2011).

BRAIN DEVELOPMENT AND CLINICAL MANIFESTATION OF DEVELOPMENTAL DISORDERS

The high developmental activity in the brain during the first postnatal years makes it difficult to detect developmental disorders at early age. Of course, we do have means to determine which infants are at high risk of developmental disorders, for instance by using magnetic resonance imaging at term age and the assessment of general movements (see Chapters 2, 10, and 11). However, we cannot diagnose developmental disorders at an early age (see also Chapter 14). This has to do with two developmental phenomena (Hadders-Algra 2018a): (1) The brain may find functional solutions for early developmental disruption. This implies that early dysfunctions may dissolve – even without professional early intervention. (2) The protracted course of brain development explains why it takes developmental time before neurodevelopmental disorders become clinically manifest. For instance, CP is generally first diagnosed from about the end of the first postnatal year onwards, whereas in some children it may take several years before the clinical picture is established (Granild-Jensen et al. 2015). The timing of the manifestation of the clinical signs of cerebral palsy most likely is related to the developmental changes in the corticospinal tract. The clinical signs of learning disorders, ASD, and DCD emerge later, in general during preschool age or early school age.

THEORIES ON MOTOR DEVELOPMENT

Concepts on motor behaviour and motor development largely changed during the last century. The earlier view that motor behaviour was primarily organised in chains of reflexes was replaced by the notion that spontaneous, intrinsic activity is a quintessential feature of the brain (Hadders-Algra 2018c). Concurrently, the ideas on motor development changed. During major part of the past century the Neural Maturationist Theories guided developmental thinking. These theories considered motor development basically as an innate, maturational process, resulting in an orderly genetic sequence in the emergence of behavioural patterns. This induced the recognition of general developmental rules, such as the cranio-caudal and the proximal-to-distal sequences of development. The idea was that the developmental changes were brought about by maturationally induced increases of cortical control over reflexes.

However, during the last two decades of the last century, it became clear that motor development is largely affected by experience. This knowledge is integrated in the two currently dominating theories, the Dynamic Systems Theory and the Neuronal Group Selection Theory (NGST; Hadders-Algra 2018c).

Dynamic Systems Theory

Dynamic systems theory is a complex systems theory, based on the principles of non-equilibrium thermodynamics (Thelen 1995). Indeed, motor development may be regarded as a complex system in which many intrinsic and extrinsic factors play a role. Examples of intrinsic factors are the child's muscle strength, body weight, postural support, mood, and brain development. External factors are task requirements and specifics of the environmental situation such as housing conditions, the presence of stimulating caregivers, and the presence of toys. According to the laws of non-equilibrium dynamics, the system of motor development is continuously searching for a stable situation at low energy costs, namely an equilibrium. It always finds a situation of equilibrium. This may mean, for example, that the infant discovers how to reach successfully towards an object. Owing to the fact that the factors contributing to the situation change over time, for example the infant grows, is gaining weight and body length, or his nervous system develops new functions, the system is pushed out of equilibrium. A re-entry into the cycle of 'disequilibrium – search for a new equilibrium' follows, or, in clinical terms, a period of 'transition'. After the transition, the system finds a new equilibrium. The infant of the above example may now also have discovered how the reaching hand may grasp and hold an object. The sequence of events described in the Dynamic Systems Theory suggests that development is a self-organizing process (Thelen 1995).

Dynamic Systems Theory makes it clear that development is not dictated by endogenously determined maturational processes. In addition, the theory highlights that non-neural factors of the infant, such as body size or the presence of an inherent disease (e.g. a complex congenital heart disease), and environmental factors, such as housing conditions or the presence of affectionate caregivers, affect motor development. Finally, Dynamic Systems Theory is able to explain that continuous changes in specific components induce discontinuous changes in motor behaviour, namely that development proceeds by means of transitions.

Neuronal Group Selection Theory

According to the NGST, motor development is characterized by two phases of variability, primary and secondary variability (Edelman 1989; Hadders-Algra 2018c). In the first phase, the typically developing infant tries out all movement options available. The movements are brought about by activity of the primary neural networks that are largely based on genetic information. Motor behaviour in this phase is characterized by variation with no or marginal capacities for adaptation (Fig. 3.3; Video 3.1). The ample and varied spontaneous activity is especially used to prepare the nervous system for the accurate and integrated use of afferent, perceptual information to adapt motor behaviour in a later phase.

Gradually, the infant obtains the ability to select the most efficient movement strategies from his repertoire. The infant enters the phase of secondary variability, which is characterized by variation and increasing adaptability (Video 3.2). The transition from the phase of primary variability to that of secondary variability occurs at function-specific ages. For instance, the transition occurs already prior to term age in the development in sucking, whereas in the development of heel-toe gait it usually happens in the first half of the second postnatal year (Hadders-Algra 2018c). The process of selection of the best adapted strategies is based on the infant's own trial and error activities and the associated afferent information. The infant with his changing body proportions explores his capacities in continuous interaction with the environment. In other words, the infant's own movements and own exploration assist in the building of internal frames of reference (internal models) of the body, his movements, and the external world. The infant moves from a motor control that is mainly based on feedback to control that largely relies on feedforward mechanisms or anticipatory control. The process of finding the optimal strategies through trial and error activities may be enhanced when the infant engages in play with others (e.g. caregivers or siblings). In these play situations the infant does not only learn from his own trial and error attempts, but he also profits from the actions performed by others due to the neural mirroring mechanisms.

In infants with an early lesion of the brain variation and adaptability are impaired. The lesion reduces the infant's repertoire (Fig. 3.4; Video 3.3) and interferes with the infant's ability to select the best strategy from the repertoire. The latter is brought about by three mechanisms. First, the exploratory drive of children with an early lesion is often reduced (Landry et al. 1993). Second, children with an early lesion of the brain have virtually always deficits in the processing of sensory information. Third, the presence of a reduced repertoire may hamper strategy selection, when the brain lesion has erased the typical best strategy and the child is forced to select a 'second best' strategy. Impaired variation is suggestive of a structural deficit of the brain (i.e. of disrupted connectivity). However, impaired adaptability may reflect a brain lesion, but it more often is a marker of minor degrees of dysfunction of the brain (e.g. of an altered setting of the dopaminergic systems) (Hadders-Algra 2010; Video 3.4).

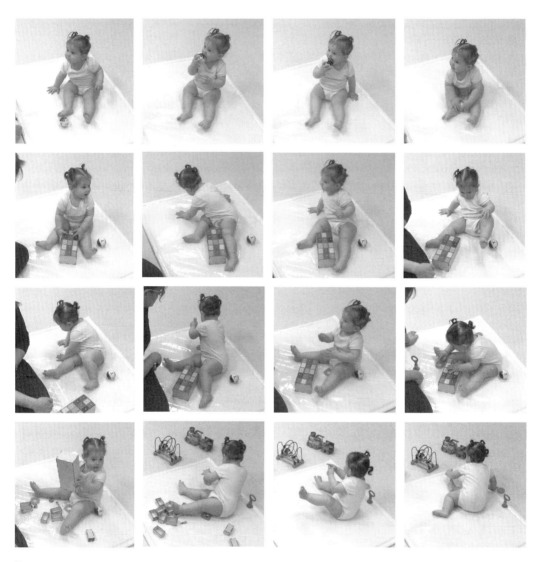

Figure 3.3 Variation in sitting. Variation in sitting movements while playing in a 10-month-old infant. The infant was born at term and had an uneventful prenatal, perinatal, and neonatal history. The figure is based on frames from 4 minutes of video recording. Published with permission of the parents.

Developmental Theories and Early Detection

The Dynamic Systems Theory and NGST share the opinion that motor development is a non-linear process with phases of transition, a process that is affected by a multitude of factors. The factors consist of features of the child, such as body weight, muscle power, or the presence of a cardiac disorder, and components of the environment, such as housing conditions, the composition of the family, and the presence of toys. Both theories (and the Neural Maturationist Theories) view a delay in the development of motor milestones as sign of increased risk of a developmental motor disorder. Due to the acknowledgement of the multifactorial origin of motor development, both theories recognize that motor development is

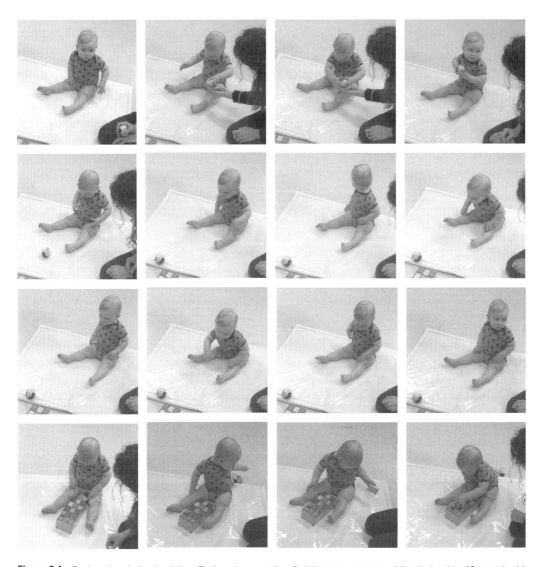

Figure 3.4 Reduced variation in sitting. Reduced repertoire of sitting movements while playing in a 10-month-old infant. The impaired variation is especially clear in the legs; on each frame leg posture is virtually identical. The infant was born at term and had an uneventful prenatal, perinatal, and neonatal history. Nevertheless, he presented with an atypical neurological condition. The figure is based on frames from 4 minutes of video recording. Published with permission of the parents.

characterized by large interindividual variation. This interindividual variation implies that delayed development of a single milestone has limited clinical value. However, delay in the attainment of multiple milestones suggests an increased risk of developmental pathology (Hadders-Algra 2018c).

The Dynamic Systems Theory and NGST differ, however, in their opinion on the role of genetically determined neurodevelopmental processes (Fig. 3.5). Genetic factors play a limited role in the former theory, whereas in NGST genetic information, epigenetic cascades, and experience play

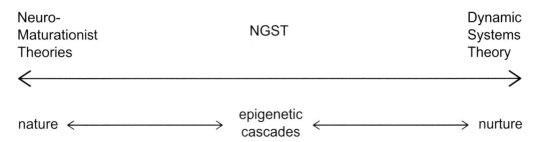

Figure 3.5   Schematic representation of nature and nurture in motor development theories.

equally prominent roles. The latter corresponds well to current insights in the complexities of genetic and epigenetic control of neural development (Hadders-Algra 2018c). Due to the integration of the specific characteristics of the developing nervous system, NGST pays explicit attention to variation (the size of the motor repertoire) and adaptability. It is getting increasingly clear that these motor properties have diagnostic value (see Chapters 10 and 11). For instance, the assessment of movement variation is the basic ingredient of the general movements assessment, an assessment with a powerful prediction of CP.

Text Box 3.2 Debate on the Diagnosis of Cerebral Palsy in Early Infancy

Due to the improved abilities to predict CP in infants who started postnatal life in the neonatal intensive care unit, it is increasingly strongly advocated to diagnose cerebral palsy in the first half of the first year post-term (Novak et al. 2017). It is undoubtedly true that it is possible to predict CP in some young infants with certainty. For instance, infants with cystic periventricular leukomalacia who demonstrate consistently so-called cramped-synchronized general movements up to and including the corrected age of 3 months will get the diagnosis of bilateral spastic CP (see Chapter 10). However, these infants are the exception to the rule. Most children diagnosed with CP have a different start of life. For example, a substantial proportion of children diagnosed with CP have an uneventful prenatal, perinatal, and neonatal history, implying that the event that resulted in CP has passed unnoticed. Other children with CP have been admitted to the neonatal intensive care unit, but their neuroimaging only showed a minor lesion of the brain. In addition, it should be realized that a considerable proportion of children with a lesion of the brain at early age is not diagnosed with CP in later life.

Thus, in general the best we can do is to detect infants at high risk of CP. This implies that we usually cannot offer caregivers of young infants the desired certainty of the diagnosis. However, this may not necessarily be a bad thing. The early diagnosis of CP only informs the family about the diagnosis; it does not provide the family with information about the child's function in later life, which varies largely among children with CP. Function in daily life of children with CP is determined in particular by their abilities in the domains of cognition, communication, and prosocial behaviour (Morris et al. 2006; Tseng et al. 2011). The child's capacities in these domains are not clear in early infancy. In other words, even when the diagnosis of CP is disclosed to caregivers of young infants, they will face uncertainty about the child's later life, just as the caregivers of infants having been labelled as high risk of a developmental disorder (see Chapter 14).

Essential in early detection and early intervention in infants at high risk of CP or with the early diagnosis of CP are: (1) the comprehensive, honest and respectful information of caregivers throughout the infant's development, including an early – but not too early – disclosure of the diagnosis of CP (Shevell and Shevell 2013; Novak et al. 2019); (2) the provision of early intervention that is tailored to the infant's and the family's opportunities and challenges, and that helps families to cope with life's uncertainties (see Chapters 12 and 14).

Developmental Theories and Early Intervention

The recognition of the multifactorial origin of motor development induces agreement between Dynamic Systems Theory and NGST on the importance of experience and context in early intervention. Yet, the suggestions for early intervention provided by NGST are more specific than those generated by the Dynamic Systems Theory. For instance, knowledge of an infant's repertoire reductions may result in the advice of the early application of assistive devices (see Chapters 14 and 15). In addition, knowing that an infant has impaired adaptability, suggests that the infant needs about ten times more active practice than the typically developing infant.

CONCLUDING REMARKS

The high developmental activity in the brain during the first postnatal year has important implications for early detection and early intervention. For early detection, the young brain offers specific opportunities but no certainties. In many infants, the high neurodevelopmental activity precludes a final diagnosis of cerebral palsy during the first year (for a discussion see Text Box 3.2). This, however, does not interfere with the provision of early intervention – all infants in whom a high risk of a developmental disorder is detected have the right for early intervention. The effect of early intervention is considered to be best when provided during the early phases of development.

REFERENCES

Black MM, Walker SP, Fernald LCH, et al. (2017) Early childhood development coming of age: science through the life course. *Lancet* **389** (10064): 77–90. doi: 10.1016/S0140-6736(16)31389-7.

Chawanpaiboon S, Vogel JP, Moller AB, et al. (2019) Global, regional, and national estimates of levels of preterm birth in 2014: a systematic review and modelling analysis. *Lancet Glob Health* 7: e37–e46. doi: 10.1016/S2214-109X(18)30451-0.

Dan B, Mayston M, Paneth N, Rosenbloom L (2014) *Cerebral Palsy: Science and Clinical Practice.* London: Mac Keith Press.

Edelman GM (1989) *Neural Darwinism. The Theory of Neuronal Group Selection.* Oxford: Oxford University Press.

Fritz SL, Rivers ED, Merlo AM, Reed AD, Mathern GD, De Bode S (2011) Intensive mobility training post-cerebral hemispherectomy: early surgery shows best functional improvements. *Eur J Phys Rehabil Med.* **47**: 569–577.

Granild-Jensen JB, Rackauskaite G, Flachs EM, Uldall P (2015) Predictors of early diagnosis of cerebral palsy from national registry data. *Dev Med Child Neurol* **57**: 931–935. doi: 10.1111/dmcn.12760.

Hadders-Algra M (2010) Variation and variability: key words in human motor development. *Phys Ther* **90**: 1823–1837. doi: 10.2522/ptj.20100006.

Hadders-Algra M (2018a) Early human brain development: starring the subplate. *Neurosci Biobehav Res* **92**: 276–290. doi: 10.1016/j.neubiorev.2018.06.017.

Hadders-Algra M (2018b) Neural substrate and clinical significance of general movements: an update. *Dev Med Child. Neurol* **60**: 39–46. doi: 10.1111/dmcn.13540.

Hadders-Algra M (2018c) Early human motor development: from variation to the ability to vary and adapt *Neurosci Biobehav Rev* **90**: 411–427. doi: 10.1016/j.neubiorev.2018.05.009.

Hadders-Algra M, Huisjes HJ, Touwen BC (1988) Perinatal correlates of major and minor neurological dysfunction at school age: a multivariate analysis. *Dev Med Child Neurol* **30**: 472–481.

Hoerder-Suabedissen A, Molnár Z (2015) Development, evolution and pathology of neocortical subplate neurons. *Nat Rev Neurosci* **16**: 133–146. doi: 10.1038/nrn3915.

Holmes JM, Levi DM (2018) Treatment of amblyopia as a function of age. *Vis Neurosci* **35**: E015. doi: 10.1017/S0952523817000220.

Kal HB, Struikmans H (2005) Radiotherapy during pregnancy: fact and fiction. *Lancet Oncol* **6**: 328–333.

Kolb B, Harker A, Gibb R (2017) Principles of plasticity in the developing brain. *Dev Med Child Neurol* **59**: 1218–1223. doi: 10.1111/dmcn.13546.

Kostović I, Sedmak G, Vukšić M, Judaš M (2015) The relevance of human fetal subplate zone for developmental neuropathology of neuronal migration disorders and cortical dysplasia CNS. *Neurosci Ther* **21**: 74–82. doi: 10.1111/cns.12333.

Landry SH, Garner PW, Denson S, Swank PR, Baldwin C (1993) Low birth weight (LBW) infants' exploratory behavior at 12 and 24 months: effects of intraventricular hemorrhage and mothers' attention directing behaviors. *Res Dev Disabil* **14**: 237–249.

Miller SL, Huppi PS, Mallard C (2016) The consequences of fetal growth restriction on brain structure and neurodevelopmental outcome. *J Physiol* **594**: 807–823. doi: 10.1113/JP271402.

Morris C, Kurinczuk JJ, Fitzpatrick R, Rosenbaum PL (2006) Do the abilities of children with cerebral palsy explain their activities and participation? *Dev Med Child Neurol* **48**: 954–961.

Mwaniki MK, Atieno M, Lawn JE, Newton CR (2012) Long-term neurodevelopmental outcomes after intrauterine and neonatal insults: a systematic review. *Lancet* **379**: 445–452. doi: 10.1016/S0140-6736(11)61577-8.

Novak I, Morgan C, Adde L, et al. (2017) Early, accurate diagnosis and early intervention in cerebral palsy: advances in diagnosis and treatment. *JAMA Pediatr* **171**: 897–907. doi: 10.1001/jamapediatrics.2017.1689.

Novak I, Morgan C, McNamara L, Te Velde A (2019) Best practice guidelines for communicating to parents the diagnosis of disability. *Early Hum Dev* **139**: 104841. doi: 10.1016/j.earlhumdev.2019.104841.

Ouyang M, Kang H, Detre JA, Roberts TPL, Huang H (2017) Short-range connections in the developmental connectome during typical and atypical brain maturation. *Neurosci Biobehav Rev* **83**: 109–122. doi: 10.1016/j.neubiorev.2017.10.007.

Rennie JM, Robertson NJ (2014) Pathways involving hypoxia-ischaemia. In: Dan B, Mayston M, Paneth N, Rosenbloom L, editors, *Cerebral Palsy: Science and Clinical Practice*. London: Mac Keith Press, pp. 109–130.

Shevell AH, Shevell M (2013) Doing the 'talk': disclosure of a diagnosis of cerebral palsy. *J Child Neurol* **28**: 230–235. doi: 10.1177/0883073812471430.

Stanley F, Blair E, Alberman E (2000) *Cerebral Palsies: Epidemiology and Causal Pathways*. London: Mac Keith Press.

Tseng MH, Chen KL, Shieh JY, Lu L, Huang CY (2011) The determinants of daily function in children with cerebral palsy. *Res Dev Disabil* **32**: 235–245. doi: 10.1016/j.ridd.2010.09.024.

Thelen E (1995) Motor development. A new synthesis. *Am Psychol* **50**: 79–95. doi: 10.1037//0003-066x.50.2.79.

Van Wassenaer-Leemhuis AG, Jeukens-Visser M, Van Hus JW, et al. (2016) Rethinking preventive post-discharge intervention programmes for very preterm infants and their parents. *Dev Med Child Neurol* **58** (Suppl 4): 67–73. doi: 10.1111/dmcn.13049.

Volpe JJ (2009 Brain injury in premature infants: a complex amalgam of destructive and developmental disturbances, *Lancet Neurol* **8**: 110–124. doi: 10.1016/S1474-4422(08)70294-1.

Wagenaar N, Nijboer CH, van Bel F (2017) Repair of neonatal brain injury: bringing stem cell-based therapy into clinical practice. *Dev Med Child Neurol* **59**: 997–1003. doi: 10.1111/dmcn.13528.

Williams PTJA, Jiang YQ, Martin JH (2017) Motor system plasticity after unilateral injury in the developing brain. *Dev Med Child Neurol* **59**: 1224–1229. doi: 10.1111/dmcn.13581.

SUGGESTIONS FOR FURTHER READING

Ismail FY, Fatemi A, Johnston MV (2017) Cerebral plasticity: windows of opportunity in the developing brain. *Eur J Paediatr Neurol* **21**: 23–48. doi: 10.1016/j.ejpn.2016.07.007.

Lagercrantz H, Hanson MA, Ment LR, Peebles DM (2010) *The Newborn Brain. Neuroscience and Clinical Applications*, 2nd edn. Cambridge: Cambridge University Press.

Stanley F, Blair E, Alberman E (2000) *Cerebral Palsies: Epidemiology and Causal Pathways*. London: Mac Keith Press.

Volpe JJ, Inder TE, Darras BT, et al. (2018) *Volpe's Neurology of the Newborn*, 6th edn. Philadelphia, PA: Elsevier.

PART III
Typical Motor Development

Sensory, Language, Cognitive, and Socio-Emotional Development

Hayley C Leonard

SUMMARY POINTS

- Motor skills are tightly linked with sensory, language, cognitive, and socio-emotional development.
- Individuals with motor disorders may therefore have difficulties in a range of other domains and those with other diagnoses may present with atypical motor skills.
- Understanding the relationships between domains throughout development will promote more targeted and effective interventions.

INTRODUCTION

Within a book dedicated to early detection and intervention for motor disorders, some readers may be surprised at the inclusion of a chapter considering sensory, language, cognitive, and socio-emotional development. This surprise may stem from an historic disconnect between research into motor development and other domains, with the motor system viewed as separate from, or less important than, other cognitive skills within the discipline of Psychology (Rosenbaum 2005). However, the inclusion of such a chapter indicates that there is a shift in our appreciation of the motor system as central to the study of behaviour. Our actions are the means through which we interact with the world and, as such, are in fact the behaviours observed in assessments of 'psychological' functions.

The current chapter aims to highlight the rich interconnections between motor skills and other domains within a highly complex system. It begins by introducing an important theoretical framework that emphasizes the integration of different domains for moment-to-moment and long-term learning. It considers influences on and the effects of motor development. The next sections outline key aspects of sensory, language, cognitive, and socio-emotional development in the first 2 years of life, ensuring that the motor system is kept in mind as an integral factor throughout this discussion. Finally, it considers lessons that can be learned from the research to help us better understand atypical development, including implications for early detection and intervention.

EMBODIED COGNITION AND DYNAMIC SYSTEMS

Within the last few decades, the study of developmental change has increasingly been informed by questions of *how* development occurs (Spencer et al. 2011). These more detailed explorations of developmental processes have highlighted that behaviour results from complex interactions between systems from moment to moment. Furthermore, it has revealed that the brain should not be seen as the composer of the music and conductor of the orchestra, with the body merely the musician producing the notes. As proposed in the *embodiment hypothesis*, 'intelligence emerges in the interaction of an organism with an environment and as a result of sensory-motor activity' (Smith 2005, p. 279). Using our orchestra analogy, the music would therefore emerge naturally through interactions between the conductor, the individual musicians, and their specific instruments. It would change from moment to moment, if different musicians with different instruments were present, and if there was a different purpose for the composition. These small individual variations could still lead to an overall long-term change in the way in which the musicians later play their instruments or work with others when composing a piece. In the same way, an infant's long-term development can be seen to be the result of continuous short-term changes that are different depending on the constraints and opportunities provided by the infant's own body, as well as the physical and social environment.

The constraints on motor development in particular have been detailed by Adolph and Hoch (2019) and are presented in Figure 4.1. Here, we can see that the reaching action produced by the infant is influenced by the infant's own body (the strength in the neck to hold up his head) and the physical environment (stimulating toys in the environment). A further influence of culture may also be evident: medical advice in the UK to place infants on their fronts for some time during the day (known as 'tummy time') may have provided an opportunity for the infant to produce that motor action. Other cultures

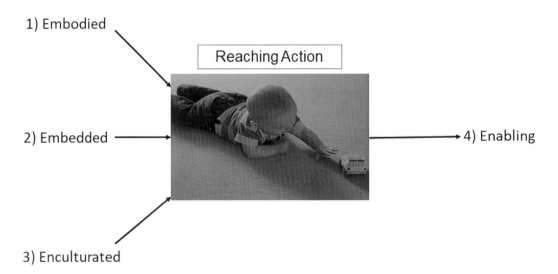

Figure 4.1   Influences on and results of an infant's reaching action, in line with Adolph and Hoch (2019). Actions are embodied (constrained by the infant's body state, e.g. reaching ability), embedded (dependent on the environment, e.g. toys in close proximity), enculturated (influenced by the social context and culture, e.g. infant placed on stomach for 'tummy time'), and enabling (provide opportunities for exploration and learning, e.g. grasping toys can lead to object manipulation). Note that the '4 Es' are also important for other domains, such as perceptual, language, cognitive, and socio-emotional development.

that do not adopt this practice may show variations in reaching. The action also produces opportunities for exploration that lead to long-term learning: reaching and grasping the toy would promote object manipulation and could lead to shared attention and labelling by the caregiver, which we know is an important step in vocabulary development (Camaioni 2001). Motor actions are therefore 'embodied, embedded, encultured and enabling' (Adolph and Hoch 2019, p. 1).

However, it is important to note that each other subsystem (e.g. language, perception, etc.) will have similar constraints and provide a wide range of opportunities for development. Furthermore, each of the subsystems will influence each other in these moment-to-moment changes; for example, if the infant does not have the visual acuity to see the object in front of him, he will not have the impetus to reach for it. We can thus consider behaviour to be the result of the combined effect of a number of subsystems working together, each with their own constraints and interactions with other subsystems.

This proposal fits within the Dynamic Systems Theory and Neuronal Group Selection Theory (NGST) outlined in Chapter 3. A key principle of these frameworks is that of *nested time scales*: while behavioural change occurs over different periods, each change affects the system and its constraints in the future (Smith and Thelen 2003). The milliseconds it takes for a particular set of neurons to fire will affect behaviour seconds later but will also change the way that the brain functions, and behaviour emerges, in the long term. For infants who have some disruption to their brain development, through a lesion or atypical connectivity, the variation and adaptability in brain functioning that aids the selection of the best possible motor strategy is impaired. As outlined in Chapter 3, this leads to reduced adaptability in the motor repertoire. These small changes early in the development of the motor subsystem could have long-term effects on other behaviours, such as in sensory, language, cognitive, and socio-emotional domains.

Having set up the basis for our understanding of the relationships between these different domains, the following sections will focus on the development of each of these areas in turn. While it would be impossible to cover all the relevant literature conducted in each vast area of infant research, an overview of key aspects of development will be provided and more detailed reviews identified.

SENSORY DEVELOPMENT

The development of sensory abilities is evident from birth and continues rapidly within the first year of life. As well as the individual senses of vision, hearing, touch, smell, and taste, the integration of information across these senses is of great importance to the infant's understanding of the world. The following section first provides an overview of development in each of these senses, before considering their integration and the impact this has on learning.

Visual Perception

From birth we can see that infants are not 'passive recipients of visual stimulation' (Johnson 2011, p. 516) and that they respond to different patterns in the visual environment with head and eye movements. Over the first three months of life, there is rapid development in the control of eye movements to allow infants to scan increasingly complex scenes for information that is more meaningful (i.e. not just the most visually salient information).

Nevertheless, vision in early infancy is significantly poorer than that of adults, including in the abilities to detect visual details (visual acuity), differences in luminance (contrast sensitivity), and depth perception (Johnson 2011). Figure 4.2a presents the image of a face in which the fine details and differences in luminance are blurred and difficult to resolve, as it might be seen by infants in the first few

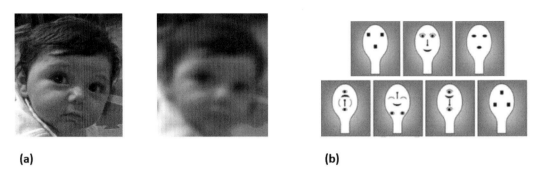

Figure 4.2 **(a)** Representation of a face as it might be seen through the constraints of the newborn visual system (right) compared to the adult visual system (left). The image is blurry and lacking in detail, although vision improves rapidly over the first year of life. **(b)** Face-like configurations (top row) are preferentially tracked by newborns over other configurations. Adapted from Johnson et al (2014) under Creative Commons CC-BY license.

months of life. Between the ages of 6 months and a year, vision will become much clearer and more adult-like (Leman et al. 2012). For depth perception, input needs to be taken from each eye and the disparity between these inputs calculated. This ability emerges at around 4 months but continues to develop to around 2–3 years of age (Johnson 2011).

The inclusion of a face stimulus above was not accidental but used to highlight one of the key visual preferences demonstrated by infants in the early neonatal period. Specifically, newborns prefer to track face compared with non-face stimuli even when they are matched for contrast and the number of elements presented within the face (Johnson et al. 2015; see Figure 4.2b). It is suggested that this initial preference towards faces is driven mainly by subcortical mechanisms that soon come under cortical control. The control of eye movements also becomes much smoother between the ages of 6 and 10 weeks, making tracking moving stimuli, such as faces, a more efficient process (Johnson 2011). Given that the faces of caregivers and others are often in the infant's visual field, at a distance suiting their visual acuity, being responsive to faces is highly adaptive. It also provides infants with plenty of experience to develop face recognition skills, which improve rapidly over the first year of life (Leman et al. 2012). Finally, a preference for faces exposes infants to a wealth of social information, which will be crucial to their own socio-emotional development. We return to this point later in the chapter.

Auditory Perception

The auditory system is functional from the gestational age of 6 months. By the end of pregnancy, the foetus demonstrates the ability to discriminate between different external sounds as well as respond to them, as evidenced by changes in physiological responses (Leman et al. 2012). While infants are thus able to detect a range of sounds from before birth, they have lower sensitivity to sounds compared to adults. Between 3 and 6 months postnatally, sounds need to be significantly louder for infants to hear them compared to adults, although the difference in detection thresholds reduces over the first 2 years of life (Fernald 2001).

Like depth perception in vision, knowing where a sound is coming from relies on integrating input from two organs (in this case, the ears), which are located on different sides of the head. Infants demonstrate this ability, known as sound localization, soon after birth by turning their head to the direction of the sound (Fernald 2001). However, the ability seems to disappear and reappear around 4 months of age. As in face perception, it is suggested that the initial behaviour is mainly controlled by subcortical mechanisms and that the behaviour gradually comes under cortical control, improving rapidly between 4 and 9 months and into the first year (Leman et al. 2012).

Auditory perception is also important for understanding the social world, particularly in the case of language. Both infants and adults are relatively more sensitive to frequencies between 2000 and 4000Hz, which is especially important for understanding speech (Fernald 2001). Infants demonstrate listening preferences for speech over non-speech at birth, and neuroimaging studies reveal that those brain areas associated with language processing in adults are activated from birth in infants (Maurer and Werker 2014). Sensitivity to language seems to be broadly tuned and to become gradually more narrowed to speech sounds related to the infant's native language over the first year (Kuhl et al. 2006; see Maurer and Werker 2014). Understanding the meaning of these sounds develops more slowly; although an infant can recognize his own name from around the age of 5 months, the ability to understand that a spoken word and picture can represent the same thing develops between 12 and 24 months (Fernald 2001). Language development is therefore clearly impacted by speech perception, and this is considered further later in the chapter.

Touch, Smell, and Taste

Touch, smell, and taste are the first senses to develop in the foetus and are functional before the gestational age of 6 months (Spence 2012), but are relatively less studied in infancy compared to visual and auditory perception. One reason for this may be the inter-relatedness of touch with vision, and of smell with taste, which means that their individual development has been neglected or considered too difficult to study. A key example is the concept of 'flavour', in which taste and smell are closely interlinked. The foetus is exposed to the taste and smell of the amniotic fluid in the womb and therefore to the flavours of the mother's diet, leading to a high sensitivity to taste and smell in newborns. While sweet flavours are preferred to sour at birth, preference for salty tastes tend to emerge around 4–6 months, with bitter flavours taking longer to appreciate (Spence 2012). Newborns can also discriminate between smells that adults rate as pleasant or aversive and, after a week outside the womb, show a preference for the smell of their mothers over strangers (Leman et al. 2012).

In terms of touch, or haptic perception, the relatively little research conducted has identified that newborns can detect differences in the contours of objects placed in their hands but occluded from vision (Streri and Féron, 2005). This sensitivity develops over the first 6 months. Investigations of infants' responses to external touches have also shown that infants up to 6 months orient towards vibrating buzzers placed on their hands, although this correct orienting is disrupted when their arms are crossed (Leman et al. 2012). Findings from these tactile stimulation studies suggest that infants' sense of their own bodies in reference to the external world is still developing after 6 months. This may rely on experience of integrating multiple sources of information from the body and through the different senses to better understand the environment and the infant's own place within it.

Multisensory Perception and Motor Development

Over the course of this section on perceptual development, it may have seemed that some senses, such as taste and smell, are more tightly linked than others. However, even if we go back to the concept of 'flavour', research has suggested that the texture, sight, and sound of food significantly influences how we taste and smell it (Spence 2012). In general, there has been a move in the more recent literature towards the idea of multisensory perception, supported by research that demonstrates the integration of a number of different senses during perceptual tasks (Lickliter and Bahrick 2000). For example, infants show a visual preference for objects they have only previously felt, and can match faces and voices based on visual and auditory synchrony. In terms of how multisensory perception develops, there have been two main approaches: that sensory modalities begin as separated and then become integrated with experience, or that they begin unified and become differentiated with age. Lickliter and Bahrick (2000) suggest that research supports a combination of the two theories: while there is extensive evidence of multisensory integration from birth that continues over development, there is also some differentiation between the senses.

Linking back to our theoretical frameworks, we can see that, within the perceptual subsystem, we can apply the same principles as we did to motor development. The senses are embodied: multisensory information is taken in through the body and the motor system is required to enable, for example, visual scanning of the environment, head movements to localize sound, hand movements to feel objects, and oral-motor control to explore the taste and smell of food. As it is in motor development, the perceptual subsystem is influenced by both body (including genetic and neural processes) and cultural contexts: it is embedded and encultured. Finally, perceptual development is enabling, with interactions between senses allowing the infant to learn about the world and his place in it. The rapid perceptual learning that occurs over the first year of life provides the basis for long-term learning in other domains, such as language, cognition, and socio-emotional development. It is to these domains that we now turn.

LANGUAGE DEVELOPMENT

Over the first 2 years of life, infants demonstrate a dramatic change in their ability to interact and communicate with those around them. Beginning with crying, vocalizations are later linked with gestures to aid communication, eventually leading to single and multiword utterances. The following section outlines key aspects of early language understanding and production, including an overview of important characteristics of the preverbal stage. Through this account, the changing relationships between language and other domains is discussed.

Preverbal Language Processing and Development

As discussed earlier in relation to auditory perception, infants demonstrate a preference for speech from birth, and this is especially the case for their mothers' voices and native languages. Further impressive newborn capacities are the abilities to detect word boundaries and word types through different acoustic cues, and to discriminate between words with different stress patterns (Gervain and Mehler 2010). These skills are important for language acquisition, providing the basis for the identification and production of single words and multiword utterances. In English, most words with two syllables are stressed on the first syllable (e.g. *in*fant), and thus being sensitive to stress patterns can give an infant clues as to where one word begins and another ends (Gervain and Mehler 2010). Infants' early abilities to discriminate relevant perceptual characteristics of speech are therefore an important foundation for understanding and producing language themselves.

In addition to correlations between perceptual and language abilities, there is also a strong link between vocal abilities and motor control in early development. Emerging motor control affects the physiology associated with vocalizations that provide the basis for language development (Iverson 2010). For example, holding the head upright changes the position of the tongue in the mouth, which aids the production of consonant-vowel pairings. Iverson and Thelen (1999) explain how vocal-motor coupling develops from early initial coordination between mouths and hands in spontaneous movements and,

Table 4.1 Early development of vocal-motor coupling
After the newborn stage, the motor behaviours highlighted precede the associated vocal behaviours, suggesting a tight link between motor and language development.

Age	Motor behaviour	Vocal behaviour
Newborn	Hand to mouth coordination	Spontaneous movements/sounds
6–8 months	Onset of reaching, rhythmical hand banging/arm waving Increase in object mouthing	Cooing, play with sounds, canonical babbling Increase in consonants during vocalizations
9–14 months	Recognitory gestures emerge and become decontextualized Communicative gestures emerge Onset of locomotion Improvement in fine motor skills and changing interactions with objects	First words emerge and become decontextualized Gains in language development (predicted by communicative gestures)
16–18 months	Synchronous gesture-word combinations	Increasing vocabulary

Sources: Iverson and Thelen (1999); Iverson (2010).

later, in directed movements with objects, to increasingly synchronous couplings such as tightly linked gestures and vocalizations (see Table 4.1). Gestures are extremely important in human communication and are seen in a simple form at around 9–12 months old. During this time period, infants begin to use recognitory gestures, which are brief actions that represent the function of particular objects (e.g. picking up a hairbrush and putting it near the hair). These early gestures demonstrate understanding of objects and their meanings or functions in a concrete sense, which lays the foundation for understanding how abstract spoken words can be associated with objects and meanings (Iverson 2010). Infants of this age also begin to use deictic gestures, such as pointing, combined with vocalizations to direct adult attention towards items of interest in the environment (Camaioni 2001). These developments in gestural use are followed by infants' first words, at around 12 months old. The rest of this section focuses on how a wider vocabulary and understanding of language develops from around this time.

First Words in Context

Infants' production of words lags well behind their language comprehension. While an infant will know an average of 900 words by the age of 24 months, they can produce only a fraction of these by the same age (Leman et al. 2012). Infants' first words tend to fall into particular categories across a range of cultures, specifically object names, those related to social interaction (e.g. 'bye-bye'), and those that highlight relational understanding, such as 'gone' or 'more' (Camaioni 2001). Single-word utterances continue for a relatively long period before words begin to be successfully combined and put into sentences at around 20 months. However, there are a number of stages that precede these successful multiword utterances, such as combining a gesture and single word to express a relationship (e.g. pointing to door and saying 'Daddy' to express that Daddy had gone). Early word combinations or sentences are often related to possessions (e.g. 'my ball') or relational understanding (e.g. 'ball gone'), as well as those related to locations and actions (Camaioni 2001). Further development of sentences and grammatical understanding take place after 24 months, and so are not within the scope of this chapter.

Given that language is essentially a social tool, it is important to consider the social context in which this impressive language development is taking place. Caregivers provide the context in which word learning and production occurs and so have a significant impact on language development. A good example of this is research that shows how the construction of language in different cultures affects the ways in which caregivers talk to their infants. While the majority of early research suggested that infants learned nouns before verbs, it seems that the relative position of nouns and verbs in a sentence within particular languages may influence the emphasis placed on them by caregivers during infant-directed speech, which affects the infant's consequent word learning (Camaioni 2001). Specifically, in Korean and Mandarin, in which verbs are more likely to be placed at the end of a sentence, caregivers tended to focus on describing actions when playing with toys with their infants; in English, in which nouns are more likely to end a sentence, caregivers focused on naming the toys during their play with their infants. Differences between these cultures are also seen in the infants' own first words, with the English infants demonstrating a focus on naming and the other cultures focusing on verbs (Camaioni 2001).

Thinking back to the 'four Es' proposed by Adolph and Hoch (2019), language development appears to be 'enculturated' and will proceed according to the cultural context. It is also 'embodied' and 'embedded', being affected by bodily and environmental constraints such as body position and the types of objects in the environment. Finally, the development of language is 'enabling': it is important for social interaction and cognitive reasoning. We come back to social development later, but now move on to a consideration of cognitive development over the first 2 years of life.

COGNITIVE DEVELOPMENT

From the previous sections, it is clear that infants use their senses to take in information about the environment and that this then affects their own behaviour and learning. The ability to process information and use it to inform behaviour continues to develop across childhood and adolescence. However, it relies on the infant attending to the relevant information in the environment, building up a representation of this information (i.e. a memory) for use in future situations, and being able to apply this knowledge to predict and interpret events. The following section provides a brief review of each of these aspects of cognitive development in turn.

Early Attention

In order to pay attention to information in the environment, infants first need to be awake and alert. Given that newborns only spend around 20% of their time in alert states, this is an important hurdle to overcome (Colombo 2001). Over the first 3 months, infants begin to have more consistent periods of alertness, which are more tightly linked to dark/light cycles and are maintained for longer. Now that he is alert, the infant can begin to make sense of his environment, exploring it by orienting towards and scanning different stimuli. In the following months, he will improve in smooth pursuit (tracking of moving objects). He can attend to more stimuli in the environment by disengaging his attention from one attractive stimulus in order to attend to something appearing in his peripheral vision (see Fig. 4.3). He will visually explore stimuli through increasing control over scanning behaviour (particularly the external contours), leading to better object recognition with age (Colombo 2001). Finally, over the course of the first year, infants begin to demonstrate greater control over their attention, no longer simply changing their attentional focus according to external influences; this is known as a shift from exogenous to endogenous control. It is demonstrated by infants' increasing abilities to sustain, shift and inhibit attention, particularly from around 6 months old (Colombo 2001; see Fig. 4.3). The developing endogenous control of attention provides the foundation for a range of other cognitive skills, including important regulatory processes known as 'executive functions', which continue to develop well into early adulthood (these are outside the scope of the current chapter; see Garon et al. [2008] for

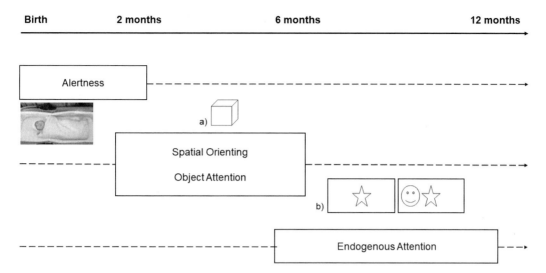

Figure 4.3   Representation of increasing attentional control over the first year. In the first 2 months, infants become gradually more alert. Over the course of the year, they become able to orient towards and visually scan objects (a) and have more control over their attention (b). Picture b represents a classic experimental visual paradigm in which a stimulus (the star) is presented to hold the viewer's attention and a second stimulus (the face) is presented either while the star remains on the screen, or after a short gap. After 6 months, infants are able to disengage their attention from the first stimulus to attend to the second stimulus when they overlap, and the speed at which they can do this increases with age. Infants can also increasingly inhibit a natural response to look towards a peripheral stimulus when it appears, demonstrating greater internal (endogenous) control over their attention.

a detailed review). Instead, we turn to memory, which is another key foundational process on which much of cognition is based.

Developing Memory

For many years, it was suggested that infants did not have the capacity to remember people, objects, and events. While the parameters of memory are certainly different in infants compared with older children and adults, more recent research has demonstrated that infants can retain increasing amounts of information over longer periods of time during the first 2 years of life (Rovee-Collier and Barr 2014). Using age-appropriate methods (see Table 4.2), research has shown that infants as young as 2 months old can remember objects that have previously been associated with a reward, as demonstrated by increased kicking in response to these objects compared with a novel object. Infants from 3 months old who have been habituated to a visual stimulus (i.e. repeatedly exposed to a stimulus until they no longer find it novel and interesting) look for longer at a new stimulus presented alongside the habituated one. Finally, from the age of 6 months, infants can reproduce a sequence of actions that were previously modelled by another individual, even after a delay (known as deferred imitation). The amount of time, or number of trials, taken to encode the initial stimulus or event and the duration of the delay over which the information can be remembered changes over the course of the first 2 years for each of these types of memory. Furthermore, for delayed imitation, the types of behaviour that infants can imitate become increasingly complex, moving from imitation of facial and body movements to actions on objects (Rovee-Collier and Barr 2014).

Table 4.2	Types of memory evident during infancy	
Method	**Example task**	**Developmental trends**
Habituation	A toy is revealed from underneath a cloth and an infant stares at the toy until it is covered again. This sequence is repeated, and the infant spends less and less time looking at the toy with each repetition; eventually, he does not look towards it at all. Decreased looking time indicates memory of the object or some aspect of it.	Infants aged 2–6 months could be habituated to a repeated visual stimulus
Operant conditioning	A mobile hung over the infant's crib is attached to the infant by a ribbon around his ankle. The infant learns that kicking causes the mobile to move and increases his kicking rate rapidly. To assess memory, infants learn this relationship with one mobile and, after a delay, are exposed to a mobile that differs in some way (e.g. colour, shape). Infants who remember the original mobile do not kick at the increased rate for the new mobile, but only for the original mobile.	At 2–3 months, infants who were trained with one mobile for 9 minutes per day for 3 days remembered the original mobile after a 24-hour delay. Using an upward extension of this task for older infants (pressing a lever to move a toy train) shows that the length of delay between training and retention increases to 8–12 weeks for 12–18-month-old infants.
Deferred imitation	A sequence of actions is conducted on objects by the experimenter and the sequence is repeated several times. After a delay, infants are provided with the same objects and their actions assessed. Infants who remember the actions reproduce the sequence on the objects, even after a delay.	At 6 months, infants can reproduce the sequence after a 24-hour delay. As seen in the reinforcement task above, infants show a linear increase up to 18 months in terms of the length of delay over which they remember (reproduce) the sequence. At 12 months, infants show deferred imitation after 1 week; at 18 months, this increases to 4 weeks. Deferred imitation can also be influenced by changing the objects and contexts in which the sequence occurs, with older infants being able to cope with more changes than younger infants.

Source: Rovee-Collier and Barr (2014).

As adults, when we discuss 'memory' as a concept, we are likely to think more about recollections of events and our own place within these events. However, infants cannot verbalize these recollections, so how can we assess whether this type of memory is evident in infancy? In terms of event memory, research has focused on presenting infants with a sequence of actions being carried out on an object (Bauer et al. 2011). Between 6 and 20 months, the duration of the delay between the presentation of an action sequence and memory of the sequence increases from around 24 hours to a year. This development can be affected by the context of the event: 18-month-olds can remember an action sequence when the same objects are used again at test, but not if one of the objects has changed. It is also likely to be related to the infant's own understanding of his place as a separate entity within the environment, with self-recognition in mirrors emerging from around 18 months (Bauer et al. 2011). Increasing understanding of the physical world may also be an important factor and is considered next.

Understanding the Physical World

As outlined at the beginning of this section, the relationship between infants' understanding of the physical world and attention and memory is, in fact, rather complex. Being able to predict the outcomes of

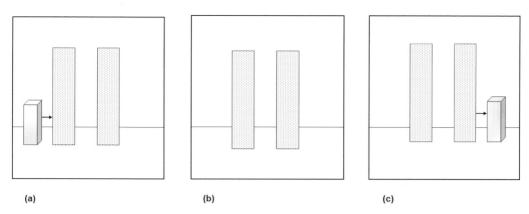

Figure 4.4 The 'violation-of-expectations' (VOE) paradigm, as used by Baillargeon and colleagues. In the first part of the test **(a)**, infants see an object being placed behind one of two screens, effectively hiding it from view **(b)**. Infants then see the same object being removed from behind the second screen, without it having appeared in between the screens or having been moved **(c)**. Infants look longer at this impossible event from as early as 2.5 months. Over the first year, they also demonstrate VOE when objects do not emerge as expected from containers, and when covered over.

particular actions relies on attention towards and memory of previous similar events; on the other hand, an increasing understanding of possible and impossible actions will affect how memory develops and the level of attention that is paid to future situations. Using a 'violation-of-expectations' (VOE) procedure, research has shown that infants as young as 2.5 months can detect when an impossible event has occurred, such as when an object is hidden behind a screen and fails to reappear (Baillargeon 2004; see Fig. 4.4). It has been suggested that very young infants thus have some understanding that objects continue to exist in time and space, which had not previously been attributed to infants before the age of 8 months. Over the first year, infants also begin to show VOE through longer looking times to impossible events when an object is placed inside a container or is covered over, based on the height and transparency of the objects involved (Baillargeon 2004). However, it is not clear from these studies whether an increase in looking time actually results from developing a lasting representation of the objects involved, or rather is driven by entirely perceptual processes occurring in the moment (Mareschal 2000). Importantly, actively reaching for objects may be more relevant for developing understanding of their properties, given that this requires the integration of both spatial and object-specific featural information. True object understanding may therefore develop later in infancy than suggested by the VOE procedure, requiring the interaction of motor and perceptual systems to build object representations (Mareschal 2000).

From the review of only a small part of the cognitive development literature above, the importance of the interaction between a number of subsystems over infancy is clear. Although the introduction of methods such as looking time procedures has meant that some milestones of development appear earlier than previously thought, it is necessary to fully investigate the mechanisms underlying these behaviours to help us to truly understand cognitive development. The important role of sensorimotor interactions with the environment should not be forgotten. Throughout this section, receiving and interpreting sensory information has been central to the behaviour measured and, even in the very basic measures of attention outlined, increasing oculomotor control was required as the infant developed. Importantly, these interactions are relevant not only for cognition, but also for many aspects of social-emotional development. The next section discusses how these apparently disparate areas of development are small parts of the same dynamic system.

SOCIO-EMOTIONAL DEVELOPMENT

The vast majority of sensory information that newborns receive during their limited alert periods is through interactions with their caregivers. These interactions are also extremely important for social and emotional development throughout infancy. From early in the infant's life, caregivers help to regulate the infant's level of arousal through play, which increases arousal and enjoyment, and through soothing distress (Bornstein and Tamis-LeMonda 2014). From around 2 months old, infants and caregivers engage in responsive exchanges through mutual gaze and sounds. Over time, different patterns of behaviour develop in both the infant and caregiver, and within the caregiver–infant dyad. The following section will provide an overview of some key aspects of this changing behaviour, including developing emotional understanding and a sense of others. It begins with an introduction to a key aspect of infancy, the attachment relationship between infant and caregiver, which is thought to provide the basis for much of the consequent socio-emotional development in later life.

Attachment

The term 'attachment' is used to describe the emotional bond between an infant and caregiver, which develops over the first year of life and continues to affect behaviour over childhood and into adulthood (Posada and Kaloustian 2010). This bond emerges gradually (see Table 4.3). Before the age of around 7 months, infants begin to build up patterns of interactions with those around them that encourage attachment, but they do not demonstrate a strong selective emotional and behavioural response to being separated from the attachment figure. Imagine a very young infant who cries or coos and is consequently picked up and held by the caregiver: the infant will learn over time the correspondence between his and the caregiver's behaviour, and that the caregiver will provide comfort or nurturance as he requires. By the age of 7 months, he has built a strong attachment with this caregiver and is consequently distressed when they are separated. Over the course of the first 2 years of life, the behavioural indicators of this attachment change but their purpose is still to seek proximity between the caregiver and infant during times of distress or anxiety (Posada and Kaloustian 2010).

Table 4.3	Stages of attachment in infancy	
Age	**Stage**	**Behaviour**
0–2 months	Pre-attachment	Does not discriminate between caregivers
2–7 months	Beginning of attachment to specific caregivers	Can discriminate between different caregivers but no strong preference expressed
7–30 months	Clear preference for attachment figure	*7–9 months* Wariness around strangers and anxiety at separation from caregiver *9–18 months* As infant begins to move around the environment independently, he balances exploration with regular returns to the caregiver for reassurance and comfort *18 months +* Behaviours still evident but reduced; attachment relationship can be increasingly regulated through improving verbal skills

Source: Posada and Kaloustian (2010).

The developing attachment relationship is also increasingly important once infants begin to move independently in the environment (usually from around 9 months onwards), with infants returning to the attachment figure for reassurance or comfort during exploratory episodes on their own. It is suggested that for exploration to occur, the infant needs to feel secure in his attachment figure's availability and responsiveness when he returns. Infants who do not develop this secure attachment may be less inclined to explore or may show atypical responses when attachment figures return from an absence; for example, infants may ignore or avoid them, or appear angry or distressed at the caregiver's return (Posada and Kaloustian 2010). These insecure attachments can have long-lasting effects on emotional and social development over the lifespan. It is to these two areas of development that this section now turns.

Emotional Development

One of the first emotional expressions to be shared between infant and caregiver is a smile. Over the first 8 weeks of life, smiles change from an endogenous pattern to become more coordinated with their caregivers' actions and external factors, becoming a representation of real happiness (Leman et al. 2012). Smiling increases when reinforced by reciprocal smiles and vocalizations, especially by the caregiver, and this aids the development of the attachment relationship. In terms of negative emotions, early infant cries can be seen to be associated with physiological needs, such as hunger or fatigue, rather than expressions of feelings in response to the environment. This emotional expression comes much later, with fear responses to strangers evident at around 7–9 months (notice the coincidental timing with the onset of separation anxiety and attachment development). Interestingly, once an infant begins to move independently around the environment, he also begins to express more anger, often due to being prohibited from exploring or touching aspects of the environment in which he is interested (Campos et al. 2000). He will also check back to his caregiver more often for reassurance. However, in order to gain this reassurance, he will need to be able to interpret the emotional signals provided by the caregiver. The development of this ability is outlined below.

Research with very young infants has shown that they can discriminate between facial expressions of emotion 1–2 days after birth, and that differential behavioural and brain responses to a range of expressions are evident within the first few months of life (Ramsey-Rennels and Langlois 2007). More familiar facial expressions, such as happiness, can be categorized earlier than those seen less often, such as anger. However, this is not evidence that infants actually understand the meaning of the facial expressions, nor that they are able to map them on to their own experiences of emotions; it may be that the discriminatory ability relies solely on perceptual differences between the facial expressions. Nonetheless, research does provide some indication of understanding of primary emotions in the first year: infants as young as 4–6 months respond with significantly more positive behaviours (happy facial expressions, vocalizations) to presentations of happy faces and more negative behaviours (fussing, crying) in response to angry faces; furthermore, 7-month-olds can match expressive vocalizations to the relevant facial expression (Ramsey-Rennels and Langlois 2007). As mentioned earlier, the infant's ability to understand the emotional expressions of the caregiver has important implications for his exploration of the environment. It will also provide the basis for understanding the thoughts and intentions of others, to which we now turn.

Social Cognition and Understanding

Understanding others' behaviour is an important puzzle to solve for infants and is central to being part of a social group. It is also a highly complex skill, comprising several stages of increasingly abstract concepts: the infant first needs to recognize that he and other people (e.g. the caregiver) are similar and external acts carried out by the caregiver can be imitated with his own body; next, that his specific bodily acts are related to mental experiences (such as distress at not achieving a goal); finally, that the caregiver also has mental experiences related to their observable bodily acts, which are similar to those experienced himself (Meltzoff 2011).

Given such a complex process, it was generally believed that a 'theory of mind' would require extended development. This was supported by early investigations of children's understanding of the knowledge held by others, using false belief tasks, in which a child and another viewer watch an object being hidden in one position before the object is moved to another position in sight of the child but when the other viewer is not watching the scene. When asked where the other viewer will look for the object, children younger than 4 years old are more likely to choose the new position, to which they have seen the object moved, even though the other viewer has not seen this change (Leman et al. 2012). This has long been interpreted as evidence that infants and young children do not have a sense of others' mental states before the age of 4.

However, research with infants using looking times has suggested that infants in their second year, much earlier than previously proposed, will look longer to the correct position (i.e. where the other viewer would look) in adapted false belief tasks than to the position in which they know the toy is placed (Leman et al. 2012). Additional research presenting infants with object-directed actions has suggested that, even in the first year, they have some understanding that others' have intentions and goals (Woodward et al. 2009; see Fig. 4.5). At 7 months old, infants who have been habituated to seeing a person reaching for a particular toy look for longer when the person reaches for a different toy than when the reach is directed towards the same toy in a different location. By 12 months, infants appear to understand another person's intentions in more complex action sequences on objects, and to predict a person's actions on an object from that person's previous attentional focus. Infants begin to understand that goals are not necessarily tied to one concrete action but may be tied to particular people, demonstrating surprise if a person's actions are not coherent with previous goals. While this is not the complex mental state attribution seen in older children and adults, it is nevertheless suggestive of much earlier understanding of others' minds than was previously proposed (Woodward et al. 2009). Importantly,

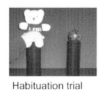

Habituation trial

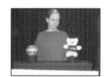

Habituation trial

New goal trial

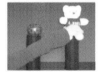

New side trial

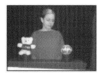

New object trial

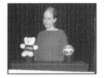

New Side trial

(a)   **(b)**

Figure 4.5 Tasks used by Woodward and colleagues revealing mental state understanding in infancy. By 7 months, infants who have been habituated to a person reaching for a particular toy look longer when the person reaches for a different toy (a new goal) than when they reach for the same toy in a different location **(a)**. By 12 months, infants show the same understanding of another person's attentional focus, not just their actions **(b)**. They not only follow the person's gaze, but look longer in the new object condition compared to the new side condition. Reproduced from Woodward et al. (2009) with permission.

social cognition, like other domains, seems to depend on infants' own interactions with the environment and experience of trying to achieve their own goals. For example, training infants to reach or to complete complex action sequences at an earlier age than is normally seen leads to earlier understanding of others' object-directed actions (Woodward et al. 2009). Taking an embodied approach to development in all the domains covered therefore appears justified. Further discussion of the key points revealed through this overview, along with their clinical implications, are discussed in the final section of this chapter.

CONCLUSIONS

I began this chapter by suggesting that some readers may be surprised at its focus on non-motor development within a book on early detection and intervention for motor disorders. However, over the course of the review, I hope that it has become clearer why the chapter is vital within such a book. Specifically, understanding the ongoing interactions between motor skills and sensory, language, cognitive, and socio-emotional development is essential for effective and timely interventions. We see this in clinical groups of individuals with motor disorders, such as developmental coordination disorder (DCD) or cerebral palsy: many of the issues that are picked up by parents, teachers, or the individuals themselves are not motor-specific, but related to these other domains. Why might this be? First, as previously mentioned, the importance of motor skills has received relatively less attention than other aspects of development and so parents and professionals may be more attuned to differences or delays in other domains. Second, the wide variation in achieving motor milestones in typical development often makes it difficult to identify potential motor delays (see Chapters 3 and 6). Furthermore, the focus of research into individual domains of development, rather than as an integrated system, has limited our ability to identify and understand the relationships across domains. Thankfully, this is beginning to change, as seen through the increasing focus on multisensory perception and greater adoption of the embodiment hypothesis. However, there is still a long way to go.

So what are the clinical implications of this approach to development? In terms of motor disorders, I believe that it is important to ensure that the individual is considered in context. This applies both to the individual's social environment and culture, which we have seen affects the development of motor and other skills, and to the motor subsystem's context within that individual body in relation to the other subsystems outlined above. While it is obviously essential to treat the motor difficulties core to the disorder, it must be understood that these difficulties have an impact on a range of other domains that cause functional limitations in everyday life. Given the tight relationships between domains and the cascading effects of early brain development on later function, it is also important to recognize that neurodevelopmental disorders that are not diagnosed on the basis of motor difficulties may also require significant motor interventions; indeed there is a high prevalence of motor problems reported across diagnostic categories, as well as a substantial number of individuals with co-occurring diagnoses. Focusing on only one area of development for intervention will therefore miss key areas of difficulty. In summary, understanding development as a dynamic system is essential to both research and practice, and will promote more targeted and effective interventions for those with motor difficulties.

REFERENCES

Adolph KE, Hoch JE (2019) Motor development: embodied, embedded, encultured, and enabling. *Annu Rev Psychol* **70**: 141–164. doi: org/10.1146/annurev-psych-010418-102836.

Baillargeon R (2004) Infants' physical world. *Curr Dir Psychol Sci* **13**: 89–94. doi: org/10.1111/j.0963-7214.2004.00281.x.

Bauer PJ, Larkina M, Deocampo J (2011) Early memory development. In: Goswami U, editor, *The Wiley-Blackwell Handbook of Childhood Cognitive Development*, 2nd edn. Chichester: John Wiley & Sons, Ltd, pp. 153–179.

Bornstein MH, Tamis-LeMonda CS (2014) Parent-infant interaction. In: Bremner JG, Wachs, TD, editors, *The Wiley-Blackwell Handbook of Infant Development*, 2nd edn. Chichester: John Wiley & Sons, Ltd, pp. 458–482.

Camaioni L (2001) Early language. In: Bremner G, Fogel A, editors, *Blackwell Handbook of Infant Development*. Oxford: Blackwell Publishers Ltd, pp. 404–426.

Campos JJ, Anderson DI, Barbu-Roth MA, Hubbard EM, Hertenstein MJ, Witherington D (2000) Travel broadens the mind. *Infancy* **1**: 149–219. doi: 10.1207/S15327078IN0102_1.

Colombo J (2001) The development of visual attention in infancy. *Annu Rev Psychol* **52**: 337–367. doi: org/10.1146/annurev.psych.52.1.337.

Fernald A (2001) Hearing, listening and understanding: auditory development in infancy. In: Bremner G, Fogel A, editors, *Blackwell Handbook of Infant Development*. Oxford: Blackwell Publishers Ltd, pp. 35–70.

Garon N, Bryson SE, Smith IM (2008) Executive function in pre-schoolers: a review using an integrative framework. *Psychol Bull* **13**: 31–60. doi: dx.doi.org/10.1037/0033-2909.134.1.31.

Gervain J, Mehler J (2010) Speech perception and language acquisition in the first year of life. *Annu Rev Psychol* **61**: 191–218. doi: org/10.1146/annurev.psych.093008.100408.

Iverson JM. (2010) Developing language in a developing body: the relationship between motor development and language development. *J Child Lang* **37**: 229–261. doi: org/10.1017/S0305000909990432.

Iverson JM, Thelen E (1999) Hand, mouth and brain. The dynamic emergence of speech and gesture. *J Consciousness Stud* **6**: 19–40.

Johnson SP (2011) Development of visual perception. *Wiley Interdiscip Rev Cogn Sci* **2**: 515–528. doi: 10.1002/wcs.128.

Johnson MH, Senju A, Tomalski P (2015) The two-process theory of face processing: modifications based on two decades of data from infants and adults. *Neurosci Biobehav Rev* **50**: 169–179. doi: org/10.1016/j.neubiorev.2014.10.009.

Kuhl PK, Stevens E, Hayashi A, Deguchi T, Kiritani S, Iverson P (2006). Infants show a facilitation effect for native language phonetic perception between 6 and 12 months. *Developmental Sci* **9**: F13–F21. doi: org/10.1111/j.1467-7687.2006.00468.x.

Leman P, Bremner AJ, Parke RD, Gauvain M (2012) *Developmental Psychology*. London: McGraw-Hill.

Lickliter R, Bahrick LE (2000) The development of infant intersensory perception: advantages of a comparative convergent-operations approach. *Psychol Bull* **126**: 260–280. doi: dx.doi.org/10.1037/0033-2909.126.2.260.

Mareschal D (2000) Object knowledge in infancy: current controversies and approaches. *Trends Cogn Sci* **4**: 408–416. doi: doi: org/10.1016/S1364-6613(00)01536-9.

Maurer D, Werker JF (2014) Perceptual narrowing during infancy: a comparison of language and faces. *Dev Psychobiol* **56**: 154–178. doi: org/10.1002/dev.21177.

Meltzoff A (2011) Social cognition and the origins of imitation, empathy, and theory of mind. In: Goswami U, editor, *The Wiley-Blackwell Handbook of Childhood Cognitive Development*, 2nd edn. Chichester: John Wiley & Sons Ltd, pp. 49–75.

Posada G, Kaloustian G (2010) Attachment in infancy. In: Bremner JG, Wachs, TD, editors, *The Wiley-Blackwell Handbook of Infant Development*. Chichester: John Wiley & Sons, Ltd, pp. 483–509.

Ramsey-Rennels JL, Langlois JH (2007) How infants perceive and process faces. In: Slater A, Lewis M, editors, *Introduction to Infant Development*, 2nd edn. Oxford: Oxford University Press, pp. 191–215.

Rosenbaum DA (2005) The Cinderella of psychology: the neglect of motor control in the science of mental life and behavior. *Am Psychol* **60**: 308–316. doi: dx.doi.org/10.1037/0003-066X.60.4.308.

Rovee-Collier C, Barr R (2014) Infant learning and memory. In: Bremner JG, Wachs, TD, editors, *The Wiley-Blackwell Handbook of Infant Development*, 2nd edn. Chichester: John Wiley & Sons Ltd, pp. 217–294.

Smith LB (2005) Cognition as a dynamic system: principles from embodiment. *Dev Rev* **25**: 278–298. doi: org/10.1016/j.dr.2005.11.001.

Smith LB, Thelen E (2003) Development as a dynamic system. *Trends Cogn Sci* **7**: 343–348. doi: 10.1016/S1364-6613(03)00156-6.

Spence C (2012) Assessing the role of visual (colour) cues on the perception of taste and flavour. In: Bremner AJ, Lewkowicz DJ, Spence C, editors, *Multisensory Development*. Oxford: Oxford University Press, pp. 63–87.

Spencer JP, Perone S, Buss AT (2011) Twenty years and going strong: a dynamic systems revolution in motor and cognitive development. *Child Dev Perspect* **5**: 260–266. doi: org/10.1111/j.1750-8606.2011.00194.x.

Streri A, Féron J (2005) The development of haptic abilities in very young infants: from perception to cognition. *Infant Behav Dev* **28**: 290–304. doi: org/10.1016/j.infbeh.2005.05.004.

Woodward AL, Sommerville, JA, Gerson S, Henderson AM, Buresh J (2009) The emergence of intention attribution in infancy. *Psychol Learn Motiv* **51**: 187–222. doi: org/10.1016/S0079-7421(09)51006-7.

SUGGESTED READINGS

Anderson DI, Campos JJ, Witherington DC et al. (2013) The role of locomotion in psychological development. *Front Psychol* **4**: 440. doi: org/10.3389/fpsyg.2013.00440.

Hadders-Algra M. (2018) Early human motor development: From variation to the ability to vary and adapt. *Neuroscience and Biobehavioural Reviews* **90**: 411–427.

Leonard, HC (2016) The impact of poor motor skills on perceptual, social and cognitive development: The case of Developmental Coordination Disorder. *Front Psychol* **7**: 311. doi: 10.3389/fpsyg.2016.00311.

Leonard HC, Hill EL (2014) The impact of motor development on typical and atypical social cognition and language: a systematic review. *Child Adol Mental H-UK* **19**: 163–170. doi: org/10.1111/camh.12055.

Thelen E (2005) Dynamic systems theory and the complexity of change. *Psychoanal Dialogues* **15**: 255–283. doi: org/10.1080/10481881509348831.

Motor Development During Foetal Life and Early Infancy

Mijna Hadders-Algra

SUMMARY POINTS

- Spontaneous movements are already emerging 7 weeks postmenstrual age.
- From 9–10 weeks postmenstrual age onwards complex and varied general movements dominate foetal motor behaviour.
- In the first 3 months after term age complex and varied general movements continue to be the most common movements.
- The last phase of general movements starts at 2 months post-term and lasts till 4–5 months post-term, when goal-directed movements take over. During this phase general movements are not only characterized by complexity and variation but also by the age-specific fidgety movements. Fidgety movements are small and elegant movements occurring irregularly all over the body. The occurrence of fidgety movements signals a major transition in the infant's development: the subcortical-cortical networks are ready to learn from the sensory information associated with the infant's activities and to move on with goal-directed actions.
- At term age infants are able to adapt sucking movements to the feeding situation.
- In the first postnatal months head control develops and precursors of goal-directed limb movements emerge.
- The 'peri-term' period is characterized by temporary physiological hyperexcitability of the nervous system, which makes young infants easily cry.

Already at an early stage of development the foetus starts to move. Ultrasound studies demonstrated that the first movements emerge at 7 weeks postmenstrual age (PMA; i.e. the age calculated from the first day of the last menstrual period of the mother; Lüchinger et al. 2008) This implies that the first movements develop before the spinal reflex pathways are completed, as these reflex circuitries emerge at week 10–11 PMA (Clowry et al. 2005). This underlines the endogenous or spontaneous nature of early human motor activity. It also implies that early motor behaviour is not primarily organized in terms of reflexes, but is based on spontaneous intrinsic activity of the nervous system (Hadders-Algra 2018a).

The current chapter discusses foetal and neonatal motor development. This means that it addresses motor behaviour in the phase of life during which spontaneous general movement activity dominates. The first section presents foetal life; the second section discusses motor behaviour in the first months after birth. In the latter section, special attention is paid to transitions in behaviour. The transition around 3 months post-term is highlighted, as it is the period in life during which the infant moves from the phase of predominant generalized movement activity to the phase in which specific goal directed movements dominate.

FOETAL MOTOR BEHAVIOUR

At 7 weeks PMA, the foetus starts to produce small sideways bending movements of the head and/or trunk. About 1 week later, also the extremities start to participate in movement activity (Fig. 5.1). The first generalized movements, involving all parts of the body, are slow, small, simple, and stereotyped (Lüchinger et al. 2008). At 9–10 weeks PMA, general movements (GMs) emerge (i.e. movements in which all parts of the body participate and during which movement direction, amplitude, and speed varies). During GMs, all possible combinations of degrees of freedom in the various body joints are explored. The emergence of complex and varied GMs coincides with the onset of synaptic activity in the transient cortical subplate (see Chapter 3). This triggered the hypothesis that the neural substrate of the varied and complex GMs initially consists of subplate activity that modulates the basic activity of the central pattern generating (CPG) networks of the GMs that are located in the spinal cord and brain stem (Hadders-Algra 2018b; Text Box 5.1). Very soon, the GMs become the most frequently used movement pattern of the foetus (De Vries and Fong 2006). They excellently express the brain's activity during the phase of primary variability (see Chapter 3) and are regarded as the cornerstone of early motor development. The latter is discussed in more detail in the next section.

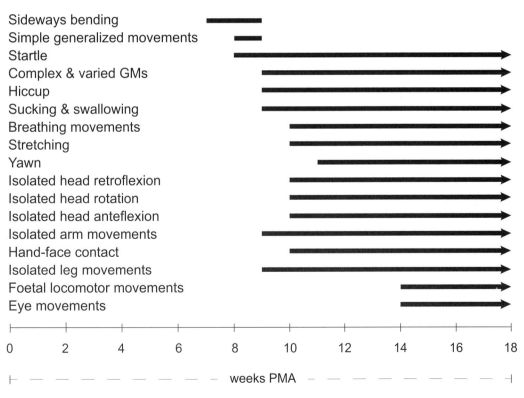

Figure 5.1 Schematic diagram on the emergence of foetal movements. The diagram is based on De Vries and Fong (2006) and Hadders-Algra (2018a). GMs = general movements; PMA = postmenstrual age.

Text Box 5.1 Central Pattern Generating Networks: The Core Module in the Organization of Motor Control

The organization of neural control of movements is best known by rhythmical movements like locomotion, respiration, sucking, and mastication. A core element in the control of these movements is the so-called central pattern generator (CPG; Fig. 5.2). A CPG is a neural network with spontaneous activity, located in the spinal cord and/or brain stem. The CPG is able to coordinate autonomously (i.e. without segmental sensory or supraspinal information) the activity of many muscles. Of course, in typical conditions the CPG network does not work autonomously but is fine-tuned to the specifics of the condition by two types of information (Frigon 2017). The first source of information originates from segmental afferent signals, for instance proprioceptive information from muscle spindles or information from pressure receptors in the skin. The segmental afferent information allows for a reactive adaptation of the output of the CPG network. The second and most important source of information originates in the complex cortical-subcortical circuitries. Activity in the latter circuitries is organized in large-scale networks, in which cortical areas are functionally connected through direct recursive interaction or through intermediary cortical or subcortical (striatal, cerebellar) structures (Bassett et al. 2015; Fuertinger et al. 2015). The supraspinal information allows – on the basis of learning processes – for the anticipatory adaptation of the output of the CPG-networks. The supraspinal networks expanded substantially during phylogeny and determine to a large extent human motor ontogeny.

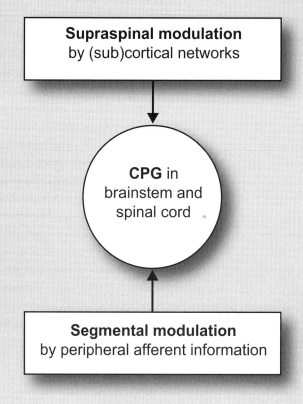

Figure 5.2 Schematic diagram of the CPG-model of motor control.

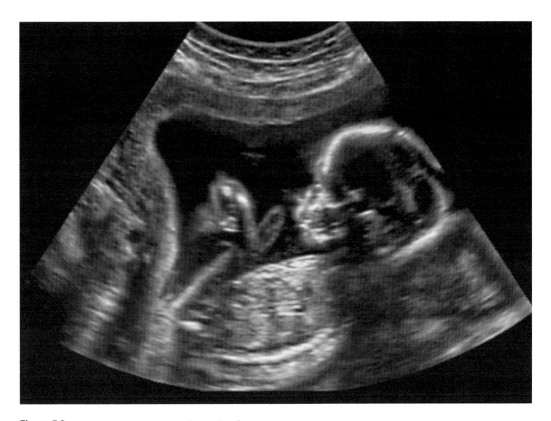

Figure 5.3 Foetal hand movement directed to face.

Other early emerging movement patterns are the startle (i.e. the abrupt and short movement starting in the limbs and involving all parts of the body), the hiccup, the sucking and swallowing movements, and the breathing movements (Fig. 5.1). From 9 weeks PMA onwards, the foetus also generates isolated arm movements and isolated leg movements (De Vries and Fong 2006). Starting at week 14 PMA, the lower extremity movements may participate in the pattern of foetal locomotion (Hadders-Algra 2018a).

The upper extremities may be involved in hand–face contact from 10 to 12 weeks PMA and in thumb sucking from 15 weeks PMA (Hepper 2013). Throughout gestation, hand motility varies, with about one-third to half of the hand movements being directed to mouth, face, or head (Sparling et al. 1999; Fig. 5.3). With increasing foetal age, the hand movements towards the head gradually change: increasingly often the lower and perioral parts of the face become the hand's target. In addition, hand movements directed to the eye get a slower end-velocity than the movements directed to the mouth. This suggests that some adaptation of the hand movement to the delicacy of its target occurs (Zoia et al. 2013; Reissland et al. 2014).

Isolated head movements (i.e. rotation, retroflexion, and anteflexion) emerge at 10 weeks PMA. As mentioned above, sucking and swallowing movements emerge early, but their incidence in the first half of gestation is low (De Vries et al. 1985). Moreover, the first jaw, lip, tongue, and pharynx movements are relatively simple. They gradually become more complex, and – from about 28 weeks PMA – also include the anterior-posterior movements of the tongue needed for successful sucking (Miller et al. 2003). Foetal sucking and swallowing is clearly associated with hand–face contact.

It should be noted that the age of emergence of the various foetal movements varies substantially between foetuses. Nevertheless, at about 16 weeks PMA all foetuses have accomplished the development of the entire foetal motor repertoire (Fig. 5.1; De Vries and Fong 2006). This repertoire continues to be present throughout gestation and largely resembles the repertoire of the full-term newborn. Two differences between the motor behaviour of the foetus and that of the newborn deserve attention. First, the foetus is able to anteflex the head in supine position, whereas the newborn, who is exposed to the forces of gravity, is unable to perform this action. Second, the foetus exhibits episodic breathing, which implies that the foetus interchanges bouts of 10–30 minutes of breathing movements with equally long periods without these movements (De Vries et al. 1982). It is evident that the newborn infant needs to transform this breathing pattern immediately into the continuous breathing required for survival.

The amount of foetal movements varies enormously, both intra- and inter-individually (De Vries and Fong 2006). Yet, in general, the incidence of movements gradually decreases with increasing gestational age (Robles de Medina et al. 2003).

NEONATAL MOTOR BEHAVIOUR

In the young infant GMs are – just as in the foetus – the most frequently occurring movement pattern. Therefore, this section starts with the discussion of the development of GMs. Next, early development of specific motor behaviour is addressed.

General Movements

Typical GMs consist of movements in which all parts of the body participate. They are characterized in particular by movement complexity and variation. Complexity denotes the spatial variation of movements. It is brought about by the independent exploration of degrees of freedom in all body joints. The continuously varying combinations of flexion–extension, abduction–adduction and endorotation–exorotation generate a flow of changes in movement direction of the participating body parts. GM variation represents the temporal variation of movements. It means that over time, the infant continues to explore the movement possibilities that the body offers. Movement complexity and variation are tightly intertwined, actually implying that the primary parameters of GM quality evaluate two aspects of movement variation. This corresponds to the notion that variation is a hallmark of the typically developing brain (Hadders-Algra 2018b).

The previous section recounted that complex and varied GMs emerge early during ontogeny. During foetal life, the basic features of GMs remain identical. However, shortly before term age (i.e. around 36–38 weeks PMA) a transition in movement form occurs. This transition occurs both inside the uterus and – in preterm infants – outside the womb. After the transition, the GMs remain complex and varied, but they get a 'writhing' appearance, implying that they impress as forceful and tense. In addition, trunk movements are smaller than previously (Videos 5.1 and 5.2). Some 10 weeks later, another transition in GM form occurs. Around the age of 2 months post-term the forceful writhing appearance disappears and so-called fidgety GMs emerge. Also, fidgety GMs are characterized by complexity and variation (Fig. 5.4), but the GM's basic movement melody now consists of a continuous stream of small and elegant movements occurring irregularly over the body (Einspieler et al. 2005; Hadders-Algra 2018b; Video 5.3). Fidgety movements are most prominently present between 11 and 16 weeks post-term (Hadders-Algra 2018b). The developmental changes in typical GMs are summarized in Table 5.1.

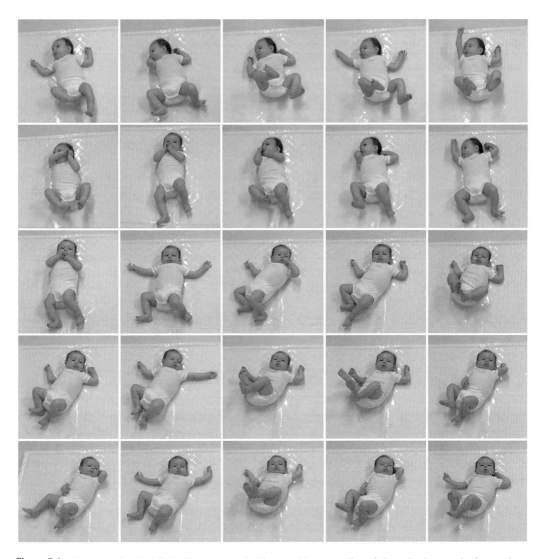

Figure 5.4 Example of typical GMs. Frames sampled from a video-recording of about 2 minutes; the frames have an interval of about 5 seconds. The figure illustrates the movement complexity and variation of typical GMs in a full-term-born infant aged 3 months. In each frame the infant's body parts show a different configuration. Figure reproduced from Hadders-Algra (2018b) with permission.

Interestingly, the ages of transition in GM form are only to a limited extent affected by environment and practice. For instance, low risk preterm infants reach the fidgety phase only about one week earlier than typically developing full-term infants, despite their advantage of several weeks of additional extra-uterine experience (Cioni and Prechtl 1990). This underscores the notion that GM development is largely based on endogenous neural processes.

In all GM phases movement complexity and variation remain GMs' primary characteristics. It has been hypothesized that complexity and variation initially is generated by cortical subplate activity. When the subplate starts to dissolve from about 28 weeks PMA, its function in the generation of movement

Table 5.1   Developmental changes in typical GMs

Age	GM form	Description
9–10 to 36–38 wk PMA	Foetal/preterm GMs	Complex and varied movements, including prominent trunk movements
36–38 wk PMA to 6–8 wk CA	Writhing GMs	Complex and varied movements with a forceful appearance
2–5 mo CA, particularly 2–4 mo CA	Fidgety GMs	Complex and varied movements with a basic melody of tiny, elegant movements occurring all over the body

CA = corrected age, i.e. weeks post-term; mo = months; GMs = general movements; PMA = postmenstrual age; wk = weeks; see Videos 5.1, 5.2, and 5.3.

complexity and variation is gradually taken over by the cortical plate ('subplate and cortical plate modulation hypothesis'; Hadders-Algra 2018b). This process of reallocation of function is completed in the primary sensory and motor cortices at 3 months post-term (i.e. in the last phase of GMs with its characteristic fidgety movements) (Hadders-Algra 2018b; Fig 5.5). Yet, the neurodevelopmental changes underlying GM development do not only involve a reallocation of the substrate of complexity and variation from subplate to cortical plate, but they also involve maturational changes in the cortical networks. The latter implies that the activity in the cortical networks gets fragmented (a process called 'sparsification'), meaning that the activity gets less intensive and occurs in more limited groups of neurons (Leighton and Lohmann 2016). This process presumably starts at the end of gestation, but it is obscured by the transiently present physiological 'hyperexcitability' of the nervous system around term age. It has been surmised that this 'hyperexcitability' – caused by a specific neurotransmitter setting (see Chapter 3) – facilitates the transition from the foetal episodic breathing pattern to the continuous breathing needed for postnatal survival. Presumably, the relatively high motoneuronal excitability is the neural correlate of the writhing character of the GMs around term age (see also Text Box 5.2). When the physiological 'hyperexcitability' disappears, the 'sparcified' activity of the cortical networks in the primary sensory and motor cortices is able to manifest itself in the form of the tiny fidgety movements ('sparsification hypothesis'; Hadders-Algra 2018a,b; Fig. 5.5).

The emergence of the tiny fidgety movements signals that the nervous system is increasingly prepared to make sense of its own actions and of the environment (Leighton and Lohmann 2016). It is also the phase that functional connections between corticospinal tract fibres and spinal motoneurons show signs of activity-dependent reorganization (Ritterband-Rosenbaum et al. 2017). This means, that from the fidgety GM phase onwards, the nervous system is ready for full engagement in goal directed motor activities.

Early Specific Motor Behaviour After Birth

Apart from the frequently occurring GMs, the young infant also shows specific motor behaviours. An example is nutritive sucking and swallowing, which postnatally has to be combined with respiration. This is a challenging task, which is not well mastered in preterm infants aged 32–33 weeks PMA. The preterm infant explores its sucking and swallowing movements. From about 36 weeks PMA, sucking and swallowing movements become increasingly adapted, the sucking rhythm stabilizes, and sucking is less often interrupted by breathing bursts (Gewolb and Vice 2006). In other words, sucking and swallowing have reached the phase of secondary variability (see Chapter 3). After term age, sucking gets increasingly

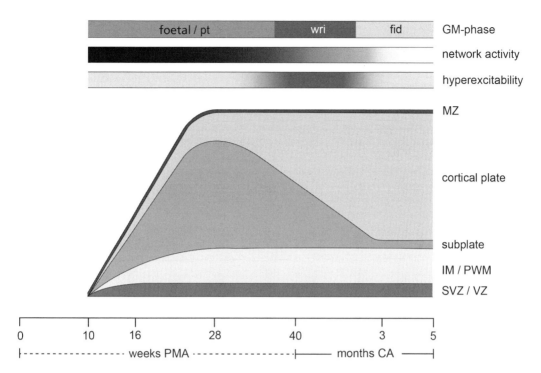

Figure 5.5   Schematic presentation of the neural processes underlying GM ontogeny. The bottom line denotes age, first in weeks PMA, after term (40 weeks) in months corrected age (CA). Above the age line the developmental changes in the human cortex are depicted. SVZ / VZ represents the subventricular and ventricular zones where the neurons and glial cells are generated; IM / PWM denotes the intermediate zone (IM) that gradually develops into the periventricular white matter (PWM); MZ is the marginal zone. The diagram illustrates that the modulating activity of the subplate is gradually taken over by the cortical plate (the *subplate and cortical plate modulation hypothesis*). The following three timelines represent from bottom to top: the physiological 'hyperexcitability' of the nervous system, in which the intensity of the grey shading represents the degree of hyperexcitability; cortical network activity that emerges across the brain from 9–10 weeks PMA, gradually increases (indicated by increasing shading) to be full-blown present (in the subplate) at mid-foetal age; next it gradually moves from global and widespread activity to local and limited activity ('sparsification'; indicated by the diminution of the dots; the *sparsification hypothesis*); on top the developmental changes in GMs. Figure reproduced from Hadders-Algra (2018b) with permission.

efficient. This is, for instance, reflected in a doubling of milk intake – the volume of milk per suck – in the first post-term month (Qureshi et al. 2002; Hadders-Algra 2018a).

The young infant's facial motility is characterized by variation. How well the newborn infant is able to imitate facial expressions is debated. Most likely this capacity is limited to the imitation of tongue protrusion (Meltzoff et al. 2018). Between 5 and 10 weeks post-term, social smiles emerge; the infant learns to select the smile and other communicative expressions from its repertoire of facial movements in response to another human's face (Fig. 5.6; Hadders-Algra 2018a). The young infant explores his vocal capacities by means of sounds called protophones. Initially, the repertoire of protophones is relatively small. It gradually expands and gets more complex. Between 3 and 5 months, the infant increasingly often selects the vowels belonging to the adult repertoire (Nathani et al. 2006).

Text Box 5.2 Peri-term Physiological 'Hyperexcitability': Behavioural Parallels

In the period that ranges from about 36 weeks PMA to 4–6 weeks post-term the human nervous system is characterized by a temporarily different setting of various neurotransmitter systems (overexpression of noradrenergic α2-receptors and glutamatergic NMDA-receptors, relatively high serotonergic innervation, and high dopaminergic turnover; see Chapter 3). This neural setting of 'physiological hyperexcitability' is associated with an increased motoneuron excitability. This is reflected in the writhing aspect of the GMs and the phenomenon of 'physiological hypertonia' of the full-term neonate. The latter term has been used to describe that the resistance to passive movements in infants around term age is higher than that in younger and older infants (Amiel-Tison and Grenier 1983).

From 6–8 weeks CA onwards, the 'physiological hyperexcitability' gradually disappears, which is reflected by the emergence of fidgety GMs. The gradual reduction in nervous system excitability is associated with an increase in autonomic stability (Mulkey and du Plessis 2019). It is also paralleled by a decrease in the prevalence of excessive infant crying (Reijneveld et al. 2001). This implies that a considerable proportion of excessive infant crying is 'cured' by the changes occurring in the developing brain.

Conceivably, the peri-term motoneuronal 'hyperexcitability' assists survival after birth around term age. Support for this assumption may be found in the prevalence of apnoea of prematurity, which rapidly decreases between 33 and 36–37 weeks PMA, that is, when the 'hyperexcitability' emerges (Stokowski 2005; Nagraj et al. 2020) – and that of sudden infant death syndrome, that peaks at 2–4 months when the 'hyperexcitability' has just disappeared (Task Force on Sudden Infant Death Syndrome and Moon 2011).

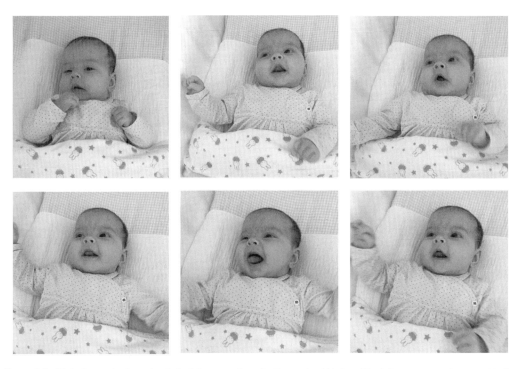

Figure 5.6 Variation and adaptation in facial expression of a 3-month-old infant. The infant communicates with the caregiver. Published with permission of the parents.

After birth, the forces of gravity challenge the infant's postural control. Full-term neonates are able to keep the head upright for a few seconds when held in a sitting position. In preterm infants, anti-gravity head control starts to develop from about 32 weeks PMA, so that low-risk preterm infants have achieved at term age the same level of head control as their term-born peers. The ability to balance the head continues to improve so that around 3 months post-term most infants are able to keep the head in the midline in supine, and can balance the head when held in a sitting position (Hadders-Algra 2018a; Video 5.4).

In the first 2–3 months post-term, babies – like foetuses – direct about one third or half of their spontaneous hand movements to the face. These movements are not guided by visual information. Yet, infants aged only a few days or weeks post-term are also able to control their arm movements to some extent on the basis of visual information. They may produce arm movements in response to an object, especially when they fixate the object and when they are put in a sitting position with ample neck and trunk support (Von Hofsten 1982; Amiel-Tison and Grenier 1983). These 'prereaching' arm movements can especially be observed at 2–3 months post-term (Video 5.5). From 4 months onwards (i.e. when GM activity fades), reaching movements become more efficient and start to result in successful grasping (Hadders-Algra 2018a).

In neonatal term infants, stepping movements may be elicited. In the absence of specific training or of support by water buoyancy (Thelen and Cooke 1987), the stepping movements disappear around the age of 2–3 months (Forssberg 1985) – a disappearance that may be related to the disappearance of the perinatal neural 'hyperexcitability'. However, when neonatal stepping is trained daily, the stepping movements can be elicited until its replacement by supported locomotion.

CONCLUDING REMARKS

From early foetal age, motor behaviour is typified by its spontaneous, complex, and varied character. This indicates that from early age motor behaviour is affected by activity from subcortical-cortical networks. Early movements especially serve exploration and further sculpting of the nervous system; they are not adapted to the situation. However, from the last trimester of gestation onwards the foetus develops some capacities to adapt specific movements (e.g. arm movements and sucking and swallowing movements) to the situation. Yet, these adaptive capacities are limited. The ability to learn to adapt movements to the context first starts to bloom after the period of fidgety GMs. The latter movements signal a major transition in the infant's development; they indicate that the subcortical-cortical networks are now ready to learn from the sensory information associated with the infant's activities and to move on with goal-directed actions.

REFERENCES

Amiel-Tison C, Grenier A (1983) *Neurologic Evaluation of the Newborn and the Infant.* New York: Masson Publishing USA Inc.

Bassett DS, Yang M, Wymbs NF, Grafton ST (2015) Learning-induced autonomy of sensorimotor systems. *Nat Neurosci* **18**: 744–751. doi: 10.1038/nn.3993.

Cioni G, Prechtl HF (1990) Preterm and early postterm motor behaviour in low-risk premature infants. *Early Hum Dev* **23**: 159–191.

Clowry GJ, Moss JA, Clough RL (2005) An immunohistochemical study of the development of sensorimotor components of the early fetal human spinal cord. *J Anat* **207**: 313–324.

De Vries JI, Fong BF (2006) Normal fetal motility: an overview. *Ultrasound Obstet Gynecol* **27**: 701–711.

De Vries JIP, Visser GHA, Prechtl HFR (1982) The emergence of fetal behaviour. I. Qualitative aspects. *Early Hum Dev* **7**: 301–322.

De Vries JIP, Visser GH, Prechtl HFR (1985) The emergence of fetal behaviour. II. Quantitative aspects. *Early Hum Dev* 12: 99–120.

Einspieler C, Prechtl HFR, Bos AF, Ferrari F, Cioni G (2005) *Prechtl's Method on the Qualitative Assessment of General Movements in Preterm, Term and Young Infants.* London: Mac Keith Press.

Forssberg H (1985) Ontogeny of human locomotor control. I. Infant stepping, supported locomotion and transition to independent locomotion. *Exp Brain Res* 57: 480–493.

Frigon A (2017) The neural control of interlimb coordination during mammalian locomotion. *J Neurophysiol* 117: 2224–2241. doi: 10.1152/jn.00978.2016.

Fuertinger S, Horwitz B, Simonyan K (2015) The functional connectome of speech control. *PLoS Biol* 13: e1002209. doi: 10.1371/journal.pbio.1002209.

Gewolb IH, Vice FL (2006) Maturational changes in the rhythms, patterning, and coordination of respiration and swallow during feeding in preterm and term infants. *Dev Med Child Neurol* 48: 589–594.

Hadders-Algra M (2018a) Early human motor development: from variation to the ability to vary and adapt. *Neurosci Biobehav Rev* 90: 411–427. doi: 10.1016/j.neubiorev.2018.05.009.

Hadders-Algra M (2018b) Neural substrate and clinical significance of general movements: an update, *Dev Med Child. Neurol* 60: 39–46. doi: 10.1111/dmcn.13540.

Hepper PG (2013) The developmental origins of laterality: fetal handedness. *Dev Psychobiol* 55: 588–595. doi: 10.1002/dev.21119.

Leighton AH, Lohmann C (2016) The wiring of developing sensory circuitries – from patterned spontaneous activity to synaptic plasticity mechanisms. *Front Neural Circuits* 10: 71.

Lüchinger AB, Hadders-Algra M, Van Kan CM, De Vries JIP (2008) Fetal onset of general movements. *Pediatr Res* 63: 191–195.

Meltzoff AN, Murray L, Simpson E, et al. (2018) Re-examination of Oostenbroek et al. (2016): evidence for neonatal imitation of tongue protrusion. *Dev Sci* 21: e12609. doi: 10.1111/desc.12609.

Miller JL, Sonies BC, Macedonia C (2003) Emergence of oropharyngeal, laryngeal and swallowing activity in the developing fetal upper aerodigestive tract: an ultrasound evaluation. *Early Hum Dev* 71: 61–87.

Mulkey SB, du Plessis AJ (2019) Autonomic nervous system development and its impact on neuropsychiatric outcome. *Pediatr Res* 85: 120–126. doi: 10.1038/s41390-018-0155-0.

Nagraj VP, Lake DE, Kuhn L, Moorman JR, Fairchild KD (2020) Central apnea of prematurity: does sex matter? *Am J Perinatol*, epub ahead of print. doi: 10.1055/s-0040-1713405.

Nathani S, Ertmer DJ, Stark RE (2006) Assessing vocal development in infants and toddlers. *Clin Linguist Phon* 20: 351–369.

Qureshi MA, Vice FL, Taciak VL, Bosma JF, Gewolb IH (2002) Changes in rhythmic suckle feeding patterns in term infants in the first month of life. *Dev Med Child Neurol* 44: 34–39.

Reijneveld SA, Brugman E, Hirasing RA (2001) Parental reports of excessive infant crying: the impact of varying definitions. *Pediatrics* 108: 893–897.

Reissland N, Francis B, Aydin E, Mason J, Schaal B (2014) The development of anticipation in the fetus: a longitudinal account of human fetal mouth movements in reaction to and anticipation of touch. *Dev Psychobiol* 56: 955–963. doi: 10.1002/dev.21172.

Ritterband-Rosenbaum A, Herskind A, Li X, et al. (2017) A critical period of corticomuscular and EMG-EMG coherence detection in healthy infants aged 9–25 weeks. *J Physiol* 595: 2699–2713. doi: 10.1113/JP273090.

Robles de Medina PG, Visser GH, Huizink AC, Buitelaar JK, Mulder EJ (2003) Fetal behaviour does not differ between boys and girls. *Early Hum Dev* 73: 17–26.

Sparling JW, Van Tol J, Chescheir NC (1999) Fetal and neonatal hand movement. *Phys Ther* 79: 24–39.

Stokowski LA (2005) A primer on apnea of prematurity. *Adv Neonatal Care* 5: 155–170. doi: 10.1016/j.adnc.2005.02.010.

Task Force on Sudden Infant Death Syndrome, Moon RY (2011) SIDS and other sleep-related infant deaths: expansion of recommendations for a safe infant sleeping environment. *Pediatrics* 128: e1341–1367. doi: 10.1542/peds.2011-2285.

Thelen E, Cooke DW (1987) Relationship between newborn stepping and later walking: a new interpretation. *Dev Med Child Neurol* 29: 380–393.

Von Hofsten C (1982) Eye-hand coordination in newborns. *Dev Psychol* **18**: 450–461.

Zoia S, Blason L, D'Ottavio G, Biancotto M, Bulgheroni M, Castiello U (2013) The development of upper limb movements: from fetal to post-natal life. *PLoS One* 8: e80876. doi: 10.1371/journal.pone.0080876.

SUGGESTIONS FOR FURTHER READING

Einspieler C (2012) *Fetal Behaviour. A Neurodevelopmental Approach.* London: Mac Keith Press.

Lagercrantz H, Hanson MA, Ment LR, Peebles DM (2010) *The Newborn Brain. Neuroscience and Clinical Applications,* 2nd edn. Cambridge: Cambridge University Press.

Prechtl HFR (1984) *Continuity of Neural Functions from Prenatal to Postnatal Life.* Oxford: Blackwell Scientific Publications.

Motor Development Between 3 Months and 2 Years

Mijna Hadders-Algra

SUMMARY POINTS

- Motor development between 3 months and 2 years is characterized by variation.
- Typical milestone development markedly varies, therefore delayed attainment of a single milestone is clinically irrelevant.
- Infants learn by trial and error experience to select situation-specific and efficient movement strategies.
- Active exploration, probing, and trying out activities promote infant motor development: practice matters!

Motor development in infancy is characterized by rapid developmental changes and large variation. These features turn early detection of developmental disorders into a challenge. Yet, these same characteristics also offer opportunities for early intervention.

This chapter reviews motor development between the ages of 3 months and 2 years. This means that it starts when the general movements are gradually replaced by goal-directed movements (see Chapter 5). The first section addresses general principles of motor development. Next, sections follow on gross motor development (the abilities to maintain and change body position and to move around), fine motor development (the abilities to carry, move, and handle objects), and oral motor development (the abilities to drink, eat, and communicate).

GENERAL PRINCIPLES IN MOTOR DEVELOPMENT

Chapter 3 mentioned that the concepts on motor behaviour and motor development changed substantially during the last century. The earlier views that (a) motor behaviour is primarily organized in chains of reflexes, and (b) motor development consists primarily of the enrolling of an endogenous, programmed script, have been discarded (Hadders-Algra 2018). Currently, two theoretical frameworks are dominant, the Dynamic Systems Theory and the Neuronal Group Selection Theory (NGST – for details see Chapter 3). These frameworks share the opinion that motor development is a non-linear and multifactorial determined process with phases of transition. The factors that may play a role are child-related factors, such as body weight or the presence of bronchopulmonary dysplasia, and environmental factors, such as the composition of the family, housing conditions, and the presence of toys (Adolph and Hoch 2019). This implies that both the Dynamic Systems Theory and the NGST acknowledge the importance of experience and context. However, the two theories differ in opinion on the role of genetically determined neurodevelopmental processes. Genetic factors play only a limited role in the Dynamic Systems Theory, whereas in NGST genetic information, epigenetic cascades, and experience are important (Edelman 1989; Hadders-Algra 2018). The latter corresponds well to current insights in the complexities of genetic and epigenetic mechanisms in the development of the nervous system (Bale 2015). As the NGST also offers more specific suggestions for early detection and early intervention than the Dynamic Systems Theory (see Chapter 3), I will use the NGST as framework of reference. Key notions in NGST are *variation* (i.e. the presence of a repertoire of options to achieve a specific goal), and *adaptability* (i.e. the capacity to select from the repertoire the most efficient strategy in a specific situation) in order to adapt motor behaviour (Hadders-Algra 2010, 2018).

The continuous interaction between child and environment generates a large heterogeneity in developmental trajectories, as both the child's repertoire of motor possibilities and the environment vary widely across children. The result is a large variation in the ages at which children achieve developmental milestones (Table 6.1, Fig. 6.1). Due to the large inter-individual variation in milestone achievement, the presence of a delayed achievement of a single milestone generally has no clinical significance. Yet, a delayed achievement of multiple milestones may be a sign of a developmental disorder (Hadders-Algra 2018).

The Pivotal Role of Play

Spontaneous activity is a quintessential characteristic of the nervous system (Hadders-Algra 2018). It generates the drive of the infant and child to explore their own body, including its motor capacities, and the material and personal environment. This implies that motor, cognitive, and social development are tightly intertwined (Bornstein et al. 2013; Adolph and Hoch 2019; see Chapter 4). The brain's drive to explore is especially expressed during play, that is, in locomotor play (with or without other individuals), object play, and social play (Pellegrini 2013; see Text Box 6.1).

Play serves practice by provision of continuous opportunities for exploration of the motor repertoire by means of trial and error. This allows the child to discover his own adaptive strategies. The drive to play, to explore, and to move is reflected by the high number of movements young children typically produce per day (see Text Box 6.2). The number of movements that infants produce largely varies, both on a day-to-day basis within infants, but also between infants. Despite

Table 6.1 Variation in age of achievement of motor milestones – the WHO Motor Development Study

Milestone	Age (months): percentiles at which milestone was achieved				
	1st	**10th**	**50th**	**90th**	**99th**
Sitting without support	3.8	4.6	5.9	7.5	9.2
Standing with assistance	4.8	5.9	7.4	9.4	11.4
Hands-and-knees crawling	5.2	6.6	8.3	10.5	13.5
Walking with assistance	5.9	7.4	9.0	11.0	13.7
Standing alone	6.9	8.8	10.8	13.4	16.9
Walking alone	8.2	10.0	12.0	14.4	17.6

The WHO Motor Development Study was a longitudinal study of children aged 4–24 months in Ghana, India, Norway, Oman, and the USA (n = 816; WHO Multicentre Growth Reference Study Group 2006).

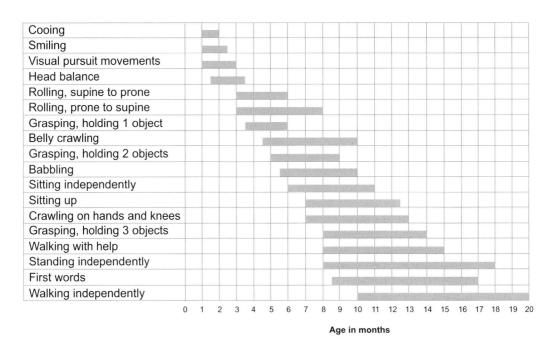

Figure 6.1   Interindividual variation in the emergence of motor milestones. Schematic representation of the ages at which some motor skills emerge during infancy. The length of the bars reflect the inter-individual variation. Adapted from the study of Touwen carried out in the Netherlands in the 1970s (Hadders-Algra 2018). Note that the Dutch data are not identical to those of the WHO Multicentre Growth Reference Study Group (2006). Figure reproduced from Hadders-Algra (2018) with permission from Elsevier Science Publishers.

the intra-individual variation, Shida-Tokeshi et al. (2018) showed that higher rates of arm movements were associated with greater developmental progress in the cognitive and language domains. This finding underscores two notions, that is, (a) the intertwinement of the various developmental domains, and (b) practice matters!

Text Box 6.1 Play and the Brain

Pellegrini (2013) defined play as follows: 'The behaviour must be voluntary, observed in a "relaxed field", the behaviour is not functional in the immediate observed context, the behaviours are repeated but the behavioural elements are exaggerated, segmented, and non-sequential in relation to functional behaviour.' Play is relatively rare in the animal kingdom; it is found in particular in species of primates that have to navigate more complex social systems, such as chimpanzees, spider monkeys, and some species of macaques (Pellis et al. 2015). Play behaviour is associated with the presence of an extended juvenile period, suggesting that a prolonged period of play practice affords opportunities to experiment with a variety of motor, cognitive, and social strategies that might be useful in later life (Pellegrini 2013). Interestingly, Kerney et al. (2017) demonstrated that in primates (including *homo sapiens*) the time budget spent in play correlates with the relative size of the main components of the cortico-cerebellar system. This suggests that play and the cortico-cerebellar system co-evolved in primates, which may have served the development of sophisticated cognitive and behavioural abilities in these species.

> **Text Box 6.2** 'Move It Out' – The High Number of Movements During Infancy
>
> The development of wearable movement sensors allowed researchers to study how many movements infants produce per day in their daily context. Shida-Tokeshi et al. (2018) longitudinally studied arm movements in typically developing infants aged 1–7 months. The study indicated that infants generate (during waking time) 4500 to 12000 arm movements per day, with movement rates ranging from 500 to 1500 movements per hour. Smith et al. (2015), who performed a longitudinal study in typically developing infants aged 1–12 months, focussed on leg movements. They reported that the infants produced on average 31000 leg movements per day, amounting to a movement rate of 3730 movements per hour. Both studies reported a large variation, both within and between subjects. For instance, an infant could produce on one day about 20000 leg movements and on another day 41000. Between the infants, the rate of arm movements could vary from about 4500 to 12000 per day, whereas the rate of leg movements could range from about 13000 to 50000 per day.
>
> These high numbers are comparable to those reported by Adolph et al. (2012), who counted in typically developing toddlers (12–19 months) the number of video-recorded steps and falls during a period of spontaneous play (15–60 minutes) in a laboratory setting. The results showed that toddlers on average take 2400 steps per hour, implying that they produce about 14000 steps per day. The study also indicated that newly walking toddlers fall about 17 times per hour, implying – by extrapolation – about 100 falls per day.
>
> It is interesting to note that the number of movements that infants generate per day largely exceeds the number of movements that adults make nowadays – at least when we refer to the number of steps produced. Adults generate on average 6000 steps per day, which is considerably less than the often recommended 10000 (Choi et al. 2007).

GROSS MOTOR DEVELOPMENT

Gross motor development comprises two elements: it involves the development of the ability to maintain body position (i.e. postural control) and the development of the capacity to move around by changing body position or location. This section addresses both elements separately. However, it is good to realize that the ability to move around is largely dependent on the skills to control posture.

Development of Postural Control

During the first two post-natal years the child's ability to control posture increases tremendously. This is, for instance, reflected by the development of the ability to sit, stand, and walk.

Before birth, little postural control is required. The foetus floats in the amniotic fluid, and the uterine walls provide ample support, in particular during the last phases of pregnancy. This situation changes postnatally: the all-round support is missing and the forces of gravity affect the infant much stronger than in the womb.

At term age the infant has some capacities to deal with the forces of gravity, for instance, the infant is able to produce general movements in all directions (see Chapter 5). Yet, the ability to balance the head in sitting position is limited: full-term infants can keep the head upright for just a few seconds. The ability to balance the head in supported sitting rapidly improves during the first postnatal months, so that around the age of 3 months infants can stabilize the head on the trunk, be it with an occasional wobble (Video 5.4; Hadders-Algra 2018).

The observation that young infants are able to balance their head while receiving full trunk support, whereas they are unable to balance the trunk when put in an independently sitting position, has generated the idea that postural control develops in a cranio-caudal order. However, the development of postural muscle coordination is at variance with this notion.

In the development of postural muscle coordination, two levels of control can be distinguished: (1) the basic organization of direction-specific adjustments, and (2) fine-tuning of the direction-specific muscle activity to the specifics of the situation (see Text Box 6.3). A postural perturbation study showed that infants aged 1 month -- the youngest infants studied – exhibited consistent direction-specific postural adjustments (Hedberg et al. 2004). This suggests that the basic level of control has an innate origin. The direction-specific muscles are recruited with large variation (i.e. with variation in which direction-specific muscles participate and when and how much they are activated).

The fine-tuning of the direction-specific activity starts around 3 months. The first way to adjust postural muscle activity consists of the selection of which muscles will contribute to the direction-specific adjustment. Focus is on the number of muscles recruited, not on the order of recruitment. In the following months, the other ways to adjust postural muscle activity emerge, and around 9 months the infant is able to use to some extent the most subtle form of adaptation that consists of adjustment of the degree of muscle contraction to the requirements of the situation.

Text Box 6.3 The Organization of Postural Control in Human Adults

Organization of Postural Muscle Activity

Postural muscle activity is organized into two levels of control. The first and basic level of control consists of direction-specificity. This means that the direction of body sway determines on which side of the body the postural muscles are primarily activated. When the body sways backward the muscles on the body's ventral side are primarily recruited; when a forward body-sway occurs the dorsal muscles are primarily activated (Fig. 6.2). The latter happens, for instance, during reaching forward. To cope with a specific direction of sway, the body has multiple direction-specific muscles at its disposal. For instance, direction-specific muscles on the dorsal side of the body are the neck and trunk extensors, the hamstrings, and the gastrocnemius muscles. The direction-specific muscles may be recruited in isolation or in combination. The net result of this organization is the presence of a repertoire of postural adjustments for each direction of sway.

At the second level of control, the direction-specific muscle activity is fine-tuned to the specifics of the situation. This may be achieved in multiple ways, that is, (a) by selecting one or more of the direction-specific muscles; (b) by recruitment (or not) of antagonistic muscles; (c) by the timing of the recruitment of the direction-specific muscles; this is a means to change recruitment order (e.g. from top-down to bottom-up); (d) by recruiting direction-specific muscle activity prior to the planned movement (e.g. reaching), that is, generating anticipatory postural activity; (e) by the timing of the recruitment of the antagonistic muscles, so that the

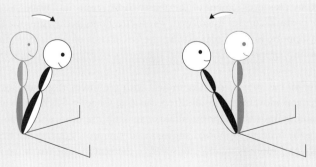

Figure 6.2 Direction-specific postural muscle activity. Schematic representation of direction-specific postural muscle activity: the direction of body sway determines the primary recruitment of postural muscles. During forward body sway (left panel) the dorsal muscles (black) are primarily activity; during backward sway (right panel) the ventral muscles (black).

degree of coactivation can be modulated; and (f) by the most subtle form of fine-tuning, that is, the adaptation of the degree of muscle contraction that is reflected by the amplitude of the electromyographic (EMG) signal).

Frames of Reference Used in Postural Control

Posture has to be controlled against a stable frame of reference (Assaiante et al. 2005). In adults, the reference frame may consist of the feet (during standing), pelvis or head (during sitting, standing, and walking). The nature of the task, including the size of the support surface, determines which reference frame is selected. For instance, when balance is really at stake, a reference frame near the support surface is selected (the pelvis during sitting, the feet during standing). However, during most movements, the risk of losing balance is less high; in these situations the position of the head in space forms the frame of reference. This underscores the notion that, in general, safeguarding the position of the head in space is postural control's major goal. Actually, this appears to be an ancient concept, as Plato (427–347 BCE) wrote in the *Timaeus*: 'Holding on and supporting itself with these limbs, it [the body] would be capable of making its way through all regions, while carrying at the top the dwelling place of that most divine, most sacred part of ourselves [i.e. the head]' (44e–45a).

During infancy, recruitment order is characterized by variation. Within the variation, minor developmental trends can be distinguished: in early infancy a slight preference for top-down recruitment is present: at this age, the head is the frame of reference (see Text Box 6.3). When the infant is able to sit independently, bottom-up recruitment is preferred, suggesting that the pelvis becomes the reference frame. During preschool and school-age, recruitment order of the direction-specific muscles during sitting is again characterized by variation. First at the end of school-age, the adult's flexible preference for top-down recruitment in sitting emerges. Also during standing and walking the frames of reference are age-dependent. At early standing and walking age the frame of reference is near the (relative) support surface, and consists of the feet during standing and the pelvis during walking. This reflects that during infancy and preschool age keeping balance during standing and walking is perceived as a difficult task (see Text Box 6.3). With increasing age, children are increasingly better to select during standing and walking the head as a frame of reference, also in difficult balancing situations (Assaiante et al. 2005).

After being able to balance the head on the trunk, the next major observable milestone of postural control is being able to sit independently. It is achieved – with large interindividual variation – around 6 months (median age; see Table 6.1). The capacity to sit independently develops gradually. In the beginning, infants need ample postural support when put in a sitting position (i.e. they need support that stabilizes the trunk up to a high thoracic level). With increasing age and experience, less support is needed, for example, the supporting hands may be lowered to a lower thoracic level and finally may let go – the infant is able to sit independently (Rachwani et al. 2015). Note that the lowering of the external support from a high thoracic level to lower parts of the trunk does not imply that postural control develops in a cranio-caudal order. It means that the infant is increasingly better able to control larger parts of the body.

When infants have just mastered the skill of sitting independently, they sit rather unstable; the swaying body explores all sitting configurations (Video 6.1). This implies that their sitting behaviour is characterized by variation without adaptation. It is the phase of 'sitting, yet cannot be left alone' (Piper and Darah 1994). Relatively soon, however, infants learn to stabilize their sitting posture and adapt it to the specifics of the situation. They are able to integrate sitting behaviour in play activities (see Fig. 3.3 and Video 6.2; Hadders-Algra 2018).

The next two clearly observable milestones reflecting postural development are the abilities to stand and walk alone. These abilities emerge – with large variation – around 11 and 12 months respectively (median ages; Table 6.1). Balance in these two conditions is more challenged than in the sitting position, due to the relatively small basis of support during standing and walking. To cope with the challenge, the infants adopt an *en bloc* strategy, in which all direction-specific neck and trunk muscles

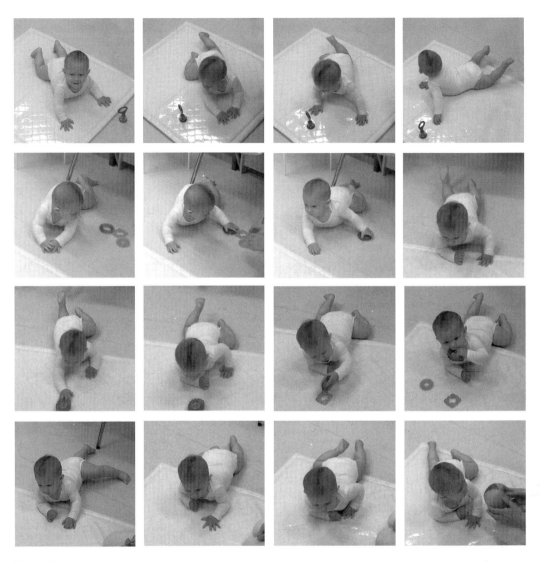

Figure 6.3 Variation during abdominal crawling. Variation in the movements of the neck, trunk, and limbs during abdominal crawling (also called belly crawling) in a 7-months-old infant. The infant was born at term and had an uneventful prenatal, perinatal, and neonatal history. The figure is based on frames from 2 minutes of video recording. Published with permission of the parents.

are activated in concert. It means that the infant freezes the degrees of movement freedom in neck and trunk. Freezing of the degrees of freedom is a well-known strategy to simplify control, especially in high constraint conditions (Assaiante et al. 2005; Hadders-Algra 2018). The dominance of the *en bloc* strategy emerges around 9 months and disappears at 2½ years of age. The walking skills improve considerably during the first months of independently walking (see next section). This is largely facilitated by the rapid improvement in anticipatory postural adjustments during the first months of walking experience (Hadders-Algra 2018).

Multiple studies demonstrated that the development of postural control is experience-dependent. For instance, Lobo and Galloway (2012) showed that 3 weeks of activities, that started at the age of 2 months and were provided by the parents for 15 minutes per day during daily care giving, promoted the infants' motor development throughout the entire first year. The training activities consisted, for instance, of placing the infant in a prone position while encouraging him to lift the head; pulling the infant up and lowering him down slowly between supine and sitting; and placing the infant in supported sitting position and allowing him to experience swaying of the head and trunk. Another example is the study of Hadders-Algra et al. (1996) in infants just learning to sit independently. The study demonstrated that challenging postural control in a sitting position (by playfully presenting toys at locations that were relatively far from the body) three times per day for 5 minutes over a period of 3 months, was associated with an acceleration of the ability to fine-tune postural muscle activity by 2 months.

In summary, starting from an innate basis, postural control mechanisms exhibit substantial developmental changes with increasing age and increasing experience. With increasing postural capacities, the child is able to balance an increasingly larger chain of body parts against gravity. The central goal of postural control is keeping the head stable in space; this governs the order of postural development. The increasing control first allows the child to balance the head on the supported body, next to balancing head and trunk during sitting (with its large base of support) and finally the lower limbs, trunk, and head during standing and walking (on the small support surface formed by the feet). This 'head first' principle does not imply a strict rule of cranio-caudal development. Rather, the mastery of postural control follows the principles of variation and selection allowing for adaptation. Which pattern is selected depends on the current frame of reference, which is task specific. In young infants who are not able to sit independently the frame of reference is the head – muscles are recruited with a minimal preference for a cranio-caudal order. In the initial phases of learning to sit independently or learning to stand independently, the support surface is the reference frame – muscles are recruited with a preference for a caudo-cranial order. After these initial phases recruitment order is entirely task specific and adaptive, with a general preference for a cranio-caudal sequence ('head first' principle). Meanwhile children also learn to further fine-tune postural activity by adapting the degree of contraction of postural muscles to the specifics of the situation.

Development of Locomotor Behaviour

By the age of 3 months, most infants no longer show neonatal stepping movements (see Chapter 5). In general, their first means to move around consists of rolling movements from supine to prone and vice versa, and exploratory movements in prone (from 4–5 months onwards). Most typically developing infants aged 3 months and over are able to take elbow support and to balance the head in prone position. They gradually learn to use their hands and arms for object manipulation in this position and discover how they can displace themselves. The displacement usually starts with pivoting (moving by means of lateroflexion of the trunk around the umbilical axis). From about 7 months onwards, this is followed by abdominal or belly crawling (i.e. the type of crawling with which the infant propels himself forward through the environment while the belly remains in contact with the support surface) (Piper and Darrah 1994). During this phase, the infant explores all possible combinations of movements that the various joints in the limbs, the neck and trunk can make. Progression in prone is characterized by variation without adaptation (Fig. 6.3). This experiential activity mostly results in the development of crawling on hands and knees – on average from about 8 months onwards (see Video 3.1). Soon after the infant has discovered this strategy, it becomes the favourite way to move around – the infant has selected an efficient and adaptive way to move around (see Video 3.2).

With increasing age and growing experience crawling proficiency improves (i.e. the steps become larger and velocity increases). The crawling experience also allows the infant to learn about ground surfaces and obstacles (i.e. about affordances in general) (Adolph and Hoch 2019). Thus – as in any motor skill – practice matters. Yet, the initiation of the 'back-to-sleep' campaign in the nineties of last century – recommending sleeping in supine instead of in prone position in order to prevent sudden infant death syndrome – induced a tendency in caregivers to place the infant also during waking hours only sporadically in prone position. The longitudinal study of Kuo et al. (2008) showed that spending less time on the tummy was associated with a later onset of crawling milestones. Yet, tummy time was not related to the age at which other motor skills emerged or to gross and fine motor developmental scores at the age of 2 years. This also means that infants who show a typical development but skip crawling and move around by bottom shuffling have a good developmental prognosis. Bottom shuffling that presents as an isolated 'sign' often runs in families. It should be realized, however, that among bottom shufflers the prevalence of children with a developmental disorder is higher than among infants who do not consistently bottom shuffle. Yet, in the bottom shufflers with a developmental disorder, bottom shuffling is usually accompanied by other stereotypies. The way in which infants move around in prone is not only determined by their genes and the integrity of their brain but also by their body proportions. For instance, infants with achondroplasia, who have a disproportionate stature with marked shortening of the limb segments and a large head, may show 'snow ploughing' (i.e. a means of prone progression during which the infants support themselves by the feet, the hands, and the large head) (Ireland et al. 2012).

The majority of infants achieve the ability to walk independently between 10 and 14 months (Table 6.1) Early walking is characterized by a large variation within and between infants. Infants frequently fall during this early, exploratory walking phase (see Text Box 6.2, Fig. 6.4, Video 6.3). However, after about 2–3 months of walking experience, infants have learned to select their preferred pattern of walking, both in terms of kinematics and muscle activation patterns (Bisi and Stagni 2015; Hadders-Algra 2018). The processes of adaptive selection are accompanied by improved walking proficiency, that is, selection of the heel-strike pattern that characterizes efficient adult gait, a decrease in step width, and increases in step length and walking velocity (Fig. 6.4, Video 6.4; Bisi and Stagni 2015; Hadders-Algra 2018).

FINE MOTOR DEVELOPMENT

Fine motor function comprises the ability to reach for objects, to lift, carry, and manipulate them. Typically, these actions are performed by the upper extremities. The fine motor functions generally include a transport component that moves the hand from the starting position to the object (reaching) and a manipulative component in which the object is grasped (manipulation). In adults, both components are highly coordinated (Hadders-Algra 2018).

Development of Reaching

Reaching towards an external object requires the infant to locate the object in space and to translate this information into an upper extremity movement towards the object. Generally, but not necessarily, target location is based on visual information.

Term newborn infants already have the capacity to move their arms in response to an object, especially when they fixate the object and when they are put in a sitting position with ample neck and trunk support. These 'prereaches' may consist of oscillating or flapping movements of the arms not clearly directed to the object, or of movements that bring the hands to the mouth (Video 6.5; Hadders-Algra 2018). Around 3 months, the prevalence of 'prereaching' movements increases, and object presentation increasingly often elicits real reaches (i.e. movements in the direction of the object). At this age, reaching movements usually do not end in grasping of the object; the reaching is not yet successful. Successful

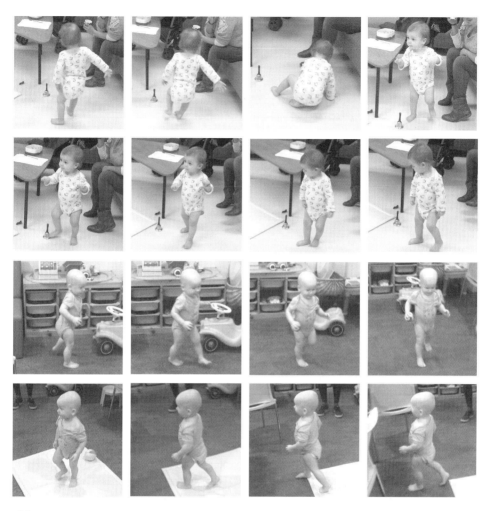

Figure 6.4 Variation without and with adaptation during walking. Upper half: variation in and little adaptation of movements during walking in a 14-month-old infant. The infant has difficulties in adjusting his movements during walking and therefore easily falls down (frames 1–3); in addition, his steps largely vary in width and length. The infant was born at term, had an uneventful prenatal, perinatal, and neonatal history, and had 4 weeks of walking experience. Lower half: variation and adaptation during walking in a 17-month-old infant. The infant shows an efficient walking pattern; he was born at term, had an uneventful prenatal, perinatal, and neonatal history, and had 6 months of walking experience.

reaching emerges between 4 and 5 months. The development of successful reaching and grasping is promoted by the rapid developmental changes occurring in the visual system that result in improved visual acuity and stereopsis (Braddick and Atkinson 2011).

The development of reaching and grasping may be facilitated by active trial and error reaching experiences. When the active practice of reaching is combined with the application of 'sticky mittens' (the combination of Velcro mittens and Velcro-covered toys), this also enhances the development of successful reaching (Libertus and Needham 2010). It is, however, debated how much of this effect can be attributed to the 'sticky mittens', the active practice of the reaching movements, or their combination (Hadders-Algra 2018).

The first successful reaching movements are characterized by variation: variation in trajectory, in movement velocity, movement amplitude, and movement duration (Video 6.6). The early reaching repertoire contains mostly reaches that consist of multiple submovements (movement units; Von Hofsten 1991; see Text Box 6.4). However, the reaching repertoire also comprises movements that are launched straightforwardly to the object ('lucky shots'; Video 6.7). With increasing age and increasing experience, the infant's ability to select a straight movement toward the object improves (Video 6.8). Initially – between 4 and 6 months – reaching performance improves quickly. Thereafter, further fine-tuning occurs at a slower pace (see Text Box 6.4).

Text Box 6.4 The Organization and Development of Reaching Movements

In healthy adults reaching movements are characterized by a bell-shaped velocity profile; it consists of one acceleration and one deceleration (Fig. 6.5). This indicates that the movement is programmed as a single movement unit by means of feedforward control. In the reaching literature the part of a reaching movement consisting of one acceleration and one deceleration is called a movement unit.

Reaching movements of infants who have just learned to reach and grasp are in general (but not always) characterized by multiple movement units (Fig. 6.5; Von Hofsten 1991). This indicates that the infants cannot program the entire reaching movement in advance; they have to implement trajectory corrections while reaching. This means that at early age feedback mechanisms play a prominent role in the control of reaching. When reaches at 4 months of age are performed in supine position, they consist of four to seven movement units (median values). However, reaches performed at the same age in a semi-reclined or upright sitting position consist of only three to five movement units. This indicates that for young typically developing infants reaching in a supine position is more challenging than reaching in a supported sitting position. Most likely, the difference in performance can be attributed to the forces of gravity that counteract reaching movements in supine more than those performed in sitting.

In the following 2 months, the number of movement units decreases significantly to 2.5–4 and the positional advantage of sitting over a supine position disappears. In this age period (i.e. between 4 and 6 months) object size and rigidity affect the kinematics of reaching: reaching movements consists of more movement units when the object is large and rigid than when the object small or soft. After the age of 6 months, infants are increasingly more often able to select an efficient, straightforward reaching movement consisting of one movement unit. Therefore, the median number of movement units in sitting position decreases to two at the end of the first year. The adult level of consistent reaches with one movement unit is achieved at the age of 2 years – at least when the child sits with ample postural support. When children reach during sitting without postural support, the adult level of reaching is first attained around the age of 7 years (Hadders-Algra 2018).

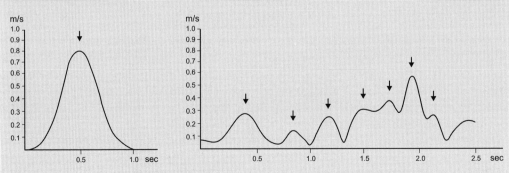

Figure 6.5   Velocity profiles of reaching movements. Left: reaching movement of an adult consisting of one movement unit (one acceleration and one deceleration). The reaching movement lasts about 1 second. Right: reaching movement of a 4-month-old infant with seven movement units; the reaching movement lasts about 2.5 seconds.

Infants' reaching movements consist of a mix of bilateral and unilateral movements with a varied unilateral preference. Already at the age of 6 months infants are able to adjust the unilateral or bilateral nature of reaching movements to the size of the object: when presented with a relatively large ball, they prefer bilateral reaches. At an early age, the preference for unilateral or bilateral reaches also depends on the infant's position: in supine, semi-reclined sitting or prone-reclined position infants generally use bilateral reaches, whereas in the supported upright sitting position unilateral reaches dominate. Infants who have mastered the ability to sit independently favour unilateral reaches in all conditions: within their varied reaches they prefer right-hand grasps (about 50%) to left-hand grasps and bimanual grasps (each about 25%; Hadders-Algra 2018). The varied hand preference persists till 2½ to 4 years of age, when children gradually develop a consistent hand preference.

Development of Manipulation

During early grasping (4–5 months) the palmar grasp is mostly observed, that is, the grasp in which the whole palmar surface and all fingers (with or without the little finger; Fig. 6.6A) are used. Nevertheless, when small objects (1–2cm) are presented to 4-month-olds they may show a large variation of grips, varying from the palmar grasp to movements with only thumb and index finger. After the age of 6 months, the frequency of grasping movements with only thumb and index finger increases. Grasping gets increasingly adapted to the form of the object (Fig. 6.6). The thumb and index finger movements get more tweaked to fine manipulative tasks: at 6–9 months the scissor grasp (with extended thumb and index finger; Fig. 6.6C) dominates, at 9–14 months the inferior pincer grasp (with extend thumb and flexed index finger; Fig. 6.6D), and from about 14 months the pincer grasp (with flexion of thumb and index finger; Fig. 6.6E) is frequently observed (Hadders-Algra 2018). Concurrent with the development of the ability to adjust finger movements to the specifics of the manipulative task, the ability to adapt the configuration and orientation of the hand while reaching to the specifics of the target object (shape and orientation) also improves (Video 6.8; Hadders-Algra 2018). In the second postnatal half year, infants also develop so-called role-differentiated bimanual manipulation. This means that each hand is able to perform a different but complementary action to handle an object, for example, an activity barbell. Yet, at the age of 13 months role-specific bimanual actions only form 20% of the infant's play actions with toys promoting such actions (Hadders-Algra 2018).

A substantial body of research addressed the question of how finger movements are adjusted during an object lifting task (Forssberg 2014). One-year-old infants are able to adjust lifting movements to some extent to the object's weight on the basis of prior trial and error experience. However, they do not use the precise and efficient coordination of the adult with a parallel preprogramming of the grip force and load force (grip-lift synergy). The 1-year-olds generate the grip force and load force sequentially and produce downward directed load forces in the prelifting phase (i.e. before lifting the object the children first push the object to the support surface). The development of the subtle parallel programming of the grip and load forces takes many years; it reaches its adult form between 8 and 11 years. The development of the coordination of the forces during object lifting illustrates the protracted developmental course of manual skills in general. For example, it is well known that the ability to perform a peg-board task, a rapid tapping task, or the finger-opposition task improves considerably during the preschool and school-age period. Physiological studies demonstrated that the developmental changes in fine manipulative abilities are accompanied by a substantial decrease in corticomotoneuronal delay. This indicates that developmental changes in the corticospinal tract contribute to the development of fine motor skills (Hadders-Algra 2018).

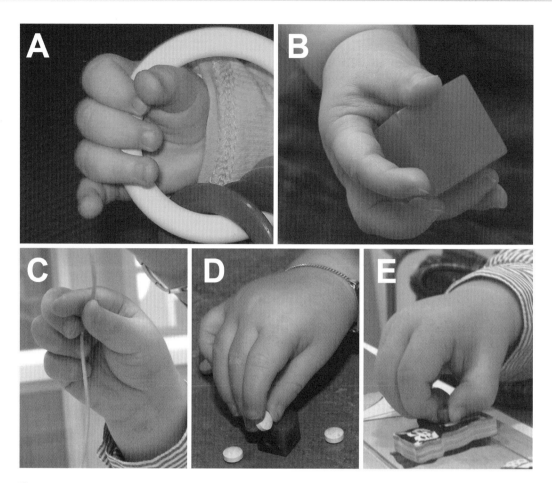

Figure 6.6   Various forms of infant grasping. **A** Palmar grasp; **B** radial palmar grasp; **C** scissor grasp; **D** inferior pincer grasp; **E** pincer grasp.

ORAL MOTOR DEVELOPMENT

Oral motor behaviour basically serves two functions: the ingestion of food by means of sucking, biting, chewing, and swallowing, and communication by means of vocalizations or spoken words.

Development of Oral Motor Behaviour Involved in Food Intake

Gradually, it has become clear that oral motor behaviour during infancy is not organized by means of reflexes, but with the help of Central Pattern Generating networks located in the brainstem (see Text Box 5.1). These networks are modulated by supraspinal activity and exhibit experience-dependent plasticity (Hadders-Algra 2018).

At the age of 3 months post-term, the infant has ample experience with sucking and is able to drink his human milk or infant formula in an efficient way (see Chapter 5). From 4 to 6 months other types of food are introduced: semisolid foods (e.g. pureed food) presented on a spoon. The infants explore and transport the food by means of sucking and munching. From about 6 months of age, chewing movements emerge. It allows the infant to deal with solid food. At 7 months, the chewing rate and the number of chewing cycles are already adapted to the texture of the food (puree or semisolid). The chewing rate does not change with increasing age, but chewing efficiency improves between 6 and 24 months: less chewing cycles and less time is needed to grind food. This is accompanied by an increasingly better lip control, increased efficiency of tongue movements, and a decreased involvement of the perioral structures in the act of swallowing. But also during preschool age, chewing efficiency continues to improve (Hadders-Algra 2018).

Development of Oral Motor Behaviour Involved in Communication

Social smiling emerges between 5 and 10 weeks post-term. When the infant gets older, non-communicative facial movements increase and become increasingly coupled. The latter is especially observed at the end of the first year in the movements of the lower lip and jaw, and this improved muscle coordination is considered to assist speech development (Hadders-Algra 2018).

From early postnatal age onwards, infants do not only produce non-speech utterances, such as crying, laughing, hiccups, and burps but also precursors of speech, the so-called protophones. With increasing age, the repertoire of protophones gradually expands, and the protophones themselves become more complex. Between 3 and 5 months, infants increasingly often select from the varied infant vowel repertoire the vowels that have adult-like frequency characteristics (Video 6.9). This selection requires sensory feedback. In typically developing infants, the sensory feedback predominantly consists of auditory information, which is enhanced by concomitant visual feedback. Probably, vowel selection is enhanced by imitation of adult speech (Kuhl and Meltzoff 1996). In this respect, it is interesting to note that, especially at early age, human faces constitute a substantial proportion of the visual scenes of an infant's waking hours, thereby offering ample opportunity for communicative interaction (Hadders-Algra 2018).

Between 5 and 10 months of age, canonical (or reduplicated) babbling develops (e.g. /dada/ or /mama/), and a bit later, and temporally largely overlapping with the former, variegated babbling (e.g. /kadabyda/). The importance of auditory feedback in this phase and the preceding one is reflected by the finding that infants with severe hearing impairment reach the stage of canonical babbling later. In addition, their babbling utterances are shorter than those of typically developing infants (Oller and Eilers 1988). In the typical babbling phase so-called perceptual attunement also occurs, a form of perceptual selection or narrowing. This process of selection proceeds as follows. Before the age of 8 months, infants are able to distinguish many of the 800 worldwide available phonemes (the basic sounds of a language; each language has a unique set of about 40 phonemes; Kuhl 2010). However, around 10–12 months infants are no longer able to discriminate non-native consonants that do not exist in their own language. For instance, the difference between 8-month-old Japanese babies are able to distinguish the /r/ and the /l/ – consonants that are pronounced similarly in the Japanese language – but they have lost this ability at 10–12 months; the perception of the difference between these consonants has disappeared from their repertoire (Kuhl 2010).

From about 12 months, the first words emerge; the acquisition of the first words is a slow process, but from 18 months onwards vocabulary development dramatically accelerates (Kuhl 2010). Studies on oral motor coordination showed that speech at 12 months is associated with a pronounced jaw displacement, accompanied by excessive compression of the lips during oral closure, and a large variation in lip movements. At 2 years, the lip movements become relatively larger and the jaw movements smaller. The lip movements are highly synchronized. This synchronization, which differs from the adult lip coordination, may be viewed as a strategy to simplify the motor action. It disappears at preschool age (Hadders-Algra 2018).

CONCLUDING REMARKS

In the age period between 3 months and 2 years, motor development is characterized by variation. With increasing age, brain development and increasing trial and error experience the infant learns to select from his motor repertoires efficient task-specific strategies. Also, the infants abilities to vary improve – which is presumably related to the increasing emergence of the permanent circuitries in the cortical plate of the frontal, parietal, and temporal association cortices during the first postnatal year (Hadders-Algra 2018). As a result, by the age of 12–18 months most typically developing infants have achieved the milestones of independent walking, the use of the pincer grasp, and the first words. It takes, however, many years of additional exploration, experience, and developmental changes in the brain, before the adult configuration of secondary variability is achieved, with its ability to produce complex skilled movements, its efficient adaptability, and its freedom to vary.

REFERENCES

Adolph KE, Cole WG, Komati M, et al. (2012) How do you learn to walk? Thousands of steps and dozens of falls per day. *Psychol Sci* **23**: 1387–1394. doi: 10.1177/0956797612446346.

Adolph KE, Hoch JE (2019) Motor development: embodied, embedded, enculturated and enabling. *Annu Rev Psychol* **70**: 141–164. doi: 10.1146/annurev-psych-010418-102836.

Assaiante C, Mallau S, Viel S, Jover M, Schmitz C (2005) Development of postural control in healthy children: a functional approach. *Neural Plast* **12**: 109–118.

Bale TL (2015) Epigenetic and transgenerational reprogramming of brain development. *Nat Rev Neurosci* **16**: 332–344. doi: 10.1038/nrn3818.

Bisi MC, Stagni R (2015) Evaluation of toddler different strategies during the first six months of independent walking: a longitudinal study. *Gait Posture* **41**: 574–579. doi: 10.1016/j.gaitpost.2014.11.017.

Bornstein MH, Hahn CS, Suwalsky JT (2013) Physically developed and exploratory young infants contribute to their own long-term academic achievement. *Psychol Sci* **24**: 1906–1917. doi: 10.1177/0956797613479974.

Braddick O, Atkinson J (2011). Development of human visual function. *Vision Res* **51**: 1588–1609. doi: 10.1016/j.visres.2011.02.018.

Choi BC, Pak AW, Choi JC, Choi EC (2007) Daily step goal of 10,000 steps: a literature review. *Clin Invest Med* **30**: E146–151.

Edelman GM (1989) *Neural Darwinism. The Theory of Neuronal Group Selection.* Oxford: Oxford University Press.

Forssberg H (2014) Neural basis of motor control. In: Dan B, Mayston M, Paneth N, Rosenbloom L, *Cerebral Palsy – Science and Clinical Practice.* London: Mac Keith Press, pp. 199–224.

Hadders-Algra M (2010). Variation and variability: key words in human motor development. *Phys Ther* **90**: 1823–1837. doi: 10.2522/ptj.20100006.

Hadders-Algra M (2018) Early human motor development: from variation to the ability to vary and adapt. *Neurosci Biobehav Rev* **90**: 411–427. doi: 10.1016/j.neubiorev.2018.05.009.

Hadders-Algra M, Brogren E, Forssberg H. (1996) Training affects the development of postural adjustments in sitting infants. *J Physiol* **493**: 289–298.

Hedberg A, Forssberg H, Hadders-Algra M (2004) Postural adjustments due to external perturbations during sitting in 1-month-old infants: evidence for the innate origin of direction specificity. *Exp Brain Res* **157**: 10–17.

Ireland PJ, Donaghey S, McGill J et al. (2012) Development in children with achondroplasia: a prospective clinical cohort study. *Dev Med Child Neurol* **54**: 532–537. doi: 10.1111/j.1469-8749.2012.04234.x.

Kerney M, Smaers JB, Schoenemann PT, Dunn JC (2017) The coevolution of play and the cortico-cerebellar system in primates. *Primates* **58**: 485–491. doi: 10.1007/s10329-017-0615-x.

Kuhl PK (2010) Brain mechanisms in early language acquisition. *Neuron* **67**: 713–727. doi: 10.1016/j.neuron.2010.08.038.

Kuhl PK, Meltzoff AN (1996) Infant vocalizations in response to speech: vocal imitation and developmental change. *J Acoust Soc Am* **100**: 2425–2438. doi: 10.1121/1.417951.

Kuo YL, Liao HF, Chen PC, Hsieh WS, Hwang AW (2008) The influence of wakeful prone positioning on motor development during the early life. *J Dev Behav Pediatr* **29**: 367–e76. doi: 10.1097/DBP.0b013e3181856d54.

Libertus K, Needham A (2010) Teach to reach: the effects of active vs passive reaching experiences on action and perception. *Vision Res.* **50**: 2750–2757. doi: 10.1016/j.visres.2010.09.001.

Lobo MA, Galloway JC (2012) Enhanced handling and positioning in early infancy advances development throughout the first year. *Child Dev* **83**: 1290–1302. doi: 10.1111/j.1467-8624.2012.01772.x.

Oller DK, Eilers RE (1988) The role of audition in infant babbling. *Child Dev* **59**: 441–449.

Pellegrini AD (2013) Play. In: Zelazo PD, editor, *The Oxford Handbook of Developmental Psychology, Volume 2: Self and Other.* Oxford: Oxford Handbooks Online. doi: 10.1093/oxfordhb/9780199958474.013.0012.

Pellis SM, Burghardt GM, Palagi E, Mangel M (2015) Modeling play: distinguishing between origins and current functions. *Adapt Behav* **23**: 331–339. doi: 10.1177/1059712315596053.

Piper MC, Darah J (1994) *Motor Assessment of the Developing Infant.* Philadelphia: WB Saunders Company.

Rachwani J, Santamaria V, Saavedra SL, Woollacott MH (2015) The development of trunk control and its relation to reaching in infancy: a longitudinal study. *Front Hum Neurosci* **9**: 94. doi: 10.3389/fnhum.2015.00094.

Shida-Tokeshi J, Lane CJ, Trujillo-Priego IA, et al. (2018) Relationships between full-day arm movement characteristics and developmental status in infants with typical development as they learn to reach: an observational study. *Gates Open Res* **2**: 17. doi: 10.12688/gatesopenres.12813.1.

Smith BA, Trujillo-Priego IA, Lane CJ, Finley JM, Horak FB (2015) Daily quantity of infant leg movements: wearable sensor algorithm and relationship to walking onset. *Sensors (Basel)* **15**: 19006–19020. doi: 10.3390/s150819006.

Von Hofsten C (1991) Structuring of early reaching movements: a longitudinal study. *J Mot Behav* **23**: 280–292.

WHO Multicentre Growth Reference Study Group (2006) Relationship between physical growth and motor development in the WHO Child Growth Standards. *Acta Paediatr Suppl* **450**: 96–101.

SUGGESTIONS FOR FURTHER READING

Campos JJ, Anderson DI, Barbu-Roth MA, Hubbard EM, Hertenstein MJ, Witherington D (2000) Travel broadens the mind. *Infancy* **1**: 149–219.

Corbetta D, DiMercurio A, Wiener RF, Connell JP, Clark M (2018) How perception and action fosters exploration and selection in infant skill acquisition. *Adv Child Dev Behav* **55**: 1–29. doi: 10.1016/bs.acdb.2018.04.001.

Hadders-Algra M, Brogren Carlberg E (Eds) (2008) *Postural Control: A Key Issue in Developmental Disorders.* London: Mac Keith Press.

Newell KM, Scully DM, McDonald PV, Baillargeon R (1989) Task constraints and infant grip configurations. *Dev Psychobiol* **22**: 817–831.

Sporns O, Edelman GM (1993) Solving Bernstein's problem: a proposal for the development of coordinated movement by selection. *Child Dev* **64**: 960–981.

PART IV

Atypical Motor Development

Atypical Motor Development of the Foetus and Young Infant

Mijna Hadders-Algra

SUMMARY POINTS

- Atypical foetal motor development is mainly manifested in impairments in quantity and quality of general movements (GMs).
- Atypical GMs are characterized by (1) a marked reduction in movement complexity and variation (poor repertoire) and (2) failure to develop age-specific fidgety movements.
- Atypical GMs that combine poor repertoire and absence of fidgety movements reflect a serious impairment of brain integrity; they have a high predictive value for cerebral palsy.
- Other signs of atypical motor development in early infancy, such as atypical sucking and swallowing, 'transient dystonia', and deformational plagiocephaly, often have a transient nature.

The most frequently occurring movements of the foetus and young infant are the general movements (GMs; see Chapter 5). Dysfunction of the young brain is well expressed in these movements. This chapter starts with the presentation of atypical foetal motility, including atypical foetal GMs. The following section discusses atypical GMs in young infants after birth. Next, sections on (a) atypical sucking and swallowing; (b) atypical control of head movements; and (c) atypical muscle tone regulation follow.

ATYPICAL FOETAL MOTILITY

Ultrasound studies on the effect of adverse conditions during prenatal life on foetal movements focused on the quantity of movements rather than on movement quality. The underrepresentation of studies using movement quality is explained by the technical problem of sonography: in the second half of gestation a single camera only can view a part of the foetus (Hayat et al. 2018).

De Vries and Fong (2007) reviewed the literature on atypical movements in foetuses with a congenital disorder of the brain or the musculoskeletal system. Some studies described the quality of foetal movements, but their use of subjective, non-standardized terminology precluded a systematic review. Yet, a review of the quantity of movements was possible. Foetuses with musculoskeletal disorders mostly presented with hypokinesia, whereas foetuses with congenital disorders involving the brain (e.g. anencephaly or trisomy 18) presented with either hypokinesia or hyperkinesia. A recent study indicated that hyperkinesia sometimes may be an expression of prenatal epilepsy (Whitehead et al. 2019).

Other conditions may also result in changes in the quantity of foetal motility (Visser et al. 2010). For instance, intra-uterine growth retardation may result in reduced foetal motility. However, maternal stress during pregnancy may also affect the quantity of foetal movements. The effect of maternal stress is not uniform: general maternal stress is associated with increased foetal motility, whereas specific pregnancy related stress (worries about pregnancy) – and its related increase in maternal cortisol – is associated with a decrease in foetal motility. Also, prenatal exposure to drugs may alter the quantity of foetal movements. For instance, exposure to betamethasone (applied to enhance foetal lung maturation in imminent preterm birth) is associated with reduced foetal motility, whereas caffeine and selective serotonin reuptake inhibitors (used as anti-depressant) are associated with an increase in foetal movements.

Foetuses with anencephaly do not only present with hyperkinesia – their movement quality is also abnormal. Their GMs are stereotyped, large and abrupt (De Vries and Fong 2007; Visser et al. 2010). Also, intra-uterine growth retardation may affect GM quality. Sival and colleagues (1992) reported that a deterioration in foetal health as reflected by the foetal heart rate pattern (presence of decelerations or reduced heart rate variability) was associated with poor repertoire GMs. The long-term outcome of their relatively small group of foetuses with abnormal GMs was heterogeneous; it varied between death, disability, and typical developmental outcome. Reissland and Francis (2010) reported that foetal stress, which was defined by the presence of foetal hiccups, back arch, and rhythmic mouth movements, was associated with jerky arm movements. Loss of movement fluency, such as jerkiness or abruptness, as an isolated sign generally is an expression of a minor impairment of the nervous system rather than being an indicator of serious brain dysfunction (Hadders-Algra 2018). The jerky nature of foetal movements in situations of stress corresponds to the accumulating literature that indicates that exposure to prenatal stress is associated with a non-optimal neurological condition later in life (Beijers et al. 2014).

Recently, Hayat et al. (2018) introduced the technique of recording foetal movements by means of magnetic resonance cine sequences (cine MR). In contrast to sonography, cine MR in the second half of pregnancy is not hampered by a limited field of view. Hayat et al. demonstrated that it is possible to record GMs and to reliably classify their quality. In addition, they showed that foetuses with various sonographic abnormalities, including malformations of the brain, had more frequently abnormal GMs than low-risk foetuses. However, the presence of abnormal GMs did not predict developmental outcome at the age of 1–2 years.

ATYPICAL GMs IN YOUNG INFANTS

Atypical GMs may manifest themselves in two different components of GM development: (1) a reduction in movement complexity and variation (poor repertoire); (2) failure to develop fidgety movements.

Poor Repertoire: Marked Reduction in Movement Complexity and Variation

Atypical GMs are primarily characterized by a marked reduction in movement complexity and variation (Einspieler et al. 2005; Hadders-Algra 2018; Video 7.1). This holds true for atypical GMs in all GM phases, including the preterm, writhing, and fidgety phases (see Chapter 5). Up until now, it has not been possible to develop a clinical tool that is able to quantify movement complexity and variation with standardized, objective measures. GM quality is assessed by the so-called Gestalt perception of the human observer. This means that the assessor needs to integrate movement information over time and space (i.e. occurring in all parts of body) in order to arrive at a single repertoire conclusion. As a

Table 7.1 Most commonly used terminology to describe GM complexity and variation

GM complexity & variation	Classification according to		GM quality
	Typical brain function		
	Prechtl	Hadders-Algra	
+++	Normal	Normal-optimal	**Typical**
++		Normal-suboptimal	
+		Mildly abnormal	
	Atypical brain function		
±	Poor repertoire, chaotic	Definitely abnormal	**Atypical**
–	Cramped, synchronized	Definitely abnormal with cramped synchronized	

+++ = Abundant complexity and variation; ++ = sufficient complexity and variation; + moderate reduction in complexity and variation; ± = marked reduction in complexity and variation; – = absence of complexity and variation.

result, GMs with atypical complexity and variation have been described in various ways (Table 7.1). Notwithstanding the minor variations in terminology, firm consensus exists about the fact that a marked reduction in movement complexity and variation (Table 7.1) reflects atypical brain function and has clinical relevance (Fig. 7.1; Einspieler et al. 2005; Hadders-Algra 2018). Increasing evidence indicates

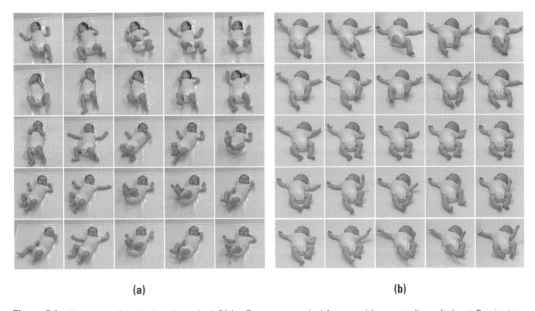

(a)   (b)

Figure 7.1 Example of typical and atypical GMs. Frames sampled from a video-recording of about 2 minutes; the frames have an interval of about 5s. The figure on the left illustrates the movement complexity and variation of typical GMs in a full-term-born infant aged 3 months. In each frame the infant's body parts show a different configuration (figure similar to Fig. 5.3). The figure on the right represents atypical GMs characterized by a marked reduction of movement complexity and variation of a full-term infant aged 3 months. He was later was diagnosed with bilateral spastic CP, Gross Motor Function Classification System level III. Figures reproduced from Hadders-Algra (2018b) with permission from John Wiley & Sons.

that GMs with atypical complexity and variation are associated with impaired connectivity in the large cortico-subcortical networks, in which the periventricular white matter plays a dominant role (Hadders-Algra 2018). This neural evidence supports the hypothesis that movement complexity and variation are generated by the cortical subplate – and at fidgety GM age – by the cortical plate, as the efferent connections of these structures transmitting the information to the CPG network of the GMs run through the periventricular white matter (see Chapter 5). The idea that GMs manifesting a marked reduction in complexity and variation reflect compromised interconnective integrity of complex cortical-subcortical networks explains why GMs with atypical complexity and variation are not only associated with CP but also with cognitive impairment, attention deficit and hyperactivity disorder, and minor neurological dysfunction (Hadders-Algra 2007; Einspieler et al. 2016).

Two major forms of reduction in movement complexity and variation in GMs can be distinguished (Table 7.1): (1) poor repertoire or definitely abnormal GMs that show a markedly reduced complexity and variation; and (2) cramped-synchronized GMs that are characterized by a suddenly occurring *en bloc* movement, in which trunk and limbs stiffly move in utter synchrony; these movements are totally devoid of complexity and variation, and indicate a severe loss of supraspinal movement control (Hadders-Algra 2007).

At the lower end of the spectrum of typical GM complexity and variation a subgroup of GMs with mildly reduced movement complexity and variation can be distinguished (mildly abnormal GMs; Table 7.1). These movements are associated with perinatal risk factors, but as a single sign they have a limited capacity to predict developmental outcome (see Text Box 7.1).

Failure to Develop Fidgety Movements

Atypical GMs may also manifest themselves in a failure to develop fidgety movements in the age period of 2–5 months corrected age (CA). Yet, the failure to develop fidgety movements has only clinical

---

Text Box 7.1 Mildly Impaired GMs

Mildly impaired GMs may manifest as a moderate reduction in movement complexity and variation (usually in combination with a lack of movement fluency) and as mild impairments in fidgety movements.

GMs with a moderate reduction in movement complexity and variation have been labelled *mildly abnormal GMs* (Video 7.2). These movements represent the lower end of the quality spectrum of typical GMs. Mildly abnormal GMs reflect typical but non-optimal brain function (e.g. an altered setting of the mono-aminergic systems). Mildly abnormal GMs are associated with a less optimal concurrent neurological condition and with an increased risk of attention deficit hyperactivity disorder (ADHD) and minor neurological dysfunction, such as fine manipulative disability or coordination problems. However, clinically these associations have limited value (Hadders-Algra 2007; Wu et al. 2020a).

Yet, mildly abnormal GMs are a sensitive tool to monitor brain function in young infants. For instance, it has been shown that parental subfertility, preterm birth, intra-uterine growth retardation, moderate degrees of hyperbilirubinaemia, and non-optimal nutritional status are associated with an increased prevalence of mildly abnormal GMs (Hadders-Algra 2007; Middelburg et al. 2010).

Two forms of *mildly impaired fidgety movements* have been distinguished, a quantitative and a qualitative variant. The former manifests as a sporadic presence of fidgety movements, the latter as fidgety movements with an abnormal quality. The amplitude and speed of these abnormal fidgety movements is exaggerated (Einspieler et al. 2005). They generate the impression of 'break dance' fidgety. Both forms of mildly impaired fidgety movements are associated with mildly abnormal GMs. Mildly impaired fidgety movements are not associated with the infant's current neurological condition (Wu et al. 2020a). The clinical significance of mildly impaired fidgety movements is debated (Hamer et al. 2011; Einspieler et al. 2016; Wu et al. 2020a), but its predictive value is considered to be limited (Einspieler et al. 2016).

significance when it is associated with a marked reduction in movement complexity and variation (Wu et al. 2020b). The failure to develop fidgety movements reflects a reduction of supraspinal inhibition (Hamer et al. 2011). This, in turn, interferes with the typical maturational process of 'sparcification' of the cortical networks (see Chapter 5). It implies an interruption of the typical developmental process during which the nervous system is shifting its major source of input from endogenous neural information to afferent information from the external world.

Also, fidgety movements may present with mild impairments and mild deviations in quantity or quality. The former have been termed sporadic fidgety movement, the latter abnormal fidgety movements. Mildly impaired fidgety movements are associated with GMs with moderately reduced complexity and variation. The clinical significance of mildly impaired fidgety movements is debated (see Textbox 7.1).

Combining the Two Atypical GM Features

The combination of both atypical GM features (i.e. a reduction in movement complexity and variation and a failure to develop fidgety movements) suggests that not only the interconnectivity of the cortico-subcortical networks is impaired, but also that supraspinal inhibition is reduced (Hamer et al. 2011; Hadders-Algra 2018). Infants who pair a marked reduction in movement complexity and variation with the absence of the age-specific fidgety movements have the highest risk of cerebral palsy (Video 7.1; Prechtl et al. 1997; Einspieler et al. 2005; Hadders-Algra 2018). Infants who combine a marked reduction in complexity and variation with the presence of age-specific fidgety activity do have an increased risk of cerebral palsy but a lower risk than the group with the double risk including absent fidgety movements (Video 7.3; Hadders-Algra 2018). Infants with complex congenital heart disease, in particular those who suffered prolonged periods of hypoxaemia, are at particular risk of showing this combination of signs (i.e. a marked reduction in complexity and variation in the presence of fidgety movements) (Huisenga et al. 2020). Interestingly, the presence or absence of fidgety movements is not associated with cognitive outcome at school age, whereas the degree of movement complexity and variation is (Butcher et al. 2009). This suggests that movement complexity and variation are stronger markers of complex network integrity than the presence of fidgety movements.

Fluency of GMs

The large majority of atypical GMs are non-fluent (i.e. they are jerky, abrupt, tremulous, or stiff). However, also, typical GMs in the lower end of the quality spectrum are non-fluent. This corresponds to the notion that the absence of movement fluency as a single sign is not an indicator of serious brain dysfunction but rather a sign of non-optimal typical brain function (Hadders-Algra 2007).

For further details on the clinical application of the assessment of the quality of GMs (general movement assessment) see Chapter 10.

ATYPICAL SUCKING AND SWALLOWING

Typically, sucking, and swallowing movements become increasingly adapted to the feeding situation from 36 weeks PMA onwards. In addition, the sucking rhythm stabilizes, and sucking is less often interrupted by breathing bursts. During the first months, post-term sucking becomes increasingly efficient (see Chapter 5).

Preterm neonates are often hampered by impaired sucking. The impairments may consist of disorganization or dysfunction. Two types of disorganization may be distinguished: (1) arrhythmic movements, with arrhythmic movements of jaw and tongue, and (2) dyscoordination between sucking and swallowing. Dysfunctional sucking implies the presence of abnormal jaw and tongue movements that interfere with sucking (Palmer et al. 1993).

Impaired sucking of preterm infants frequently persists until term age; at that age, the majority of preterm infants still show disorganized sucking, usually consisting of arrhythmic movements (Da Costa et al. 2010). This means that preterm infants have difficulties in selection the most efficient sucking movements (impaired adaptability, see Chapter 3). During the first weeks post-term, the sucking pattern of preterm infants gradually normalizes, so that at 8–10 weeks CA the majority of preterm infants show typical and efficient sucking movements. The normalization of sucking behaviour is associated with a rapid decrease in the need of supplementary tube feeding (Da Costa et al. 2010). The presence of dyscoordinated or dysfunctional sucking patterns or inefficient sucking between term age and 10 weeks CA is associated with non-optimal motor, cognitive, and language development at 1 and 5 years (Medoff-Cooper et al. 2009; Wolthuis-Stigter et al. 2017).

ATYPICAL CONTROL OF HEAD MOVEMENTS

It is first after birth that impairments in the control of head movements become clearly expressed (i.e. when the infant has to counteract the forces of gravity). Atypical control of the movements of the head is expressed as impairments in the abilities that young infants typically are able to perform in supine, prone, and sitting position. Impaired head control in supine means that the infant has difficulties in moving the head in all directions and shows a strong preference for a specific side position (see Text Box 7.2).

In a prone position, impaired head control results in an impaired ability to lift the head from the support surface and a head position preference. During the pull-to-sit manoeuvre, the infant is unable to align the head with the trunk: the infant shows a head lag or an active retroflexion of the head. Finally, an impaired head control manifests itself in difficulties keeping the head upright when held in a sitting position. The clinical knowledge that an impaired control of head movements is a manifestation of neurological impairment resulted in the inclusion of head control items in all common infant neurological assessment methods (e.g. Dubowitz et al. 1999).

ATYPICAL MUSCLE TONE REGULATION

Muscle tone refers to the muscles' resistance to stretch during passive movements. It depends on the motoneuronal excitability and on the elastic properties and flexibility of the ligaments and joints. In young infants, impaired muscle tone virtually always has a neurological cause. Low muscle tone (hypotonia) may be caused by impairments in the muscles, nerves, spinal cord, or brain. High muscle tone (hypertonia) or muscle tone with sudden changes between hypertonia and hypotonia result from brain dysfunction.

Knowledge on the prevalence of impaired muscle tone in young infants is limited. The prevalence of impaired muscle tone in the various parts of the body at term age varies in late preterm and full-term infants between 25% and 50% (Romeo et al. 2013). Infants born preterm or with a low birthweight often show 'transient dystonia' (i.e. they show impaired muscle tone regulation consisting of sudden

Text Box 7.2 Head Position Preference and Deformational Plagiocephaly

Typically, the full-term newborn infant is able to move the head in all directions. Nevertheless, the neonate has – just as the near-term foetus – a slight preference for keeping the head in the right-side position. This means that a slight head position preference belongs to typical infant behaviour and that a strong head position preference is a sign of impaired head control. If an infant's head preference is not opposed but rather facilitated by daily care giving routines, the head position preference tendency will increase. Examples of caregiving routines that promote a head preference position are a consistent positioning of the infant during feeding or dressing, so that it favours the head preference side (Boere-Boonekamp and Van der Linden-Kuiper 2001; Van Vlimmeren et al. 2007).

Boere-Boonekamp and Van der Linden (2001) reported the prevalence of head preference positions (Fig. 7.2) in the general Dutch population: 10% at 8 weeks, 11% at 8–16 weeks, and 3% 16–26 weeks. Persistent head position preferences are associated with the development of deformational plagiocephaly (i.e. an asymmetrical distortion of the skull) (Fig. 7.3). Little information on the prevalence of deformational plagiocephaly in the general population is available. Van Vlimmeren et al. (2007) and Ballardini et al. (2018) reported the prevalence in full-term infants: 22% in 7-week-old infants and 38% in 3-month-old infants respectively. Nuysink et al. (2013), who longitudinally studied deformational plagiocephaly in preterm infants born before 30 weeks of gestation, reported prevalences of 30% at term age, 50% at 3 months CA and 23% at 6 months CA. In 65% to 75% of the infants the right side is the preferred side. The available data suggest that the prevalence of deformational plagiocephaly peaks around 2–4 months and decreases to about 1% at the age of 5 years.

The aetiology of deformational plagiocephaly is not well understood. A recent systematic review concluded that most studies addressing this issue were highly selective, therewith precluding pertinent conclusions (De Bock et al. 2017). The factor that has been associated most consistently with deformational plagiocephaly

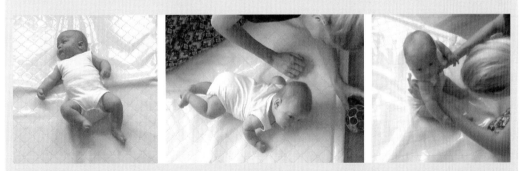

Figure 7.2   Consistent head position preference. Infant born at 37 weeks PMA at 2 months CA. The infant has a consistent positional preference to the right side: in supine, prone, and sitting.

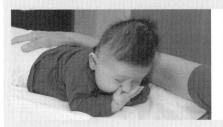
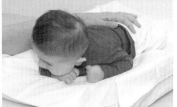
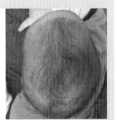

Figure 7.3   Deformational plagiocephaly.

is male sex. But the role of preterm birth, supine sleeping position, and the amount of daytime tummy time are disputed (De Bock et al. 2017).

More consensus exists on the co-morbidity of deformational plagiocephaly with developmental delay (De Bock et al. 2017; Martiniuk et al. 2017). In addition, deformational plagiocephaly may be associated with impaired muscle tone regulation: infants with deformational plagiocephaly may present with a slightly lower tone or a slightly higher tone (Fowler et al. 2008). The delayed development and the impaired muscle tone regulation indicate that deformational plagiocephaly is not an isolated phenomenon. It rather is a sequel and concomitant of a non-optimal neurological condition.

For early intervention in infants with head position preference and deformational plagiocephaly see Chapter 13.

changes in muscle tone or hypertonia in combination with predominant patterns of hyperextension of neck and trunk and extension of the legs). The transient dystonia usually decreases in the second half year of post-term life (Pedersen et al. 2000).

The significance of impaired muscle tone depends on the presence of accompanying neurological signs – muscle tone being one of the domains of the neurological examination (see Chapter 10). Nevertheless, a finding of the Generation R study, a Dutch population-based cohort that follows children from foetal life onwards, deserves attention. The study indicated that infants who had a low muscle tone at 2–5 months of age were consistently at increased risk of internalizing behavioural problems during preschool and school age – even when social and family conditions had been taken into account (Serdarevic et al. 2017). It is conceivable that the association is brought about by subtle genetic variations giving rise to and interacting with altered settings of neurotransmitter systems, such as the monoaminergic systems.

CONCLUDING REMARKS

The most prominent manifestations of atypical motor development during foetal life consist of impairments in the quantity and quality of GMs. Atypical motor development in young infants is especially expressed in (1) atypical quality of general movements; (2) atypical sucking, and swallowing; (3) atypical control of head movements; and (4) atypical muscle tone regulation. Many of these signs of atypical motor development have a transient nature (i.e. they disappear at older infant ages). The transient nature of the signs can be attributed to the major reorganizational processes occurring in the brain during infancy, especially around the age of 3–4 months CA (see Chapter 3). This is the major reason that atypical sucking and swallowing, deformational plagiocephaly, and transient dystonia in young infants are relatively poor predictors of developmental outcome. In contrast, the presence of atypical GMs – consisting of the combination of reduced complexity and variation (poor repertoire) and the absence of the age-specific fidgety movements – in infants aged 3–5 months CA is a major predictor of cerebral palsy.

REFERENCES

Ballardini E, Sisti M, Basaglia N, et al. (2018) Prevalence and characteristics of positional plagiocephaly in healthy full-term infants at 8–12 weeks of life. *Eur J Pediatr* **177**: 1547–1554. doi: 10.1007/s00431-018-3212-0.
Beijers R, Buitelaar JK, De Weerth C (2014) Mechanisms underlying the effects of prenatal psychosocial stress on child outcomes: beyond the HPA axis. *Eur Child Adolesc Psychiatry* **23**: 943–956. doi: 10.1007/s00787-014-0566-3.

Boere-Boonekamp MM, Van der Linden-Kuiper LT (2001) Positional preference: prevalence in infants and follow-up after two years. *Pediatrics* **107**: 339–343.

Butcher PR, Van Braeckel K, Bouma A, Einspieler C, Stremmelaar EF, Bos AF (2009) The quality of preterm infants' spontaneous movements: an early indicator of intelligence and behaviour at school age. *J Child Psychol Psychiatry* **50**: 920–930. doi: 10.1111/j.1469-7610.2009.02066.x.

Da Costa SP, van der Schans CP, Zweens MJ, et al. (2010) The development of sucking in preterm, small-for-gestational age infants. *J Pediatr* **157**: 603–609. doi: 10.1016/j.jpeds.2010.04.037.

De Bock F, Braun V, Renz-Polster H (2017) Deformational plagiocephaly in normal infants: a systematic review of causes and hypotheses. *Arch Dis Child* **102**: 535–542. doi: 10.1136/archdischild-2016-312018.

De Vries JI, Fong BF (2007) Changes in fetal motility as a result of congenital disorders: an overview. *Ultrasound Obstet Gynecol* **29**: 590–599.

Dubowitz LMS, Dubowitz V, Mercuri E (1999) *The Neurological Assessment of the Preterm and Full-term Newborn Infant,* 2nd edn. London: Mac Keith Press.

Einspieler C, Prechtl HFR, Bos AF, Ferrari F, Cioni G (2005) *Prechtl's Method on the Qualitative Assessment of General Movements in Preterm, Term, and Young Infants.* London: Mac Keith Press.

Einspieler C, Bos AF, Libertus ME, Marschik PB (2016) The general movement assessment helps us to identify preterm infants at risk for cognitive dysfunction. *Front Psychol* **7**: 406. doi: 10.3389/fpsyg.2016.00406.

Fowler EA, Becker DB, Pilgram TK, Noetzel M, Epstein J, Kane AA (2008) Neurologic findings in infants with deformational plagiocephaly. *J Child Neurol* **23**: 742–747. doi: 10.1177/0883073808314362.

Hadders-Algra M (2007) Putative neural substrate of normal and abnormal general movements. *Neurosci Biobehav Rev* **31**: 1181–1190. Epub 2007 May 5.

Hadders-Algra M (2018) Neural substrate and clinical significance of general movements: an update, *Dev Med Child. Neurol* 60: 39–46. doi: 10.1111/dmcn.13540.

Hamer EG, Bos AF, Hadders-Algra M (2011) Assessment of specific characteristics of abnormal general movements: does it enhance the prediction of cerebral palsy? *Dev Med Child Neurol* **53**: 751–756. doi: 10.1111/j.1469-8749.2011.04007.x.

Hayat TTA, Martinez-Biarge M, Kyriakopoulou V, Hajnal JV, Rutherford MA (2018) Neurodevelopmental correlates of fetal motor behavior assessed using cine MR imaging. *AJNR Am J Neuroradiol* **39**: 1519–1522. doi: 10.3174/ajnr.A5694.

Martiniuk AL, Vujovich-Dunn C, Park M, Yu W, Lucas BR (2017) Plagiocephaly and developmental delay: a systematic review. *J Dev Behav Pediatr* **38**: 67–78. doi: 10.1097/DBP.0000000000000376.

Medoff-Cooper B, Shults J, Kaplan J (2009) Sucking behavior of preterm neonates as a predictor of developmental outcomes. *J Dev Behav Pediatr* **30**: 16–22. doi: 10.1097/DBP.0b013e318196b0a8.

Middelburg KJ, Haadsma ML, Heineman MJ, Bos AF, Hadders-Algra M (2010) Ovarian hyperstimulation and the in vitro fertilization procedure do not influence early neuromotor development; a history of subfertility does. *Fertil Steril* **93**: 544–553. doi: 10.1016/j.fertnstert.2009.03.008.

Nuysink J, Eijsermans MJ, Van Haastert IC, et al. (2013) Clinical course of asymmetric motor performance and deformational plagiocephaly in very preterm infants. *J Pediatr* **163**: 658–665.e1. doi: 10.1016/j.jpeds.2013.04.015.

Palmer MM, Crawley K, Blanco IA (1993) Neonatal Oral-Motor Assessment Scale: a reliability study. *J Perinatol* **13**: 28–35.

Pedersen SJ, Sommerfelt K, Markestad T (2000) Early motor development of premature infants with birthweight less than 2000 grams. *Acta Paediatr* **89**: 1456–1461.

Prechtl HFR, Einspieler C, Cioni G, Bos AF, Ferrari F, Sontheimer D (1997) An early marker for neurological deficits after perinatal brain lesions. *Lancet* **349**: 1361–1363.

Reissland N, Francis B (2010) The quality of fetal arm movements as indicators of fetal stress. *Early Hum Dev* **86**: 813–816. doi: 10.1016/j.earlhumdev.2010.09.005.

Romeo DM, Luciano R, Corsello M, et al. (2013) Neonatal neurological examination of late preterm babies. *Early Hum Dev* 89: 537–545. doi: 10.1016/j.earlhumdev.2013.01.002.

Serdarevic F, Ghassabian A, van Batenburg-Eddes T, et al. (2017) Infant neuromotor development and childhood problem behavior. *Pediatrics* 140: e20170884. doi: 10.1542/peds.2017-0884.

Sival DA, Visser GH, Prechtl HF (1992) The effect of intrauterine growth retardation on the quality of general movements in the human fetus. *Early Hum Dev* **28**: 119–132.

Van Vlimmeren LA, Van der Graaf Y, Boere-Boonekamp MM, L'Hoir MP, Helders PJ, Engelbert RH (2007) Risk factors for deformational plagiocephaly at birth and at 7 weeks of age: a prospective cohort study. *Pediatrics* **119**: e408–418.

Visser GH, Mulder EJ, Ververs FF (2010) Fetal behavioral teratology. *J Matern Fetal Neonatal Med* **23** (Suppl 3): 14–16. doi: 10.3109/14767058.2010.517717.

Whitehead CL, Cohen N, Visser GHA, Farine D (2019) Are increased fetal movements always reassuring? *J Matern Fetal Neonatal Med* Feb **22**: 1–6. doi: 10.1080/14767058.2019.1582027. E-Pub ahead of print.

Wolthuis-Stigter MI, Da Costa SP, Bos AF, Krijnen WP, Van Der Schans CP, Luinge MR (2017) Sucking behaviour in infants born preterm and developmental outcomes at primary school age. *Dev Med Child Neurol* **59**: 871–877. doi: 10.1111/dmcn.13438.

Wu YC, Straathof EJM, Heineman KR, Hadders-Algra M (2020a) Typical general movements at 2 to 4 months: movement complexity, fidgety movements, and their associations with risk factors and SINDA scores. *Early Hum Dev*, epub ahead of print. doi: 10.1016/j.earlhumdev.2020.105135.

Wu YC, Bouwstra H, Heineman K, Hadders-Algra M (2020b) Atypical general movements in the general population: prevalence over the last 15 years and associated factors. *Acta Paediatr* **109**: 2762–2769. doi: 10.1111/apa.15329.

SUGGESTIONS FOR FURTHER READING

Hadders-Algra M, Tacke U, Pietz J, Rupp A, Philippi H (2019) Reliability and predictive validity of the Standardized Infant NeuroDevelopmental Assessment neurological scale. *Dev Med Child Neurol* **61**: 654–660. doi: 10.1111/dmcn.14045.

Hamer EG, Bos AF, Hadders-Algra M (2011) Assessment of specific characteristics of abnormal general movements: Does it enhance the prediction of cerebral palsy? *Dev Med Child Neurol* **53**: 751–756. doi: 10.1111/j.1469-8749.2011.04007.x.

Huisenga DC, Van Bergen AH, Sweeney JK, Wu Y-C, Hadders-Algra M (2020) The quality of general movements in infants with complex congenital heart disease undergoing surgery in the neonatal period. *Early Hum Dev*, epub ahead of print. doi: 10.1016/j.earlhumdev.2020.105167.

Ihlen EAF, Støen R, Boswell L, et al. (2019) Machine learning of infant spontaneous movements for the early prediction of cerebral palsy: a multi-site cohort study. *J Clin Med* **9**, pii: E5. doi: 10.3390/jcm9010005.

Marcroft C, Khan A, Embleton ND, Trenell M, Plotz T (2015) Movement recognition technology as a method of assessing spontaneous general movements in high risk infants. *Front Neurol* **5**: 284. doi: 10.3389/fneur.2014.00284.

Northoff G (2013) Gene, brains, and environment-genetic neuroimaging of depression. *Curr Opin Neurobiol* **23**: 133–142. doi: 10.1016/j.conb.2012.08.004.

Rönnqvist L, Hopkins B (1998) Head position preference in the human newborn: a new look. *Child Dev* **69**: 13–23.

Straathof EJM, Heineman KR, Hamer EG, Hadders-Algra M (2020) Prevailing head position to one side in early infancy – a population-based study. *Acta Paediatr* **109**: 1423–1429. doi: 10.1111/apa.15112.

Van Vlimmeren LA, Engelbert RH, Pelsma M, Groenewoud HM, Boere-Boonekamp MM, Van der Sanden MW (2017) The course of skull deformation from birth to 5 years of age: a prospective cohort study. *Eur J Pediatr* **176**: 11–21. doi: 10.1007/s00431-016-2800-0.

Wu YC, Van Rijssen IM, Buurman MT, Dijkstra LJ, Hamer EG, Hadders-Algra M (2020) Temporal and spatial localization of general movement complexity and variation – why Gestalt assessment requires experience. *Acta Paediatr*, epub ahead of print. doi: 10.1111/apa.15300.

Atypical Motor Development Between 3 Months and 2 Years

Mijna Hadders-Algra and Lindsay Pennington

SUMMARY POINTS

- Atypical motor development may manifest itself in impairments such as atypical movement quality or atypical muscle tone, and in limitations in mobility, drinking and eating, and communication.
- Atypical motor development in early life may be a transient phenomenon, but it also may be the first stage of a permanent developmental disorder.
- Atypical motor development is often accompanied by impairments and limitations in other developmental domains, for example, impairments in the processing of sensory information, cognitive deficits resulting in limitations in learning and the application of knowledge, and behavioural dysregulation.

Atypical motor development during infancy may be an early expression of a developmental disorder. Yet, it may also be a sign of temporary impairment that is followed by typical developmental outcome. The aim of this chapter is to discuss the various ways in which atypical motor development may manifest itself between the ages of 3 months and 2 years corrected age (CA). We start with a discussion of the motor impairments that signal atypical motor development, including the impaired quality of self-produced movements, atypical muscle tone, and atypical reflexes and reactions. Next, we describe the limitations in mobility that may occur during early life. We first address the significance of a delayed attainment of milestones in the mobility domain in general, where we focus on (1) atypical gross motor development (i.e. the limitations in maintaining and changing body position and the limitations in moving around); and (2) atypical fine motor development (i.e. the limitations in carrying, moving, and handling objects). The following two sections describe the limitations in eating and drinking, and those in communication. Finally, we discuss the impairments and limitations that are often associated with atypical motor development.

IMPAIRMENTS SIGNALLING ATYPICAL MOTOR DEVELOPMENT

Impaired Movement Quality

The quality of the infant's self-produced movements provides information on the integrity of the infant's brain and the infant's developmental prognosis (Hadders-Algra 2010). The following aspects of impaired movement quality may be distinguished (Heineman et al. 2011; see Chapter 3):

- Reduced movement variation: examples are a stereotyped flexion of the elbows, stereotyped fisting and thumb adduction, stereotyped extension movements or stereotyped pedalling of the legs, or stereotyped clawing of the toes (Fig. 8.1). The presence of stereotypies suggests an impaired integrity of the subcortical-cortical networks; it is associated with an increased risk of CP (Heineman et al. 2011) and possibly also of developmental coordination disorder and autism spectrum disorder (ASD) (Hadders-Algra 2010; Elison et al. 2014). In addition, a reduced movement repertoire has been associated with limited learning opportunities (Dusing et al. 2016).
- Reduced adaptability (i.e. an impaired ability to select the best strategy from the movement repertoire available). Reduced adaptability is especially due to impaired processing of sensory information. This results in a reduced capacity to generate internal frames of reference (internal models) of the body, its movements, and the external world. This in turn limits the child's capacity to use feedforward control while moving (i.e. to select in anticipation the most appropriate movement strategy for each situation). Consequently, the child has to rely more on feedback movement control, which results in movement inefficiency. Infants with a reduced movement repertoire always have a reduced adaptability; in these infants the selection problems are aggravated by the absence of a proportion of the typical strategies – due to repertoire reduction. More often, however, a reduced adaptability is associated with a typical movement repertoire. This means that reduced adaptability is a rather unspecific sign of atypical motor development. It is, for instance, frequently encountered in infants born preterm

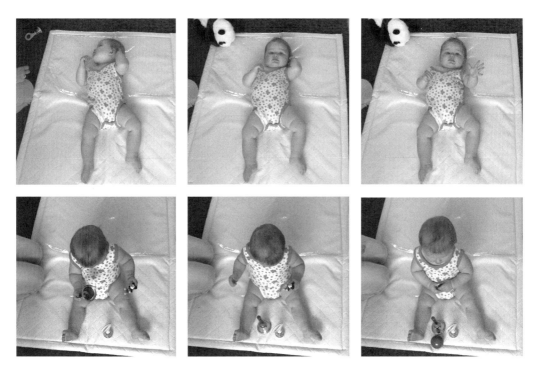

Figure 8.1   Stereotyped extension of both legs. Nine-month-old infant with stereotyped extension of both legs in supine and sitting; the frames were sampled from a video-recording (from a sequence of about 30 seconds in supine and 30 seconds in sitting).

(Hadders-Algra 2010; Heineman et al. 2010). Impaired adaptability has been associated with lower intelligence quotient (IQ) scores at school age (Wu et al. 2020).

- Asymmetry: young infants may present with a head position preference to one side that is accompanied by mild asymmetries in the movements of other parts of the body. These asymmetries are usually transient (see Chapter 7). However, asymmetries that are accompanied by other signs of neurological impairment may signal the presence of a neurological disorder, such as an obstetric brachial plexus lesion or unilateral spastic CP. The latter should be suspected especially when the asymmetry emerges after the age of 6 months (Hay et al. 2018).

- Reduced movement fluency: this may mean the presence of jerky, stiff, sluggish, or tremulous movements. Jerky, stiff, and sluggish movements denote an impaired regulation of the velocity profile of the movements, with accelerations that are either too fast (abrupt, jerky movements) or too slow (sluggish and stiff movements). Tremor means the presence of regularly oscillating movements with a frequency of 1–5 Hz and amplitudes that vary between some millimetres and some centimetres. As a single sign, non-fluent movements have limited clinical significance, but when accompanied by other neurological signs they add to the clinical picture.

Atypical Muscle Tone

Muscle tone is the resistance against passive movements (Sanger et al. 2003). Infants may present with atypical muscle tone, that is, a muscle tone that is too high (hypertonia), a muscle tone that is too low (hypotonia), or a changing, fluctuating, or varying muscle tone (dystonia). The atypical muscle tone may manifest itself in the proximal (axial) muscles of neck and trunk, in the distal muscles of the arms or legs, or be more generalized. The atypical muscle tone may be too high in some parts of the body (e.g. in the ankles), but too low in other parts (e.g. in the trunk) (Straathof et al. 2020). The presentation of atypical muscle tone may also change over the first years of life. For instance, infants later diagnosed with CP may first present with hypotonia, with hypertonia emerging in the second half of the first year or even after the first birthday (Carr 2014).

Atypical muscle tone is an unspecific sign of neurological dysfunction. Its clinical significance largely depends on the accompanying signs, such as reflex abnormalities and atypical movements and postures. Infants who are later diagnosed with CP mostly gradually develop spasticity (i.e. the muscle's high velocity-dependent sensitivity to stretch) (Sanger et al. 2003; Carr 2014).

Hypotonia is the most frequently encountered form of atypical muscle tone in infancy. Its origin is heterogeneous, both in terms of aetiology and neurological substrate (see Table 8.1). Therefore, the presence of hypotonia signals the need of further diagnostics. Hypertonia occurs less often. It is a sign of supraspinal neurological dysfunction. The dysfunction may be transient – the infant growing out of an initial hypertonia – or it may be the sign of a permanent impairment. The latter occurs especially when the infant gradually grows into a hypertonia, which generally indicates the evolution of CP (Carr 2014).

In early life, two major forms of dystonia may be distinguished: transient dystonia and dystonic CP. The latter form is relatively rare and emerges in the second or third year of life (Carr 2014). Transient dystonia is especially seen in infants born preterm. The clinical picture consists of impaired muscle tone, often consisting of a mix of a relatively mild hypertonia and a mild hypotonia, and extension patterns in neck, trunk, and legs (Ferrari et al. 2012). As the word 'transient' already indicates, this pattern disappears, usually in the second half of the first year. When the transient dystonia is not accompanied by other signs of neurological dysfunction, developmental prognosis is favourable. Yet, caregivers of preterm infants with transient dystonia need to be informed about this particular

Table 8.1   Origin of hypotonia in young children

Localization	Origin
Supraspinal[1]	– systemic disorders, e.g. sepsis, metabolic disorders
	– genetic disorders, e.g. trisomy 21, Prader-Willi syndrome
	– malformation of the brain, e.g. holoprosencephaly, cerebellar hypoplasia
	– prenatal, perinatal, or neonatal lesion of the brain
	– congenital hypotonia with favourable outcome
Spinal cord, nerves, muscles[2]	– spinal cord, e.g. spina bifida, spinal muscular atrophy
	– nerves, e.g. hereditary motor sensory neuropathy
	– muscles, e.g. muscular dystrophy, myopathies

[1] Little is understood of the mechanisms involved in the supraspinal origin of hypotonia; this holds true for hypotonia at any age. Atypical information carried by any of the descending motor pathways may be involved. The atypical descending information results in a reduction of the typical activity of the spinal stretch reflexes (gamma loop). It is well known that cerebellar dysfunction may result in hypotonia, in particular hypotonia of the axial muscles. But, for instance, also aberrant information of the mono-aminergic systems may result in hypotonia. In addition, hypotonia may be an acute sign of a lesion of the spinal cord.

[2] Impaired function of any part of the motor unit may result in hypotonia, e.g. impaired function of the spinal motor neuron, the peripheral nerve, the neuromuscular junction, and the muscle. Hypotonia caused by impaired motor unit function is always accompanied by some degree of muscle weakness and a varying degree of reduction of stretch reflex activity.

Further information: see Bodensteiner (2008), Harris (2008), Robinson (2013).

behaviour. The reason is twofold. First, transient dystonia may interfere with caregiver–infant interaction, as caregivers may erroneously interpret the extension pattern as the infant signalling rejection of the caregivers' attempts to interact or of activities the caregivers and children are engaging in. Second, transient dystonia may affect infant development, as extension of neck and trunk interferes with proper feeding and – through shoulder retraction – with the development of eye–hand coordination. Therefore, it is recommended to provide caregivers with information how they can create conditions that prevent extension patterns.

Atypical Reflexes and Reactions

Typical motor development is dominated by self-produced motor behaviour and not by reflex or reactive movement patterns (see Chapter 6). This does not mean that reflex circuitries do not play a role in typical behaviour. Reflex circuitries constitute the basic building blocks of neural organization. Examples are the circuitries involved in the knee jerk (as an example of monosynaptic reflexes), the withdrawal response, and the asymmetrical tonic neck reflex (as examples of polysynaptic reactions). Over the lifespan, these circuitries are integrated in daily motor behaviour (see e.g. Bruijn et al. 2013). Yet, typically they do not dominate motor activities.

The various forms of reflexes and reactions are summarized in Table 8.2. Neurological impairment is generally expressed in the reflexes and reactions. This is the reason that infant neurological assessments test a variety of reflexes and reactions. An isolated atypical finding in one or two reflexes or reactions usually has no clinical significance. It is the number of atypical responses that matters and – more important – whether the atypical responses are accompanied by other signs of neurological impairment, such as atypical postures and movements and atypical muscle tone.

Table 8.2 Reflexes and reactions in young children

Category	Impairment	Significance
Monosynaptic tendon jerks, e.g. – biceps reflex – knee jerk – Achilles tendon reflex	1. low threshold, increased reflexogenic zone; high clonic intensity 2. high threshold, low intensity 3. absent response 4. asymmetry	– 1–4: may indicate supraspinal impairment – 2–3: may indicate motoneuron, nerve or muscle impairment – 4: may indicate in particular unilateral CP or peripheral nerve impairment (e.g. brachial plexus lesion)
Polysynaptic reactions, e.g. – withdrawal reaction[a] – foot sole reaction (FSR)[b]	– absent response – asymmetry – FSR: stereotyped tonic dorsiflexion 1st toe, or stereotyped clawing	– impairments indicate especially supraspinal dysfunction – impairments may reflect peripheral nerve lesion
Postural reactions,c including reactions to postural challenges, e.g. 1. asymmetrical tonic neck reflex (ATNR) 2. pull-to-sit[e] 3. vertical suspension[f]	1. ATNR pattern[d] present as stereotypy 2. head lags behind, active retroflexion of the head, impaired flexion of the hips 3. infant 'slips through', stereotyped extension of legs (with or without adduction ('scissoring')	– impairments indicate supraspinal dysfunction
Infantile reactions,g e.g. 1. Moro reaction[h] 2. palmar grasp reaction[i] 3. plantar grasp reaction[j]	– asymmetry – in early infancy: absent response – 1: exaggerated, tremulous response; persistent presence > 6 months CA – 2: persistent presence > 9 months CA	– impairments usually indicate supraspinal dysfunction – impairments may indicate peripheral nerve lesion

For further information see Zafeiriou (2004), Hamer and Hadders-Algra (2016).

[a]Withdrawal reaction: a nociceptive stimulus to the foot-sole elicits flexion of the leg.

[b]The foot sole reaction is elicited by stroking along the lateral side of the foot-sole (preferably from toe to heel in order to avoid a conflicting response of the plantar grasp reaction). Young infants respond with a varied dorsiflexion of the first toe; the dorsiflexion changes into the adult plantar flexion between 6 and 18 months CA.

[c]Postural reactions: note that typically postural control is not governed by reactions, but by a complex interaction between spinal and supraspinal networks (see Chapter 6).

[d]ATNR-pattern: the tendency to extend the limbs on the face side of the body and to flex the limbs on the contralateral side (see Fig. 8.2).

[e]Pull-to-sit manoeuvre: the manoeuvre starts with the infant in a supine position; the assessor takes the infant by the wrists and pulls the infant into a sitting position.

[f]Vertical suspension: the assessor holds the infant suspended in a vertical position by placing her hands in the infant's armpits.

[g]We prefer to use the term 'infantile reactions' rather than 'primitive reflexes' as the latter does not do justice to the complex organization of the young human nervous system.

[h]Moro reaction: the assessor holds the infant in supine suspension; a sudden drop of the infant's head (stimulation of neck propriocepsis and vestibulum) or a sudden lowering of the entire infant (vestibular stimulation only) results in an abduction-extension movements of both arms; this is followed by a moderate flexion-adduction movement of the arms.

[i]Palmar grasp reaction: placement of the assessor's index finger in the infants palm of the hand results in flexion of the fingers.

[j]Plantar grasp reaction: pressing the assessor's thumb on the foot-sole near the origin of the toes results in flexion of the toes.

LIMITATIONS IN MOBILITY SIGNALLING ATYPICAL MOTOR DEVELOPMENT

Delayed Attainment of the Milestones in the Mobility Domain

A delayed attainment of the milestones in the mobility domain is the best known sign of atypical motor development beyond 3 months CA (Noritz et al. 2013). Thus, it is not surprising that the assessment

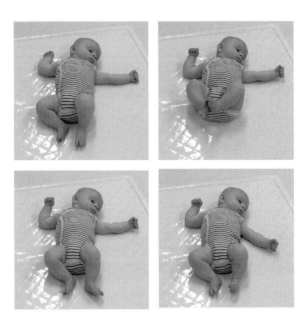

Figure 8.2 Stereotyped ATNR pattern. Infant aged 4 months with frequently occurring ATNR pattern during spontaneous motility; the frames were sampled from a video-sequence of about 1 minute.

of milestones in the mobility domain forms part and parcel of any developmental examination, such as the developmental screening of the paediatrician (Miall et al. 2016), or specialized evaluations, including the Bayley Scales of Infant and Toddler Development, the Alberta Infant Motor Scale, and the Standardized Infant NeuroDevelopmental Assessment (see Chapter 11). Yet, the delayed attainment of a single motor milestone has little clinical significance, due to the fact that typical motor development is characterized by an immense variation (see Chapter 6 and Fig. 6.1). But, when a delay occurs in multiple milestones, the chance increases that this is one of the first manifestations of a developmental disorder. The developmental tests that use the milestones are based on this principle: an accumulation of signs of slow development across the mobility skills, such as locomotion in prone, sitting, standing, walking, reaching, and grasping, increases the risk of a developmental disorder, including cerebral palsy (CP). This risk increases further if the delay in milestone attainment gets more pronounced during the course of the first year (Maitre et al. 2013). A late attainment of milestones in the mobility domain, including a delayed onset of independent walking, is not only associated with an increased risk of CP, but has also been associated with lower intelligence scores (Wu et al. 2020), ASD (Lloyd et al. 2013), and developmental coordination disorder (Faebo Larsen et al. 2013). Yet, it is important to realize that milestones in the mobility domain predict motor developmental outcome only to a limited extent. This was, for instance, illustrated by the meta-analysis of Luttikhuizen dos Santos et al. (2013) that demonstrated that the infant Bayley Psychomotor Developmental Index scores only moderately predicted motor outcome at 3–6 years. The finding that a delayed attainment of mobility milestones is only moderately predictive of later outcome illustrates that the achievement of mobility milestones is the net result of a complex interaction between the infant, including the infant's talents and resilience and the infant's impairments (e.g. brain injury, complex congenital heart defect, or chronic lung disease) and the infant's environment (see Chapter 3). In fact, one could say: developmental delay is not a diagnosis, but it is an invitation to make one.

Limitations in Maintaining and Changing Body Position and Limitations in Moving Around

An early sign of atypical motor development is a limited capacity to maintain head position for a determined period of time. Typically, infants are able to balance their head properly from about 3 months CA onwards. In young infants, a limited capacity to balance the head is a rather unspecific sign of atypical development, but with increasing age the sign gets more diagnostic significance. It is important to realize that a limited capacity to balance the head largely interferes with the infant's other activities, as it hampers, for instance, the infant's ability to visually explore the environment, to communicate with partners, and to drink and eat.

With increasing age, as the infant's postural control abilities typically improve (see Chapter 6 and Fig. 6.1), other limitations in the ability to maintain body position may emerge: infants may not, or may only with a large delay, develop the capacity to sit and to stand independently. Also, these limitations largely interfere with activities in daily life.

In the same way, limitations in the infant's abilities to get into and out of a body position and to move from one location to another may emerge. Again, the types of limitations that may be observed, are age-dependent, as the infant's abilities to roll, crawl, get into sitting and standing position, and to walk, run, and climb develop in an age-dependent sequence (see Chapter 6).

The child's limitations in maintaining and changing body position and the limitations in moving around form the basis of the Gross Motor Function Classification System (GMFCS; Palisano et al. 1997). The GMFCS is the standard way to classify gross motor function in children with CP. It is based on self-initiated movements and focusses on the performance of sitting, transfers, and mobility in the context of daily life. It distinguishes five levels for which criteria have been specified for five age bands: before 2 years (Table 8.3), 2–4 years, 4–6 years, 6–12 years, and 12–18 years. The classification system enables professionals to communicate with caregivers, as it facilitates the understanding of the child's current and future condition. The latter holds true in particular for children older than 2 years, in whom the GMFCS classification is rather stable. In children younger than 2 years, the prediction of the child's future mobility performance is less accurate, as with increasing age the child's GMFCS classification may

Table 8.3 Gross Motor Function Classification System – Expanded and Revised (GMFCS – E & R) – description of the five levels in children before their second birthday	
LEVEL I	Infants move in and out of sitting and floor sit with both hands free to manipulate objects. Infants crawl on hands and knees, pull to stand and take steps holding on to furniture. Infants walk between 18 months and 2 years of age without the need for any assistive mobility device.
LEVEL II	Infants maintain floor sitting but may need to use their hands for support to maintain balance. Infants creep on their stomach or crawl on hands and knees. Infants may pull to stand and take steps holding on to furniture.
LEVEL III	Infants maintain floor sitting when the low back is supported. Infants roll and creep forward on their stomachs.
LEVEL IV	Infants have head control but trunk support is required for floor sitting. Infants can roll to supine and may roll to prone.
LEVEL V	Physical impairments limit voluntary control of movement. Infants are unable to maintain antigravity head and trunk postures in prone and sitting. Infants require adult assistance to roll.

The Gross Motor Function Classification System – Expanded and Revised (Palisano et al. 2007) is the expanded and revised version of the original GMFCS, developed by Palisano et al. (1997); see: https://www.canchild.ca/system/tenon/assets/attachments/000/000/058/original/GMFCS-ER_English.pdf.

move one level up or one level down (Gorter et al. 2009). Application of the GMFCS also promotes communication between professionals, both in the clinical and in the research setting. Nowadays, the GMFCS is not only used in children with CP, but also in children with other diagnoses. This may be useful, but currently the scientific validation of this usage is lacking (Towns et al. 2018).

The limitations in maintaining and changing body position and limitations in moving around largely interfere with activities and participation in daily life. They also have a negative impact on cognitive and social development. Therefore these limitations form a core theme in early intervention. For early intervention, a dual strategy is recommended: (a) to provide caregivers with information how they can offer the infant opportunities to practise specific mobility activities during daily caregiving engagements; (b) to inform caregivers about the advantages of assistive devices that provide proper postural support or assist the child's mobility for promotion of the child's participation in daily life. Examples of assistive devices are simple pillows, tailor-made adaptive seating systems mounted on a wheelchair, or ride-on toy cars (see Chapter 15).

Limitations in Carrying, Moving, and Handling Objects

In typically developing infants, the ability to lift, move, handle, transfer, and put down objects emerges after the age of 3 months. Atypical motor development may manifest itself in a delay or lacking emergence of these motor activities (see Chapter 6). In addition, a consistent asymmetric performance is a red flag signalling atypical development; in particular, it may indicate the presence of unilateral CP or a brachial plexus lesion. Limitations in carrying, moving, and handling objects interfere with activities in daily life, especially with self-care activities such as eating, drinking, and dressing, and in the exploration of objects. As a result, these limitations have a negative impact on the child's cognitive and social development.

The child's limitations in carrying, moving, and handling objects forms the basis of the Manual Ability Classification System (MACS; Eliasson et al. 2006). The MACS is used to classify manual abilities of children with CP as performed in their daily life environment. Similar to the GMFCS it has five levels of performance. It has two age bands: 1–4 years (Mini-MACS; Table 8.4) and 4–18 years. No data

Table 8.4	Mini-Manual Ability Classification System (Mini-MACS) for children with cerebral palsy aged 1–4 years
LEVEL I	Handles objects easily and successfully. The child may have a slight limitation in performing actions that require precision and coordination between the hands but they can still perform them. The child may need somewhat more adult assistance when handling objects compared to other children of the same age.
LEVEL II	Handles most objects, but with somewhat reduced quality and/or speed of achievement. Some actions can only be performed and accomplished with some difficulty and after practice. The child may try an alternative approach, such as using only one hand. The child needs adult assistance to handle objects more frequently compared to children at the same age.
LEVEL III	Handles objects with difficulty. Performance is slow, with limited variation and quality. Easily managed objects are handled independently for short periods. The child often needs adult help and support to handle objects.
LEVEL IV	Handles a limited selection of easily managed objects in simple actions. The actions are performed slowly, with exertion and/or random precision. The child needs constant adult help and support to handle objects.
LEVEL V	Does not handle objects and has severely limited ability to perform even simple actions. At best, the child can push, touch, press, or hold on to a few items, in constant interaction with an adult.

The Mini-MACS is the adaptation of the Manual Ability Classification System (MACS; Eliasson et al. 2006) that has been developed for children and youth aged 4–18 years. See: https://www.macs.nu/files/Mini-MACS_English_2016.pdf.

on the stability of the MACS classification over time are available. The application of the MACS – like the application of the GMFCS – facilitates the communication between professionals and caregivers and that between professionals.

LIMITATIONS IN EATING AND DRINKING

Atypical motor development is often noted in early feeding behaviours. Breast or bottle feeding relies on finely tuned coordination of movements of the larynx, pharynx, velum, jaw, tongue, lips, and cheeks to produce rhythmical sequences of sucking, swallowing, and breathing. Infants with atypical oral motor development may have observable difficulties latching on, poor extraction of milk, and delayed and discoordinated swallow. For some infants, oral motor limitations may only become apparent during weaning when their calorific requirements can no longer be met by milk or formula alone and they transition to being spoon fed soft puree that requires oral manipulation and then onto foods that need chewing. With either milk or solid food, reduced oral motor control is suspected if children are described as 'messy eaters', have difficulty managing saliva and take more time to feed than their peers. Red flags for discoordinated swallow and aspiration include coughing; gagging; arching; wet, gurgly breathing; taking multiple swallows to clear food; watering eyes; and food refusal. Such difficulties require prompt investigation of both the oral phase and pharyngeal phase of swallowing, and the safety of oral feeding.

Several clinical assessments consider the safety and efficiency of children's eating, drinking, and swallowing and involve observation of mealtimes, examination of oral motor control, and consideration of nutritional intake. In some cases, instrumental investigation using videofluoroscopy or Fibreoptic Endoscopic Evaluation of Swallowing (FEES) is required. The Eating and Drinking Abilities System (EDACS; Table 8.5) allows description of children's performance from 3 years of age (Sellers et al. 2013). A downward extension to 18 months is currently in development.

Limitations in oral motor control that affect eating and drinking may be managed by adaptations to the texture and consistency of food, positioning of the child, utensils, and the pace of feeding. For children whose eating and drinking is considered unsafe, gastrostomy is recommended. Replacement or supplementary feeding via gastrostomy may also be advised for who are unable to consume adequate calories efficiently to ensure adequate growth and to facilitate social participation.

LIMITATIONS IN COMMUNICATION

Infants communicate using facial expression, body movement, gesture, and vocalization, and from 12 months they begin to produce spoken words (see Chapter 6). Atypical motor development can affect each of these modes of communication. Red flags for atypical vocal and speech development can be

Table 8.5   Eating and drinking abilities classification system

LEVEL I	Eats and drinks safely and efficiently.
LEVEL II	Eats and drinks safely but with some limitations to efficiency.
LEVEL III	Eats and drinks with some limitations to safety; may be limitations to efficiency.
LEVEL IV	Eats and drinks with significant limitations to safety.
LEVEL V	Unable to eat or drink safely – tube feeding may be considered to provide nutrition.

For details see Sellers et al. (2014) and https://www.sussexcommunity.nhs.uk/get-involved/research/chailey-research/eating-drinking-classification.htm.

noted in lack of vocal play in the first 6 months, absent or restricted babbling before one year of age, and a restricted repertoire of syllables and inflections in jargon that appears before real words. Children with cerebral palsy who have little or no speech at 2 years are likely to be nonspeaking at 4 years of age (Hustad et al. 2017).

At around 9–10 months of age, children develop triadic gaze, looking at their carer, a desired object and back to the carer to signal, which establishes joint attention. They also reach for objects during these episodes of joint attention and this reaching soon develops into pointing. Infants may also vocalize during these interactions. Atypical motor development affecting sitting, reaching, and pointing can disturb this interaction. Limitations make gestural signals difficult for carers to interpret. For example, if an infant reaches towards a toy but over or undershoots the target, a caregiver may understand that a different toy is being requested and hand an unwanted toy to their child. Lack of success in communication may lead to infant distress and, gradually, caregivers learn to construct interaction routines around the infant's signals that are clear and consistent. This tailoring of interaction often places young children with atypical motor development in the role of responder, making it difficult for them to become active, independent communicators. Limitations in mobility and handling objects may also restrict their exploration of their world, limit their topics of conversation, and restrict their language learning.

Communication limitations interfere with social and cognitive development. Intervention for children with a restricted range of communication signals before 2 years of age often focusses on their caregivers, helping them to recognize children's signals and creating more and varied opportunities to communicate. Provision of alternative and augmentative communication (AAC) systems, such as picture or symbol charts and books and software for tablet computers, is strongly recommended to ensure that children have access to vocabulary and expressive language learning (see Chapter 15). Similar to classifications of mobility, hand function, and eating and drinking, classification systems have been developed to describe the communication performance of children with atypical motor development, but as yet they are validated with children from aged 4 years when speech and communication are well developed (see Further Reading).

ASSOCIATED IMPAIRMENTS AND LIMITATIONS

The majority of developmental motor disorders originates from an impairment in the central nervous system. Usually, the impairment is not restricted to the networks involved in motor control but also affects networks involved in sensation, cognition, and behavioural regulation. This means that infants with atypical motor development may also have the following impairments directly resulting from the brain's compromised integrity (Dan et al. 2014):

- impaired processing of sensory information: the most frequently problems being visual impairment, including the cerebral visual impairment of children with CP, and impaired processing of somatosensory information;
- cognitive impairments, which at early age often implies a lack of exploratory drive and initiative;
- impaired behavioural regulation, including frequent crying, irritability, and attention problems;
- seizure disorder.

These impairments do not only impact mobility development; they also often give rise to limitations, such as limitations in learning and the ability to apply knowledge, limitations in self-care, and limitations in interpersonal interactions and relationships, for instance, during play. In turn, limitations in mobility may have a negative impact on cognitive and social development. This underlines the strong interrelation of the various developmental domains.

In addition, atypical motor development and its accompanying neurological deficits may secondarily result in contractures and deformities, such as hip dysplasia and scoliosis, and stunted growth (Dan et al. 2014).

Health professionals involved in the care of infants with atypical motor development should be aware of the possibility of the above mentioned additional impairments and limitations, as they may have a major impact on the infant's development and the daily life of the infant and the family. The additional impairments and limitations also have important consequences for therapeutic guidance. For instance, if an infant has a visual impairment, caregivers may be recommended to use toys that produce sound and to keep the room's furniture in a more or less fixed position. Or, if an infant has a limited exploratory drive, caregivers may be advised to assist the infant in playful exploration.

CONCLUDING REMARKS

Atypical motor development may manifest itself in various motor impairments, such as an atypical movement quality, atypical muscle tone, and atypical reflexes and reactions, and in limitations in the mobility domain, in drinking and eating, and communication. Atypical motor development in early life may be a transient phenomenon, but it may also form the first stage of a permanent developmental disorder, such as CP. In both cases, the child and the family are in need of professional guidance in the form of early intervention. The various means of early intervention are discussed in Chapters 12–15.

REFERENCES

Bodensteiner JB (2008) The evaluation of the hypotonic infant. *Semin Pediatr Neurol* **15**: 10–20. doi: 10.1016/j. spen.2008.01.003.

Bruijn SM, Massaad F, Maclellan MJ, Van Gestel L, Ivanenko YP, Duysens J (2013) Are effects of the symmetric and asymmetric tonic neck reflexes still visible in healthy adults? *Neurosci Lett* **556**: 89–92. doi: 10.1016/j. neulet.2013.10.028.

Carr L (2014) Clinical presentation. In: Dan B, Mayston M, Paneth N, Rosenbloom L, editors, *Cerebral Palsy: Science and Clinical Practice.* London: Mac Keith Press, pp. 225–239.

Dan B, Mayston M, Paneth N, Rosenbloom L, editors (2014) *Cerebral Palsy: Science and Clinical Practice.* London: Mac Keith Press.

Dusing SC (2016) Postural variability and sensorimotor development in infancy. *Dev Med Child Neurol* **58** (Suppl 4): 17–21. doi: 10.1111/dmcn.13045.

Eliasson AC, Krumlinde-Sundholm L, Rösblad B et al. (2006) The Manual Ability Classification System (MACS) for children with cerebral palsy: scale development and evidence of validity and reliability. *Dev Med Child Neurol* **48**: 549–554.

Elison JT, Wolff JJ, Reznick JS, et al. (2014) Repetitive behavior in 12-month-olds later classified with autism spectrum disorder. *J Am Acad Child Adolesc Psychiatry* **53**: 1216–1224. doi: 10.1016/j.jaac.2014.08.004.

Faebo Larsen R, Hvas Mortensen L, Martinussen T, Nybo Andersen AM (2013) Determinants of developmental coordination disorder in 7-year-old children: a study of children in the Danish National Birth Cohort. *Dev Med Child Neurol* **55**: 1016–1022. doi: 10.1111/dmcn.12223.

Ferrari F, Gallo C, Pugliese M, et al. (2012) Preterm birth and developmental problems in the preschool age. Part I: minor motor problems. *J Matern Fetal Neonatal Med* **25**: 2154–2159. doi: 10.3109/14767058.2012.696164.

Gorter JW, Ketelaar M, Rosenbaum P, Helders PJ, Palisano R (2009) Use of the GMFCS in infants with CP: the need for reclassification at age 2 years or older. *Dev Med Child Neurol* **51**: 46–52. doi: 10.1111/j.1469-8749.2008.03117.x.

Hadders-Algra M (2010) Variation and variability: key words in human motor development. *Phys Ther* **90**: 1823–1837. doi: 10.2522/ptj.20100006.

Hamer EG, Hadders-Algra M (2016) Prognostic significance of neurological signs in high-risk infants – a systematic review. *Dev Med Child Neurol* **58** (Suppl 4): 53–60. doi: 10.1111/dmcn.13051.

Harris SR (2008) Congenital hypotonia: clinical and developmental assessment. *Dev Med Child Neurol* **50**: 889–892. doi: 10.1111/j.1469-8749.2008.03097.

Hay K, Nelin M, Carey H, et al. (2018) Hammersmith Infant Neurological Examination Asymmetry Score distinguishes hemiplegic cerebral palsy from typical development. *Pediatr Neurol* **87**: 70–74. doi: 10.1016/j.pediatrneurol.2018.07.002.

Heineman KR, La Bastide-Van Gemert S, Fidler V, Middelburg KJ, Bos AF, Hadders-Algra M (2010) Construct validity of the Infant Motor Profile: relation with prenatal, perinatal, and neonatal risk factors. *Dev Med Child Neurol* **52**: e209–215. doi: 10.1111/j.1469-8749.2010.03667.x.

Heineman KR, Bos AF, Hadders-Algra M (2011) Infant Motor Profile and cerebral palsy: promising associations. *Dev Med Child Neurol* **53** (Suppl 4): 40–45. doi: 10.1111/j.1469-8749.2011.04063.x.

Hustad KC, Allison KM, Sakash A, McFadd E, Broman AT, Rathouz PJ (2017) Longitudinal development of communication in children with cerebral palsy between 24 and 53 months: Predicting speech outcomes. *Dev Neurorehabil* **20**: 323–330. doi: 10.1080/17518423.2016.1239135.

Lloyd M, MacDonald M, Lord C (2013) Motor skills of toddlers with autism spectrum disorders. *Autism* **17**: 133–146. doi: 10.1177/1362361311402230.

Luttikhuizen dos Santos ES, de Kieviet JF, Königs M, van Elburg RM, Oosterlaan J (2013) Predictive value of the Bayley scales of infant development on development of very preterm/very low birth weight children: a meta-analysis. *Early Hum Dev* **89**: 487–496. doi: 10.1016/j.earlhumdev.2013.03.008.

Maitre NL, Slaughter JC, Aschner JL (2013) Early prediction of cerebral palsy after neonatal intensive care using motor development trajectories in infancy. *Early Hum Dev* **89**: 781–786. doi: 10.1016/j.earlhumdev.2013.06.004.

Miall L, Rudolf M, Smith D (2016) *Paediatrics at a Glance.* John Wiley & Sons, incorporated, ProQuest Ebook Central.

Noritz GH, Murphy NA, Neuromotor Screening Expert Panel (2013) Motor delays: early identification and evaluation. *Pediatrics* **131**: e2016–2027. doi: 10.1542/peds.2013-1056.

Palisano R, Rosenbaum P, Walter S, Russell D, Wood E, Galuppi B (1997) Development and reliability of a system to classify gross motor function in children with cerebral palsy. *Dev Med Child Neurol* **39**: 214–223.

Robinson G (2013) The infant with hypotonia. In: Seal A, editor, *Children with Neurodevelopmental Disabilities – The Essential Guide to Assessment and Management.* London: Mac Keith Press, pp. 83–90.

Sanger TD, Delgado MR, Gaebler-Spira D, Hallett M, Mink JW; Task Force on Childhood Motor Disorders (2003) Classification and definition of disorders causing hypertonia in childhood. *Pediatrics* **111**: e89–97.

Sellers D, Mandy A, Pennington L, Hankins M, Morris C (2014) Development and reliability of a system to classify the eating and drinking ability of people with cerebral palsy. *Dev Med Child Neurol* **56**: 245–251. doi: 10.1111/dmcn.12352.

Straathof EJM, Heineman KR, Hamer EG, Hadders-Algra M (2020) Patterns of atypical muscle tone in the general infant population – prevalence and associations with perinatal risk van neurodevelopmental status. *Early Hum Dev*, epub ahead of print. doi: 10.1016/j.earlhumdev.2020.105276.

Towns M, Rosenbaum P, Palisano R, Wright FV (2018) Should the Gross Motor Function Classification System be used for children who do not have cerebral palsy? *Dev Med Child Neurol* **60**: 147–154. doi: 10.1111/dmcn.13602.

Wu Y-C, Heineman KR, la Bastide-van Gemert S, Kuiper D, Drenth Olivares M, Hadders-Algra M (2020) Motor behaviour in infancy is associated with cognitive, neurological and behavioural function of parents with reduced fertility. *Dev Med Child Neurology* **62**: 1089–1095. doi: 10.1111/dmcn.14520.

Zafeiriou DI (2004) Primitive reflexes and postural reactions in the neurodevelopmental examination. *Pediatr Neurol* **31**: 1–8.

SUGGESTIONS FOR FURTHER READING

Barty E, Caynes K, Johnston LM (2016) Development and reliability of the Functional Communication Classification System for children with cerebral palsy. *Dev Med Child Neurol* **58**: 1036–1041. doi: 10.1111/dmcn.13124.

Dan B, Mayston M, Paneth N, Rosenbloom L, editors (2014) *Cerebral Palsy: Science and Clinical Practice.* London: Mac Keith Press.

Hidecker MJC, Paneth N, Rosenbaum PL, et al. (2011) Developing and validating the Communication Function Classification System for individuals with cerebral palsy. *Dev Med Child Neurol* **53**: 704–710. doi: 10.1111/j.1469-8749.2011.03996.x.

Pennington L, Virella D, Mjøen T, et al. (2013) Development of The Viking Speech Scale to classify the speech of children with cerebral palsy. *Res Dev Disabil* **34**: 3202–3210. doi: 10.1016/j.ridd.2013.06.035.

Rosenbaum PL, Walter SD, Hanna SE, et al. (2002) Prognosis for gross motor function in cerebral palsy: creation of motor development curves. *JAMA* **288**: 1357–1363.

PART V

Diagnostics: Assessment of Neuromotor Conditions in Early Childhood

Psychometric Properties of Standardized Tests

Barbara Sargent

SUMMARY POINTS

- Standardized tests are used to identify infants at risk for neuromotor conditions, diagnose neuromotor conditions, predict future performance, determine eligibility for early intervention services, plan intervention, and monitor the effects of intervention.
- When selecting a standardized test, professionals must consider the reason for testing, the construct the test measures, the age and medical conditions of children for whom the test was developed, the psychometric properties of the test, and the time and cost to administer the test.
- Psychometric properties are the intrinsic properties of a standardized test and include validity, reliability, clinical meaningfulness, and accuracy.
- It is critical for test psychometrics that standardized tests be administered and scored using standard procedures.

Professionals working with infants and toddlers at risk for or diagnosed with neuromotor conditions make numerous clinical decisions based on information from standardized tests. These decisions include: identifying infants at risk for neuromotor conditions, diagnosing neuromotor conditions, predicting future performance, determining eligibility for early intervention services, planning intervention, and monitoring the effects of intervention (Heineman and Hadders-Algra 2008). In addition, administrative decisions about program effectiveness, the need for program change, and resource allocation can be made based on standardized test results from a cohort of children.

Selecting the most appropriate standardized test and correct interpretation is critical to informed decisions. When selecting a standardized test, professionals must consider the reason for testing, the construct the test measures, the age and medical conditions of children for whom the test was developed, the psychometric properties of the test, and the time and cost to administer the test. Professionals must also understand exactly what information the test can provide without over or under interpretation.

The current chapter provides an overview of the psychometric properties of standardized tests and general considerations regarding their interpretation. Chapters 10 and 11 provide information on specific standardized tests for infants from birth to 2 years of age.

PURPOSE OF STANDARDIZED TESTS

Standardized tests have three purposes: discriminative, evaluative, and predictive.

Discriminative measures are used to determine if a child has differences compared to a normative group. Discriminative measures are used in clinical practice to diagnose specific medical conditions, identify children who are not performing age appropriate skills, and establish eligibility for early intervention services. To be effective for discrimination, tests must have high accuracy in terms of true positive rates (sensitivity) and true negative rates (specificity).

Evaluative measures are used to quantify a child's change in performance over time by comparing the child's current performance against previous performance on the same test. Evaluative measures are used in clinical practice to measure change over time or change as the result of an intervention. To be effective for evaluating the effects of intervention, evaluative measures must be responsive to a clinical meaningful change in the outcome of interest. An evaluative test with low responsiveness may show no effect of intervention even if an effect occurred.

Predictive measures are used to estimate a child's future outcome, behaviour, or prognosis based on current performance. Predictive measures are used in clinical practice to predict future performance, for example, how atypical findings on the General Movement Assessment (Einspieler et al. 2004) at 3 months of age predict a diagnosis of cerebral palsy at 2 years of age. This information may be useful for professionals and caregivers as they plan an intervention program. To be effective for prediction, tests must have high reliability and evidence that the test can predict future outcomes of interest.

TYPES OF STANDARDIZED TESTS

Standardized tests are classified as norm referenced or criterion referenced.

A *norm referenced test* is used to compare the performance of a child to a normative sample of age-matched children from a well-defined population of children (Furr 2018). Norm referenced tests are considered *discriminative measures* since they are used in clinical practice to identify children who are performing below age level in specific domains, expressed as a standard score or percentile rank. For example, norm referenced tests are used to establish eligibility for early intervention services when the child is below a certain cut-off score, compared to the normative sample, such as two standard deviations below the mean.

Before testing a specific child using a norm referenced test, it is important to consider the characteristics of the normative sample to determine if it is appropriate to compare the child to the normative sample. For example, the most widely used standardized tests have been developed and normed in Canada and the United States, but they are used in countries throughout the world under the false assumption that development is similar across cultures (Mendonca et al. 2016). This can lead to erroneous labelling of children as developmentally delayed or early achieving if children from that culture achieve developmental milestones at different ages than the test's normative sample due to differences in environment and child-rearing practices (Mendonca et al. 2016). To prevent misinterpretation of results, characteristics of the normative sample must be carefully considered when interpreting standardized test results for a specific child.

A *criterion referenced test* quantifies how well a child performs on a specified set of knowledge, skills, or abilities (Furr 2018). Most criterion referenced tests are considered *evaluative measures* since they are used in clinical practice to determine the functional skills or abilities of a child and how these skills change over time, expressed as scaled scores. For example, if a child performs 75% of the test items, it would be interpreted as the child demonstrating knowledge of 75% of the content domain.

Since criterion referenced tests are evaluative measures, they are the most appropriate type of test to document change with intervention. However, if a child is expected to attain age appropriate skills with intervention, professionals may choose to use norm referenced tests to quantify change with intervention. An important consideration is that the results of norm referenced tests are always interpreted in reference to the normative sample. Therefore, although a child may demonstrate improved motor skills over time, a child's score on a norm referenced test may not adequately reflect the change since the child's score is interpreted in reference to age-matched children in the normative sample.

SCORES

Scores provide information about an individual child's performance compared to other children or specific criteria. The normal distribution or 'bell curve' is the basis for computing most types of standardized scores including standard scores and age equivalent scores (Fig. 9.1).

Standard scores, or *Z-scores*, provide information on the degree to which an individual child's test score is above or below the mean test score of the normative sample, expressed in standard deviations (Furr 2018). For example, a score of 0 is interpreted as perfectly average, 1 is interpreted as 1 standard deviation above the mean, and –2 is interpreted as 2 standard deviations below the mean. The strength of standard scores is that they are reported in equivalent standard deviation units. Therefore, standard

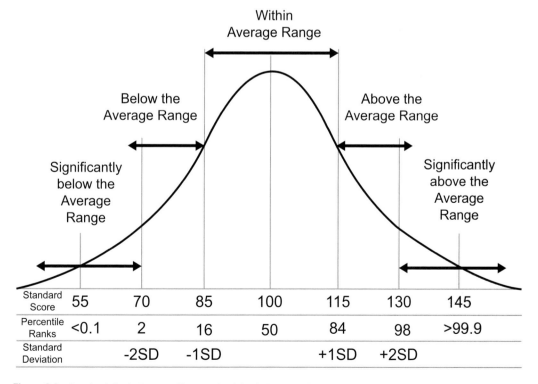

Figure 9.1   Graph of the bell curve. The graph of the bell curve illustrates how standard scores, percentile ranks, and standard deviations are computed.

scores can be compared across ages and across tests, and they indicate the magnitude of difference of the tested child's score from the mean score of the normative sample. A limitation of standard scores is that their usefulness depends on the representativeness of the normative sample. In addition, standard scores can be difficult for caregivers to understand. To improve interpretation of standard scores, they can be presented as *percentile ranks*, the percentage of scores that are below or equal to a specific test score (Furr 2018). For example, a child with a standard score of 1 has a percentile rank of 84%. This can be interpreted to caregivers as the child scored higher than 84% of the children in the normative sample.

Age equivalent scores provide an estimate of the mean age that the normative sample received the specific raw test score of the tested child. These scores should be used cautiously since they have three well-documented limitations that hinder interpretation (Conrad 2018). First, age equivalent scores do not take into consideration the range of normal performance. Therefore, it is unknown whether a child with a low score is performing within the range of normal performance or far below normal performance, except in extreme cases. Second, age equivalent scores may not provide an accurate appraisal of a child's performance, especially in children with neuromotor conditions who may have inconsistencies or gaps in performance. For example, a 3-year-old child with bilateral spastic cerebral palsy who independently walks with a walker, may receive an age equivalent of 10 months on a test of gross motor development, although his overall gross motor function may be much higher than that of a typical 10-month-old infant. In contrast, a 12-month-old child with unilateral spastic cerebral palsy may receive an age equivalent of 12 months on a test of motor development, even though his overall motor function may be much lower than that of a typical 12-month-old infant if he is not consistently incorporating the most affected limbs into his movement. Third, age equivalent scores cannot be used to document change over time because differences in age equivalent scores are due to smaller differences in raw scores over time. For example, a 2-month increase in age equivalent score for a 4-month-old infant is more significant than for a 2-year-old child.

PSYCHOMETRIC PROPERTIES

Psychometric properties are defined as the intrinsic properties of a standardized test and include validity, reliability, clinical meaningfulness, and accuracy. Common psychometric properties are defined in Table 9.1.

Validity

Validity is defined as 'the degree to which evidence and theory support the interpretations of test scores for proposed uses of tests' (American Educational Research Association 2014). This contemporary definition of validity highlights the importance of the interpretation of test scores, also referred to as construct validity. *Construct validity* is the extent to which test scores can be interpreted as reflecting a specific construct, that is, does the test measure what it purports to measure (Furr 2018). Three types of construct validity are convergent validity, discriminant validity, and construct validity using known groups. *Convergent validity* is the extent to which test scores correlate with another test known to measure the same construct and is given at the same time. For example, test scores on a neurological examination correlate with concurrent magnetic resonance imaging results. *Discriminant validity* is the extent to which test scores do not correlate with another test known to measure an unrelated construct and is given at the same time. *Construct validity using known groups* is the extent to which test scores are different for groups of children known to be different on the specific construct the test purports to measure. For

Table 9.1 Definitions of Common Psychometric Properties

Psychometric property	Definition
Validity	
Construct	Extent to which test scores can be interpreted as reflecting a specific construct
Convergent	Extent to which test scores correlate with another test known to measure the same construct and is given at the same time
Discriminant	Extent to which test scores do not correlate with another test known to measure an unrelated construct and is given at the same time
Known groups	Extent to which test scores are different for groups of children known to be different on the specific construct the test purports to measure
Content	Extent to which a test reflects the full domain of the construct it purports to measure
Criterion	Extent to which test scores are correlated with an established or gold standard test
Concurrent	Extent to which test scores are correlated with performance on a gold standard test that measures the same construct and is given at the same time
Predictive	Extent to which test scores are correlated with a specific outcome or performance on a gold standard test given at a future point in time
Reliability	
Internal consistency	Extent to which multiple items within a test measure the same construct
Test–retest	Extent to which a test produces the same result when repeatedly applied to a child who has not experienced a change in the construct being measured
Intrarater	Consistency with which a test produces the same score when used by the same test administrator with the same child
Interrater	Consistency with which a test produces the same score when used by multiple test administrators with the same child
Clinical meaningfulness	
Minimal detectable change	Smallest amount of change that is reflective of true change and not that which can be accounted for by measurement error; calculated as $SEM \times 1.96 \times \sqrt{2}$
Responsiveness	The ability of the test to detect change over time
Minimally clinically important difference	Smallest amount of change that is meaningful from the perspective of a child, caregiver, or professional
Accuracy	
Sensitivity	Ability of a diagnostic test to correctly identify children who have a specific medical condition; true positive rate; calculated as $\dfrac{number\ of\ true\ positives}{number\ of\ true\ positives + number\ of\ false\ negatives}$
Specificity	Ability of a diagnostic test to correctly identify children who do not have a specific medical condition; true negative rate; calculated as $\dfrac{number\ of\ true\ negatives}{number\ of\ true\ negatives + number\ of\ false\ positives}$.
Positive likelihood ratio	Proportion of true positives among those with positive results in a reference population; calculated as $\dfrac{sensitivity}{1 - specificity}$
Negative likelihood ratio	Proportion of true negatives among those with negative results in a reference population; calculated as $\dfrac{1 - sensitivity}{specificity}$

example, test scores on a developmental assessment differ between infants born full-term and infants born extremely preterm.

Content validity is the extent to which a standardized test reflects the full domain of the construct it purports to measure (Furr 2018). *Criterion validity* is the extent to which test scores are correlated with an established or gold standard test. Two types of criterion validity are concurrent validity and predictive validity. *Concurrent validity* is the extent to which test scores are correlated with performance on a gold standard test that measures the same construct and is given at the same time (Furr 2018). For example, how scores on the Test of Infant Motor Performance (Campbell 2005) are correlated with scores on the motor subtest of the Bayley Scales of Infant and Toddler Development, 3rd edition (Bayley 2005) at 3 months of age. *Predictive validity* is the extent to which test scores are correlated with a specific outcome or performance on a gold standard test given at a future point in time (Furr 2018), for example, how scores on the Test of Infant Motor Performance (Campbell 2005) at term equivalent predict scores on the motor subtest *of the* Bayley Scales of Infant and Toddler Development, 3rd edition (Bayley 2005) at 2 years of age. Predictive validity has two well-reported limitations. First, it only describes an association between measures and does not explain why the relationship exists. Second, the prediction of neurodevelopmental outcome is challenged by the multiplicity of factors that may influence current performance and future outcome, including the developmental changes in the young brain (see Chapter 3) and the child's environment.

Reliability

Reliability is defined as the consistency or repeatability in score production of a standardized test (Furr 2018). Reliability indicates the similarity of test results given across different contexts. Types of reliability include internal consistency, test–retest, intrarater, and interrater reliability.

Internal consistency and test–retest reliability quantify the consistency of the standardized test itself. *Internal consistency* quantifies the extent to which multiple items within a standardized test measure the same construct (Furr 2018). *Test–retest reliability* quantifies the extent to which a standardized test produces the same result when repeatedly applied to a child who has not experienced a change in the construct being measured (Furr 2018).

Intrarater and interrater reliability quantify the consistency of the raters who conducted the test. *Intrarater* reliability quantifies the consistency with which a test produces the same score when used by the same test administrator with the same child (Furr 2018). *Interrater reliability* quantifies the consistency with which a test produces the same score when used by multiple test administrators with the same child (Furr 2018).

The intraclass correlation coefficient (ICC) and Cohen's kappa are two statistical methods used to assess intrarater and interrater reliability. ICC is used for continuous data and kappa is used for nominal data. Guidelines for interpretation are not universally accepted, but a commonly reported guideline for both ICC and kappa is: <0.40 is poor, 0.40–0.59 is fair, 0.60–0.74 is good, and 0.75–1.00 is excellent (Cicchetti 1994).

Standard error of measurement (SEM) indicates the precision of an individual test score (Furr 2018). The SEM can be used to develop confidence intervals (CI) for interpreting the accuracy of a test score (Furr 2018). A 95% CI is interpreted as: with repeated testing of the child, 95% of the scores will fall within the lower and upper bounds of the interval if the child's function has not changed. While there are no generally acceptable ranges for CIs, a relatively narrow CI, versus wide CI, is interpreted as a more accurate estimate of a child's true score.

Clinical Meaningfulness

Clinical meaningfulness is defined as the standardized test's ability to provide professionals and caregivers with relevant information. Concepts related to clinical meaningfulness include floor and ceiling effects, minimal detectable change, responsiveness, and minimally clinically important difference.

A *floor effect* occurs when the scores of a group of children cluster at the bottom of the test, and a *ceiling effect* occurs when the scores of a group of children cluster at the top of the test. Floor and ceiling effects occur when there is a lack of range in the test to fully characterize a group of children (Fetters and

Tilson 2019). The *minimal detectable change (MDC)* is the smallest amount of change that is reflective of true change and not that which can be accounted for by measurement error (Fetters and Tilson 2019). *Responsiveness* is defined as a test's ability to detect change over time. One measure of responsiveness is the minimally clinically important difference (Fetters and Tilson 2019). The *minimally clinically important difference (MCID)* is the smallest amount of change that is meaningful from the perspective of a child, caregiver, or professional (Fetters and Tilson 2019).

Accuracy

Accuracy is defined as the degree to which the results of the standardized test are close to the true value of the construct being measured. Concepts related to accuracy include sensitivity, specificity, positive likelihood ratios, and negative likelihood ratios.

Sensitivity, also called true positive rate, is the ability of a diagnostic test to correctly identify children who have a specific medical condition (Furr 2018). It is measured as a proportion with a range from 0 to 1. For example, 99% of children who have cerebral palsy are identified by the test as having cerebral palsy. Clinically, a highly sensitive test rarely results in a positive result for a child that does not have the medical condition, so a negative result on a sensitive test is considered good evidence that the child does not have the medical condition. The mnemonic SN*out* is helpful to remember; when a test with high sensitivity is *negative* it helps to rule *out* the medical condition. *Specificity*, also called true negative rate, is the ability of a diagnostic test to correctly identify children who do not have a specific medical condition (Furr 2018). It is also measured as a proportion with a range from 0 to 1. For example, 99% of children who do not have cerebral palsy are identified by the test as not having cerebral palsy. Clinically, a highly specific test rarely results in a negative result for a child that has the medical condition, so a positive result on a specific test is considered good evidence that the child has the medical condition. The mnemonic SP*in* is helpful to remember; when a test with high specificity is *positive* it helps to rule *in* the medical condition. Ideally, standardized tests should have high sensitivity and specificity. However, sometimes professionals are willing to accept a lower specificity rate if the sensitivity rate is high when screening infants for certain medical conditions, such as cerebral palsy. In this case, the risk of over-identifying infants for early intervention is considered more important than under-identifying infants who may benefit from early intervention.

Likelihood ratios combine sensitivity and specificity and are used to determine how likely it is that a child has a specific medical condition after testing positive or negative on a diagnostic test (Goldstein and Bornstein 2018). The *positive likelihood ratio (LR+)* is the proportion of true positives among those with positive results in a reference population. The *negative likelihood ratio (LR–)* is the proportion of true negatives among those with negative results in a reference population. To determine the post-test probability that a child has a specific medical condition, first the pretest probability that the child has the medical condition needs to be estimated. This pretest estimation is then multiplied by the LR+ if the diagnostic test was positive or by the LR– if the test was negative to determine the post-test probability that the child has the medical condition. An important consideration is that the diagnostic test is only useful if its LR values are far from 1 because this will significantly alter the post-test probability of a diagnosis.

IMPORTANCE OF FOLLOWING STANDARD PROCEDURES

Standardized tests are developed and tested using standard procedures. Therefore, it is critical for test validity, reliability, clinical meaningfulness, and accuracy that standardized tests be administered and scored using standard procedures. This includes following instructions, using the designated testing items, and providing only the required number of demonstrations and trials. However, a common finding of surveys of rehabilitation professions in the United States and Canada is that they frequently deviate from standard procedures due to a child's cognition, sensory processing, attention span or behaviour (Stuhec and Gisel 2003; Hanna et al. 2007; Fay et al. 2018). Modifying test procedures has a negative effect on the psychometrics of the modified test, limiting the ability to interpret the results, especially in terms of standard or scaled scores. One way to address this clinically is to administer the test using standard procedures for reporting, and, if indicated, assess specific items again with modification to inform future intervention strategies.

CONCLUDING REMARKS

Professionals require a strong understanding of the psychometric properties of standardized tests to appropriately select and interpret the results of standardized tests for infants and toddlers at risk for or diagnosed with neuromotor conditions. The next two chapters will provide information on the psychometrics of specific standardized tests for infants from birth to 2 years of age.

REFERENCES

American Educational Research Association, American Psychological Association, National Council on Measurement in Education (2014) *Standards for Educational and Psychological Testing*. Washington, DC: American Educational Research Association.

Bayley N (2005) *Manual for the Bayley Scales of Infant and Toddler Development*, 3rd edn. San Antonio, TX: Psychological Corporation.

Campbell S (2005) *The Test of Infant Motor Performance. Test User's Manual. Version 2.0*. Chicago, IL: Infant Motor Performance Scales, LLC.

Cicchetti DV (1994) Guidelines, criteria, and rules of thumb for evaluating normed and standardized assessment instruments in psychology. *Psychol Assess* **6**(4): 284–290.

Conrad Z (2018) Age equivalent scores. In: Frey B, editor, *The Sage Encyclopedia of Educational Research, Measurement, and Evaluation*. Thousand Oaks, CA: SAGE Publications, Inc., p. 62.

Einspieler C, Prechtl H, Bos AF, Ferrari F, Cioni G (2004) *Prechtl's Method on the Qualitative Assessment of General Movements in Preterm, Term, and Young Infants. Clinics in Developmental Medicine No. 167*. London: Mac Keith Press.

Fay D, Brock E, Peneton S et al. (2018) Physical therapists' use and alteration of standardized assessments of motor function in children. *Pediatr Phys Ther* **30**: 318–325. doi: 10.1097/pep.0000000000000532.

Fetters L, Tilson J (2019) *Evidence Based Physical Therapy*, 2nd edn. Philadelphia, PA: F.A. Davis Co.

Furr R (2018) *Psychometrics: An Introduction*, 3rd edn. Thousand Oaks, CA: SAGE Publications, Inc.

Goldstein S, Bornstein M (2018) Sensitivity. In: Frey B, editor, *The SAGE Encyclopedia of Educational Research, Measurement, and Evaluation*. Thousand Oaks, CA: SAGE Publications, Inc., pp. 1508–1509.

Hanna SE, Russell DJ, Bartlett DJ, Kertoy M, Rosenbaum PL, Wynn K (2007) Measurement practices in pediatric rehabilitation: a survey of physical therapists, occupational therapists, and speech-language pathologists in Ontario. *Phys Occup Ther Pediatr* **27**: 25–42.

Heineman KR, Hadders-Algra M (2008) Evaluation of neuromotor function in infancy – a systematic review of available methods. *J Dev Behav Pediatr* **29**: 315–323. doi: 10.1097/DBP.0b013e318182a4ea.

Mendonca B, Sargent B, Fetters L (2016) Cross-cultural validity of standardized motor development screening and assessment tools: a systematic review. *Dev Med Child Neurol* **58**: 1213–1222. doi: 10.1111/dmcn.13263.

Stuhec V, Gisel EG (2003) Compliance with administration procedures of tests for children with pervasive developmental disorders: Does it exist? *Can J Occup Ther* **70**: 33–41. doi: 10.1177/000841740307000105.

SUGGESTIONS FOR FURTHER READING

American Educational Research Association, American Psychological Association, National Council on Measurement in Education (2014) *Standards for Educational and Psychological Testing*. Washington, DC: American Educational Research Association.

Furr RM (2018) *Psychometrics: An Introduction*, 3rd edn. Thousand Oaks, CA: SAGE Publications, Inc.

Assessments in the Neonatal Period and Early Infancy

Alicia Jane Spittle and Mijna Hadders-Algra

SUMMARY POINTS

- A range of assessment tools are available to provide insights into an infant's early motor, neurological and behavioural development.
- Early motor assessments may include assessment of both quality and quantity of movement and assist in the prediction of a range of motor outcomes from developmental delay to cerebral palsy.
- Neurological assessments include assessment of various aspects of neurological function such as tone, reflexes, orientation, along with movement quality and quantity and are predictive of cerebral palsy and atypical neurological and cognitive function long-term.
- Neurobehavioural assessments provide an insight into an infant's neurological and behavioural development and are associated with many aspects of longer-term neurodevelopment including cognitive, language, and motor outcomes.
- Longitudinal application of appropriate standardized assessments allows the assessment of the infant's developmental status, the infant's recovery from brain injury or other complications, and the infant's risk of developing a deficit.

It is well recognized that intervention in infants at high risk of developmental disorders should start as early in life as possible, as the nervous system is most plastic at early age (Chapter 3). This chapter provides an overview of the assessments available in the neonatal period (defined as from birth to 28 days, including preterm birth) and in early infancy (defined as up to 3 months' post-term age for the purpose of this chapter). The assessments provide an insight into an infant's current neurodevelopment; they are an entry point for intervention and can be predictive of future developmental outcomes.

Many assessment tools exist that assess different aspects of development during the first year of life (Noble and Boyd 2012). We focus on the instruments that are available for infants younger than 4 months corrected age (CA), including (a) motor assessments, (b) neurological assessments, and (c) neurobehavioural assessments. The specific assessment tools discussed have been selected on the basis of both their clinical utility, such as the time taken to administer, costs of the assessment, training requirements, and good psychometrics such as validity and reliability (see Chapter 9; Spittle et al. 2008; Noble and Boyd 2012).

Neonatal and early infant motor, neurological, or neurobehavioral examinations aim to assess the integrity of the infant's nervous system, both in the general paediatric population and in groups of high-risk infants, such as infants born preterm, with a low birth weight, with genetic conditions and/ or substance exposure during pregnancy (Chapter 3). The examinations assess an infant's spontaneous behavioural repertoire and responses to the extra-uterine environment to varying degrees (Majnemer and Snider 2005). Whilst formal examinations of newborns and infants have been around since the early 1900s (Brown and Spittle 2014), increased understanding of the developing nervous system over the past few decades has resulted in an increasing focus on the infant's spontaneous movements (Prechtl 1990). Furthermore, the importance of standardized assessments has been increasingly acknowledged, underlining the need of consistent procedures for administration and scoring to ensure that all infants are assessed under similar conditions (Chapter 9).

In this chapter we first address general issues that apply to all assessments at an early age, including a description of the various types of assessments and the specific considerations for assessments at an early age. Next, we describe the various instruments: that is, (a) motor assessments; (b) neurological assessments; and (c) neurobehavioural assessments. In the concluding paragraph we discuss the significance of the findings in the light of family-centred care.

DIFFERENT TYPES OF NEONATAL AND EARLY INFANT DEVELOPMENTAL ASSESSMENTS

Whilst there are similarities between different assessment tools in the neonatal period and early infancy, they can be broadly grouped into three categories described below:

- *Motor assessments* in early development focus on movement quality, quantity, and/or symmetry and may include observations of spontaneous movements and the infant's posture, along with motor responses to elicited movements. Examples include the General Movements Assessment (GMA; see also Chapter 7; Einspieler et al. 2004; Hadders-Algra 2018) and the Test of Infant Motor Performance (Campbell et al. 1995).
- *Neurological examinations* often include a motor assessment with the addition of items to assess neurological function such as dysmorphic features, cranial nerves, active and passive muscle tone and reflex testing, and some aspects of neurobehaviour such as level of alertness, and orientation to stimuli. Examples include The Hammersmith Neonatal Neurological Examination (Dubowitz et al. 1999) and the Neurological Examination of the Full-term Newborn infant (Prechtl 1977).
- *Neurobehavioural assessments* examine an infant's behaviour in more detail than traditional neurological examinations and include assessment of habituation, orientation, response to environmental stimuli including visual and auditory input and ability to self-calm. Examples include the NICU Network Neuobehaviour Scale (Lester et al. 2004) and the Neonatal Behavioral Assessment Scale (Brazelton and Nugent 2011).

CONSIDERATIONS FOR ASSESSMENTS AT EARLY AGE

What Is the Purpose of Early Assessment?

The early assessments are performed in the neonatal nursery or outpatient clinic to assist in overall management of infants and can assist clinicians and researchers in a variety of purposes (Majnemer and Snider 2005; Spittle et al. 2008; Novak et al. 2017). They serve:

- as a baseline assessment to monitor the evolution of the sequelae of brain injury: emergence of signs of recovery;
- to discriminate which infants are at greater risk for neurodevelopmental impairments, as they show signs of delayed or atypical development;
- to plan intervention by providing an understanding of the infant's strengths and weaknesses;
- to evaluate change over time in response to intervention;
- provide prognostication in conjunction with other investigations and clinical history.

Choosing the right tool is essential. The choice depends on the purpose of the assessment and thus requires an understanding of the features of the motor, neurological, and neurobehavioural examinations, including their psychometric properties.

Handling Neonates and Infants

When assessing development in the first few months of life, it's important to have a theoretical framework underpinning the assessment and neonatal practice in general. The concepts of dynamic systems theory, neuronal group selection theory (Chapter 3), family centred care (Chapter 12), behavioural states (Prechtl 1974; Brazelton and Nugent 2011) and the Synactive Theory of Newborn Behavioural Organisation and Development (Als 1982) are all key concepts that clinicians should be aware of before assessing babies at high risk of developmental impairments (Sweeney et al. 2010).

It is essential to monitor the infant's behavioural state when conducting a neonatal or infant assessment as the same stimulus can produce a different response in different states (see Text Box 10.1). Most tests are best performed between feeds, closer to the infant's next feed with the infant more likely to be in an optimal behavioural state, particularly for preterm infants and newborn term infants (Dubowitz et al. 2005).

The *Synactive Theory of Newborn Behavioural Organization and Development*, developed by Als, acknowledges the continuous interaction of the autonomic, motor, state, attention/interaction, and regulatory subsystems of the foetus and newborn with their environment (Als 1982). Through behavioural responses and interaction of these subsystems, infants may communicate how they are coping within the environment. Development of these subsystems begins as an embryo and continues into the newborn period. The aspects taken into account are:

- autonomic system: observed through vital signs, such as respiratory and cardiac function (e.g. oxygen saturation);
- motor system: observed via quality and quantity of movements in the limbs and trunk;
- behavioural state (see Text Box 10.1);
- attention-interaction system: assessed by the ability of the infant to be alert and interact with the environment and caregiver;
- self-regulation: assessed by the strategies that the infant uses to stabilize the subsystems.

Stability of function in one domain will influence the overall stability of the infant and thus is important to keep in mind when pacing the examination. If an infant is beginning to show signs that they are not coping, for instance starts to show motor signs (e.g. disorganized movements), self-regulation signs (e.g. shifting to a lower state of arousal), and/or physiological signs (e.g. oxygen desaturations), the assessment needs to be altered or ceased accordingly.

Text Box 10.1 Behavioural States in Newborn Infants

Behavioural state refers to a relatively stable condition of alertness, such as quiet sleep, rapid eye movement (REM) sleep, quiet wakefulness, active wakefulness, and crying. For the assessment of young infants, two aspects of behavioural state are important:

- Stably organized behavioural states first emerge at 36–38 weeks postmenstrual age (PMA). This means that the various parameters determining behavioural state, such as the presence of eye movements, the presence of body movements and the regularity of respiration, change synchronously when the infant moves from one behavioural state to the other. However, before 36–38 weeks PMA, the various physiological parameters act independently and their transitions are not synchronized. As a consequence, infants younger than 36–38 weeks PMA may show an 'indetermined' behavioural state. The periods with indetermined behavioural state decrease with increasing PMA (Nijhuis et al. 1982).
- Behavioural states reflect the temporary organization of the infant's brain. Consequently, the infant's neuro-mechanisms, including the infant's active and reactive behaviour, depend on the infant's behavioural state.

Worldwide, two classification systems of behavioural state are most commonly used, the one described by Heinz Prechtl (Prechtl 1974) and the one of Terry Brazelton (Brazelton and Nugent 2011); see Table 10.1.

Table 10.1 Behavioural state classification in young infants >36–38 weeks PMA

Behavioural state	Prechtl	Brazelton
Non-REM sleep: eyes closed, reg. respiration, no GMs	1	1
REM sleep: eyes closed, irreg. respiration, movements, incl. GMs	2	2
Drowsy: eyes open and close, glazed look, reg. respiration, movements	3	
Quiet wakefulness: eyes open, virtually no movements	3	4
Active wakefulness: eyes open, movements, including many GMs	4	5
Crying: eyes opened or closed, movements, crying vocalizations	5	6

GMs: general movements; irreg: irregular; reg: regular.

Who Performs the Assessment?

Different examinations need differing levels of skills to administer, with all assessments tools requiring an understanding of infant development and psychometrics to accurately interpret assessment results. Assessment of an infant in the neonatal period, especially in the neonatal intensive care unit, can be complex and, as such, specialist skills are recommended (Sweeney et al. 2010). Healthy term-born infants are more robust to assess than high-risk infants such as those born preterm or with substance exposure, and thus assessment of fragile infants should be conducted by appropriately skilled health professionals experienced in handling young infants. Traditionally neurological examinations are performed by medical professionals including paediatricians and neonatologists, whilst health professionals, such as physiotherapists, occupational therapists, psychologists, and nurses, perform a motor or neurobehaviour examination. The specific training and professional background are specific to each assessment tool and it is essential that these training procedures are adhered too, to ensure reliability and validity of the assessment. For the infants nursed in the neonatal intensive care unit, special attention should be paid to how the infant responds to different positions and handling, as the infant's physiological stability may be at stake. Nevertheless, Allinson et al. (2017), who assessed infants born <30 weeks PMA between 29 and 32 weeks PMA, demonstrated that the infants' physiological stability during a motor or neurological examination was similar to that during nursing cares. This demonstrates that these infant assessments are safe to conduct (Allinson et al. 2017).

The Challenges and Opportunities of Neuroplasticity

Early assessment is a prerequisite for early detection. Early detection, in turn, allows for the onset of intervention at an age during which the nervous system exhibits a high degree of plasticity. However, the immediate drawback of the high plasticity is that it limits the ability of early infant assessments to predict with high accuracy the infant's developmental outcome. The neuroplasticity of the developing brain provides the potential to recover from an early lesion and early dysfunction and to adapt with time to the environment. The recovery may – or may not – be facilitated by appropriate support and early intervention. Yet, the developmental changes in the nervous system, including the increasing influence of supraspinal circuitries – such as those mediated by the corticospinal tract – may also induce a deterioration of function. The infant is growing into a deficit (Van Balen et al. 2015). This stresses the need of longitudinal assessments in order to monitor the infant's developmental changes. It goes without saying that clinicians and researchers need to be considerate in how this information is communicated to families to ensure they understand the strengths and limitations of the assessment itself.

MOTOR ASSESSMENTS

There have been several systematic reviews examining the psychometrics and clinic utility of early motor assessments (Heineman and Hadders-Algra 2008; Spittle et al. 2008; Noble and Boyd 2012). These reviews varied in regards to the age of infants being assessed at 0–4 months in the review by Noble and Boyd (2012), 0–12 months in the review of Spittle et al. (2008), and 3–18 months in the review of Heineman and Hadders-Algra (2008). All reviews highlight that the best assessment will depend on the purpose of the assessment (i.e. discriminative, predictive, or evaluative). Whilst all tools were discriminative, the GMA has the best predictive validity for later motor outcome, whilst the Test of Infant Motor Performance (TIMP) had the best evaluative validity in the first 3 months post-term age.

General Movements Assessment (GMA)

General movements (GMs) are the most frequently occurring movements of the foetus and young infant involving all parts of the body. GMs gradually disappear at 3–5 months post-term, when they are replaced by goal-directed activity, such as reaching movements or attempts to roll to the side. Typical GMs are primarily characterized by movement complexity and variation (Prechtl 1990). Moreover, they show age-specific characteristics, the presence of fidgety movements at 2–5 months post-term being the most prominent one. Fidgety movements denote the irregular occurrence of small and dancing movements all over the body (see Chapter 5). Atypical GMs are primarily characterized by a reduction in movement complexity and variation. Additionally, the order of typical development may be disrupted; in particular, the infant may fail to develop fidgety movements between 2 and 5 months CA (for details, see Chapter 7).

   The properties of GMA may be summarized as follows (for details see Einspieler et al. 2004; Hadders-Algra 2004; Table 10.2 provides a quick overview):

• *Purpose of the test:* GMA is a video-based assessment of the quality of spontaneously generated GMs in supine position. GMA provides information on the current condition of the infant's nervous system and assists prediction of developmental outcome.

Table 10.2	General Movement Assessment
Purpose	Assessing the integrity of the brain of the foetus and young infant Predicting high risk of developmental disorders, including cerebral palsy
Age range/population	Foetuses, preterm and full-term neonates, infants up to and including 5 months CA
Age periods	– Foetal/preterm GMs: before 36–38 weeks PMA – Writhing GMs: from 36–38 weeks PMA to 2 months CA – Fidgety GMs: 2 to 5 months CA
Scoring	GM quality is scored on ordinal scales (for details see Chapter 7)
Format	Video-based method
Time needed	Recording of 3–10 minutes, depending on age and behavioural state of moving infant; assessment of video and scoring take 3–5 minutes
Normative sample	n = 455 infants, 3 months CA (Dutch)[a]
Reliability	Intrarater: ICC 0.89; interrater reliability: κ-values: 0.81–0.92 Stability over time: within GM phase 90% similar rating; between GM phases frequent changes in rating[b]
Validity	*Construct validity:* definitely abnormal GMs and absent fidgety associated with serious brain lesions, in particular lesions of the periventricular white matter; mildly abnormal GMs at fidgety age associated with e.g. preterm birth, hyperbilirubinaemia, infant nutrition and subfertility[c] *Predictive validity:* Atypical GMs at fidgety age lacking fidgety movements: sensitivity to predict CP 98% (95% CI 74–100%), specificity 91% (95% CI 83–93%)[d]
Training	Via introductory and advanced courses, see e.g. http://general-movements-trust.info and http://www.developmentalneurology.com/website/index.php/en
Costs	GM courses in high income countries, 2-day course 350–400€, 3.5-day course about 900€; in low and middle income countries adjusted costs. Manual: about 60€.

[a]Bouwstra et al. (2009, 2010); [b]Einspieler et al. (2004); Hadders-Algra et al. (2004); Schröder et al. (2020); [c]Hadders-Algra (2007, 2018); Peyton et al. (2017); [d]Bosanquet et al. (2013).

- *Population:* GMA is applicable to all infants up to 5 months CA. However, its predictive properties are best in high-risk infants, such as infants born preterm (Hadders-Algra 2018).
- *Description of outcome parameters:* GMA results in a classification of typical versus atypical GMs. Atypical GMs are characterized as 'poor repertoire' and/or absent or atypical fidgety movements (for details of nomenclature see Table 7.1, for video examples see Videos 5.1, 5.2, 7.1, 7.2, and 7.3).
- *Administration:* The assessment of spontaneous movements implies that assessors and caregivers refrain from interaction with the infant. In addition, the infant is not provided with toys or a pacifier, as the idea of GMA is to assess endogenously generated motor activity. A supine position is recommended as this position allows the infant to express movement complexity and variation best. GMs may also be observed when the infant lies in side-position, but this position hampers the expression of movement complexity and variation in the limbs resting on the support surface.

For GMA, a video-recording of minimally 3 minutes of a moving infant in an adequate behavioural state is required. The video is needed for a proper assessment of movement complexity and variation. The use of a tripod is recommended, but not obligatory, as mobile phones may also be used. The latter allows video-recording by caregivers in the home situation (Spittle et al. 2016a). In addition, we suggest recording the infant so that the infant's head is at the top of the screen and his/her feet at the

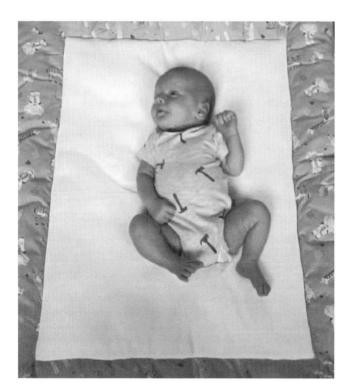

Figure 10.1   Standard situation for GMA: infant in supine position with the head on the top of the screen, dressed minimally, and no toys or pacifier.

bottom (Fig. 10.1). The off-line GMA itself also requires in general about 3 minutes. For practical details on the implementation of GMA in clinical practice see De Bock et al. (2017).

GMA only can be performed when the infant is in an adequate behavioural (i.e. Prechtl's behavioural states 2 or 4) (Table 10.1). In order to achieve these behavioural states and to avoid crying, the infant's proximal joints may be supported by nesting devices or supportive pillows. This type of support facilitates the infant's behavioural state regulation, whilst it does not affect the endogenously generated GM quality (De Graaf-Peters et al. 2006). Of course, care should be taken that the infant has sufficient space to move.

GMA is best performed with the infant wearing minimal clothing, that is, the infant's dressing is limited to a diaper or a diaper with an infant bodysuit ('onesie').

- *Psychometric properties:* Intrarater and interrater agreement of well-trained assessors indicate that GMA has an excellent reliability. However, it is gradually acknowledged that it takes considerable experience to become a skilled assessor (Marcroft et al. 2015). This has induced a worldwide search for systems that can perform automated GMA. We expect that in the near future such systems will be available. In groups of high-risk infants, GMA is a powerful tool to predict cerebral palsy (CP). Atypical GMs, especially when present in the fidgety phase, and in particular when a serious reduction in movement complexity and variation is accompanied by the absence of fidgety movements, are associated with a very high risk of CP. Atypical GMs that lack fidgety movements at fidgety age are associated with a sensitivity to predict CP of 98% (95% confidence interval (CI) 74–100%) and a specificity of 91% (95% CI 83–93%; Bosanquet et al. 2013). In groups of full-term infants with or without milder perinatal complications, GMA still predicts later outcome, but with less accuracy than that in preterm infants (Hadders-Algra 2018). GM quality, in particular a reduction of the infant's repertoire, is also associated with other neurodevelopmental outcomes, such as cognitive impairment and attention deficit hyperactivity disorder (Hadders-Algra 2018).

- *Training:* GMA cannot be learned from a textbook, the method requires supervised training. Training courses are provided at various locations around the world, see for example, http://general-movements-trust.info and http://www.developmentalneurology.com.

It should be realized that the GMA is a useful addition to the traditional neurological and/or motor examination, but is not intended to be used in isolation for diagnosing or prognosticating later neurological function.

Test of Infant Motor Performance (TIMP)

The TIMP is designed to evaluate motor control and organization of posture and movement for functional activities in preterm and term-born infants (Campbell et al. 1995). It can be used by physiotherapists, occupational therapists, and other health professions in the special care nursery and follow-up settings. The TIMP includes both observational and elicited items, with the elicited items chosen to reflect the demands placed on an infant during caregiving activities and play. A screening version of the TIMP called the TIMPSI (Test of Infant Motor Performance Screening Items) has been developed based upon the most discriminative and predictive items on the TIMP and is shorter to administer (Campbell et al. 2008). The properties of the TIMP are summarized as follows (for further details see https://www.thetimp.com/; Table 10.3 provides a quick overview).

- *Purpose of the test:* The TIMP involves both observation and handling of the infant to get a comprehensive understanding of the infant's motor function. The observational items are noted at the beginning of the assessment when the infant is supine, with the elicited items involving handling and/or interacting with the infant in a supine position, sitting, rolling, and prone position. The TIMP provides information on the infant's motor performance, it can discriminate amongst infants with varying risk for poor motor outcome (Campbell and Hedeker 2001), can evaluate change in motor performance over time and in response to intervention, and assists in prediction of outcome (Campbell et al. 2002). The TIMP can also be used as an educational tool to assist parents in understanding their child's development (Dusing et al. 2008).
- *Population:* The TIMP can be used from 34 weeks PMA for infants who are born preterm up to 16 weeks' CA. It can be used in a variety of high-risk groups, including infants born preterm, small for gestational age, cardiac conditions, down syndrome, spinal muscular atrophy, torticollis, plagiocephaly, and/or brachial plexus injury.
- *Description of outcome parameters:* The TIMP provides an overall score that can be converted to a t-score and centile rank based upon 990 infants at risk of atypical neurological outcome from the United States of America with infants of a variety of races and ethnicities. Scoring includes categories of 'average, low average, far below average', which can be used to assist in referral to early intervention.
- *Administration:* The TIMP includes 27 spontaneous items that are scored as observed (1) or not-observed (0) and 25 elicited items scored on a scale of 0–4 or 0–5 depending on the item (0 = poor performance; 4–5 = better performance). The observed items are scored at the beginning of the assessment, with the infant in a supine position and the assessor and caregivers refraining from interaction. The observed items do not only include observation of the quality of general movements but also that of isolated limb and head movements. After the observational

Table 10.3 Test of Infant Motor Performance	
Purpose	Evaluation of motor control and the organization of posture and movement for functional activities in preterm and term-born infants
Age range/population	Preterm infants from 34 weeks' and full-term neonates, infants up to 16 weeks CA
Scoring	T-scores, scoring includes categories of 'average, low average, far below average'
Format	The TIMP includes 27 spontaneous items and 25 elicited items
Time needed	Assessment and scoring take 20–40 minutes
Normative sample	n = 990 infants at risk of atypical neurological outcomes from USA[a]
Reliability	Excellent test–rest reliability and inter/intrarater reliability when used by trained assessors[b]
Validity	*Construct validity:* discriminates between low–medium risk infants (e.g. healthy term and preterm infants) versus high risk infants (e.g. infants with brain injury)[c] *Predictive validity:* associated with Bayley psychomotor scores at 6 months, AIMS scores at 12 months and Peabody scores at 3 years.[d] *Evaluative validity:* ability to show change over time in response to early intervention[e]
Training	Training options include an on-line course (https://www.thetimp.com/learn-the-tests) or a 2-day workshop with a certified instructor
Costs	On-line course: $380 USD; Manual $40 USD

[a]Campbell et al. (1995); [b]Ustad et al. (2016); [c]Campbell and Hedeker (2001); [d]Campbell et al. (2002); Kolobe et al. (2004); Kim et al. (2011); [e]Spittle et al. (2008).

part, the elicited items are administered with the assessor handling the infant. The elicited items include observing the infant's motor responses to different stimulation (including animate and inanimate objects), assessing the infant's postural and motor control responses in supine and prone positions, pulling to sit, rolling, standing, and in space (e.g. lateral tilt). The TIMP takes 20–40 minutes to perform. The score form provides detail on how the assessor should administer each item and the specific criteria that the infant has to demonstrate to score on each item. For infants assessed in the special care unit, the therapist needs to be very mindful of the handling required to complete the examination, with the examination being much easier to perform on infants closer to 3 months CA.

- *Psychometric properties:* The psychometrics of the TIMP have been studied extensively, particularly in test development and have excellent reliability (Campbell et al. 1995). It is able to discriminate motor performance in low–medium risk infants (e.g. heathy term and preterm infants) versus high-risk infants (e.g. infants with brain injury; Campbell and Hedeker 2001). It has been shown to predict 12-month motor performance on the Alberta Infant Motor Scale with sensitivity of 92% and specificity of 76% (Campbell et al. 2002). TIMP scores have also been shown to correlate highly with Bayley scores with ROC values of 0.825 for the Bayley psychomotor development index (PDI) and 0.992 for the mental development index (MDI) at 6 months (Kim et al. 2011). In addition, the TIMP has been shown to be predictive of Peabody Developmental Motor Scales scores <2SD below the mean at preschool age when used at 3 months CA with a specificity of 0.72 and specificity of 0.91 using a cut-off core of –0.5SD (Kolobe et al. 2004). The TIMP has been used as an outcome measure to assess response to interventions in several research trials, although a minimal clinical important change score has not been determined (Spittle et al. 2008).

- *Training:* Whilst official certification is not necessary to perform the TIMP, training in the assessment tool is recommended. Training options include an on-line course (https://www.thetimp.com/learn-the-tests) via nine learning modules, which includes videos and score tests or a 2-day workshop with a certified instructor.

NEUROLOGICAL ASSESSMENTS

Neonatal neurological examinations have been widely used in clinical and research settings for decades. The first neurological examinations developed in the 1920s were based upon muscle tone and postural reflexes, reflective of the understanding of infant development at the time (Hadders-Algra 2001; Brown and Spittle 2014). From the 1960s, several pioneers in the field including Prechtl (1977), Amiel-Tison (Amiel-Tison and Gosselin 2000) and the Dubowitzs (Dubowitz et al. 1999), along with their colleagues, went on to develop standardized assessments tools based upon this early work and with an understanding of the importance of performing an examination with a consistent systematic procedure. Further, these neurological assessments began to incorporate the concept of behavioural state, as there was an increased understanding that the brain, not just the spinal cord, was involved in an infant's response to the environment. This understanding implied that the young nervous system is not merely a reflexive or reactive organ but that it is a complex system generating continuously endogenous activity (Prechtl 1974, 1977).

Hammersmith Neonatal Neurological Examination

The Dubowitz Neurological Assessment of the Preterm and Full-term Infant (Dubowitz et al. 1999), also known as the Hammersmith Neonatal Neurological Examination (HNNE), is a validated tool to objectively assess the neurology of preterm and term-born newborn infants. It was designed to be easily performed and scored in clinical practice, to ensure it could be used as a routine neurological examination for newborns at risk of neurological abnormalities. The HNNE was designed to be a general neurological examination (rather than focusing on reflexes or movement alone) encompassing various aspects of neurological function, such as behaviour states, tone, reflexes, and movement quality (Dubowitz et al. 2005). It has been used in clinical and research practice for over 30 years, with updates in the late nineties to improve the reliable administration. The properties of the assessment may be summarized as follows (for details, see Dubowitz et al. 1999; Table 10.4 provides a quick overview):

- *Purpose of the test:* To record neurological function of preterm and term-born newborns and identify abnormalities and/or deviations from typical development. It can be used to document an infant's neurological maturation and recovery from a perinatal insult. It is recommended to be used in conjunction with neuroimaging and clinical history to identify infants with neurological impairments. It is primarily designed to be a discriminative test and to monitor recovery over time (Dubowitz et al. 2005), rather than to be a predictor of long-term outcome.
- *Population:* It can be used to detect atypical neurological signs in preterm and term-born infants with lesions of the central and peripheral nervous system up to 1-month post-term age, including neuromuscular disorders, neonatal encephalopathy, intraventricular haemorrhage, and periventricular leukomalacia.
- *Description of outcome parameters:* The test includes 34 items subdivided into six categories of tone, tone patterns, reflexes, movements, abnormal signs, and behaviour. In every day clinical practice,

Table 10.4	Hammersmith Neonatal Neurological Examination
Purpose	Quick, practical, and easily administered standardized general neurological examination for neonates
Age range/population	Healthy and at-risk preterm and full-term neonates, infants up to and including 10 weeks CA
Domains	Tone, motor patterns, observation of spontaneous movements, reflexes, abnormal signs, and behaviour
Scoring	Raw scores can be converted to optimality scores[a]
Format	34 items including observation of the infant and administration of items such as pull to sit, reflexes, and responses to auditory and visual stimuli
Time needed	Assessment and scoring take 10–15 min
Normative sample	Healthy term-born infants in the UK (n = 224) and in Australia (n = 201). Preterm infants in the UK (n = 380), Australia (n = 209), and Singapore (n = 212)[a]
Reliability	Interrater reliability: ICC>0.74[b]
Validity	*Construct validity:* abnormal findings on the HNNE have been related to brain injury in term and preterm infants and neuromuscular conditions. It can differentiate neurological function between term and preterm infants and infants of different cultural backgrounds. Scores improve with age[c] *Predictive validity:* optimality scores assist prediction of cognitive outcomes in preterm infants and neurological function in infants with hypoxic ischaemic encephalopathy[d]
Training	No training needed. Study of the manual recommended. Video examples available online www.hammersmith-neuro-exam.com[e]
Costs	Manual: about 95€[e]

[a]Dubowitz et al. (1998); Spittle et al. (2016b); Chin et al. (2019); [b]Dubowitz et al. (1999); McReady et al. (2000); Spittle et al. (2009); Eeles et al. (2017); [c]Mercuri et al. (1999), Guzzetta et al. (2005); Ricci et al. (2008); [d]Mercuri et al. (1999); Spittle et al. (2017); [e]Dubowitz et al. (1999).

the pattern of the examination on the scoring sheet provides a general impression of the infant and opportunity to monitor change in test items over time (Dubowitz et al. 2005). Optimality scores based on full term infants examined within the first 48 hours after birth (Dubowitz et al. 1998), term-born infants within the first month post-term (Spittle et al. 2016b) and preterm infants (Mercuri et al. 2003) are available. The examination reflects current neurological status, and caution should be taken in infants who have had a challenging start to life in predicting long-term outcomes, as a poor neurological examination may be seen in early stages of recovery but improve over time.

- *Administration:* The test should take no more than 15 minutes to administer. The test items have been chosen to be suitable to administer to preterm infants in an incubator (Dubowitz et al. 2005). Test items do not have to be administered in a particular order and it will depend on the state of the infant as to which item to begin the assessment with. In most cases, the test will involve observing the infant's spontaneous movements and posture (including abnormal signs) and then administering handling items to complete the tone and reflexes items. The infant's behaviour is then assessed briefly, examining responses to auditory and visual stimulation, along with observing the infant's cry and ease of soothing. A record sheet (proforma), with a description of the item and a stick figure is used to record the response that best describes the infant's neurological response (for each of the 34 items). Each item is given a score out of five options, which are then converted to 0 (scores <5th centile or

>95th centile), 0.5 (scores between the 5th and 10th centile or 90th and 95th centile) or 1 (scores between the 10th and 90th centile) and summed to give an optimality score.

- *Psychometric properties:* The interrater reliability of the HNNE is good to excellent including low-resource settings. The HNNE is primarily a discriminative tool and has been validated on large samples of term-born infants (Dubowitz et al. 1998) and preterm infants (Mercuri et al. 2003). It has been shown to be predictive of long-term neurological outcome in infants with hypoxic ischaemic encephalopathy and of cognitive outcomes at 2 years of age in moderate to late preterm children (Mercuri et al. 1999; Spittle et al. 2017). Yet, repeated examinations are recommended to allow for the evaluation of recovery.
- *Training:* No formal training is required (Dubowitz et al. 2005). To facilitate use, a manual and training videos are available for free at the HINE and HNNE website (www.hammersmith_neuro-exam. com). The authors have purposefully made the assessment easy to learn, administer, and score to increase accessibility of the HNNE.

NEUROBEHAVIOURAL ASSESSMENTS

Neurobehaviour is a concept that takes into account that all human experiences have a psycho-social and a biological context (Salisbury et al. 2005). Neurobehavioural examinations assess the behavioural function of an infant, in conjunction with the infant's neurological function rather than behaviour or neurology alone. For example, when assessing if an infant can fix and follow an object, there is consideration for what state the infant is in, the type of stimulation used to get the infant to fix and follow (e.g. animate vs inanimate object), how much stimulation the infant needs to do this (e.g. auditory, visual, or both) and how much support is needed (e.g. swaddling). Not surprisingly, neurobehaviour assessments have also been used as an intervention tool for parents, as they can help with demonstrating an infant's strengths and areas where the infant needs more support to do a task.

It is important to be mindful of the population that the neurobehavioural assessment has been designed for, as these type of assessments involve more handling than most motor and neurological examinations. There are neurobehavioural assessments designed specifically term-born infants (e.g. Neonatal Behavioural Assessment Scale [NBAS]), preterm infants (e.g. Assessment of Preterm Infants' Behavior [APIB]) and infants exposed to substances during pregnancy (e.g. Neonatal Intensive Care Unit Neurobehavioral Scale [NNNS]). Systematic reviews have reported numerous neurobehavioural assessments. The NNNS and APIB turned out to have strong psychometric properties (Noble and Boyd 2012; Brown and Spittle 2014) and are therefore described in detail in this chapter (Table 10.3 and Table 10.4). The NBAS is described below in brief, as it is considered as the grandfather of the APIB and NNNS; however, it lacks the psychometric robustness of the later assessments (Barlow et al. 2018).

The Neonatal Behavioural Assessment Scale (NBAS) and the Newborn Behavioural Observation (NBO) System

The NBAS was designed by Brazelton and his colleagues in the late 1970s to assess an infant's response to the extrauterine environment within a behavioural state context in term-born infants between 0 and 2 months (Brazelton and Nugent 2011).

Whilst the NBAS is one of the earliest neurobehavioural assessments, it was not designed to be used as a traditional standardized assessment tool (i.e. discriminative, evaluative, predictive; Tronick and

Lester 2013). Rather, it was designed to improve caregiver–infant interaction at the behavioural level by understanding the newborn's neurological function and ability to participate actively in interactions. It involves the examiner interacting with the infant to assess their ability to respond and recover from different stimuli, such as visual stimulation from the examiner's face to assist the caregiver's awareness and understanding of their individual newborn behaviour and ability to communicate their needs and preferences. It includes 28 behavioural items, each scored on a 9-point scale and 20 neurological items, scored on a 4-point scale.

The NBAS has been used in many clinical populations, for instance to examine the effects of preterm birth, low birth weight, prenatal substance exposure, and environmental pollutants. It also has been used to evaluate neonatal behaviour in different cultures. It can be adapted for the preterm infants; however, we recommend for preterm and/or other vulnerable infants using a more specific tool developed for these patient groups, such as the NNNS or APIB.

The Newborn Behavioural Observation (NBO) system (Nuygent 2007) is a shorter version of the NBAS involving 18 items that can be used from 36 weeks to 3 months post term.

The Neonatal Intensive Care Unit Neurobehavioral Scale (NNNS)

The NNNS is a comprehensive infant assessment tool that assesses neurological integrity, behavioural function, and stress/withdrawal signs (Lester et al. 2004). It was developed using principals of the NBAS and other neurological examinations but with the intent to be suitable for high-risk infants particularly those exposed to illicit drugs in-utero. It takes into account the infant's state of arousal and motor activity, the infant's ability to self-calm, physiological stability, and how much consoling is required during the examination. The properties of the assessment may be summarized as follows (Table 10.5 provides a quick overview):

- *Purpose of the test:* Comprehensive neurobehavioural examination that can be used as an early bio-marker for detecting at-risk infants and predicting long-term neurodevelopmental impairment, along with planning and individualizing interventions (Tronick and Lester 2013).
- *Population:* From birth in preterm infant (once medically stable) up to 1 month post term in preterm and term-born infants, particularly high-risk infants.
- *Description of outcome parameters:* The NNNS provides information on how an infant's behaviour capacity, neurological integrity and signs of stress compare to normative values. NNNS extreme scores (>90th centile or <10th centile) are indicative of less than optimal development (Provenzi et al. 2018) based on a norm-referenced population of term-born infants. It consists of 128 items that are used to calculate 13 summary scores including habituation, attention, arousal, regulation, handling, quality of movement, excitability, lethargy, non-optimal reflexes, asymmetrical reflexes, hypertonicity, hypotonicity, and a stress/abstinence scale.
- *Administration:* The NNNS has a standardized administration format. It specifies how the examiner interacts with the infant with flexibility in how the assessment is administered depending on the infant's states and behaviour. If the infant is in the appropriate state, the examination commences with assessing the infant's ability to habituate to a variety of stimuli. This is followed by administration of reflex and postural items and then orientation items. The orientation items are comprehensive and include animate and inanimate stimuli, along with noting the amount of support the infant needs to perform the task. Following administration of the items, the examiner completes a test form and items are entered into an Excel program to create scores for each subscale. Scores can be compared with normative data (Fink et al. 2012).

Table 10.5 The NICU Network Neurobehavioural Scale (NNNS)	
Purpose	Evaluation of the neurological integrity, behavioural functioning, and stress responses in healthy and at-risk infants
Age range/population	Preterm and high-risk term neonates
Domains	Habituation, attention, arousal, regulation, handling, quality of movement, excitability, lethargy, non-optimal reflexes, asymmetry, hypotonia, stress abstinence
Scoring	Summary scores per domain; scores <10th centile or >90th centile indicate poor performance
Format	Standardized format, including documentation of stress signs, states of arousal, self-regulation strategies and response to comforting by the examiner during the examination. In total, 115 items
Time needed	Assessment takes about 20 minutes, scoring 30–60 additional minutes
Normative sample	Healthy term-born infants in the USA (n = 334) at term and at 1 month (n = 99) and in Australia (n = 201) at 38–42 weeks' GA[a]
Reliability	Interrater reliability: ICC > 0.85[b]
Validity	*Construct validity:* preterm birth, sex, substance exposure in-utero, caesarean section, neonatal and intrapartum risk factors, age at testing and ethnicity influence test scores[c] *Predictive validity:* NNNS scores correlate with later behaviour, cognitive, language, and motor outcomes[d]
Training	Certification is required to administer the NNNS. Training is tailored to the experience of the clinician, taking between 2 and 5 days
Costs	Training: $1800 USD

[a]Fink et al. (2012); Spittle et al. (2016b); Provenzi et al. (2018); [b]Fink et al. (2012); Eeles et al. (2017); [c]Salisbury et al. (2005); Brown et al. (2006, 2009; Tronick and Lester (2013); [d]Liu et al. (2010); El-Dib et al. (2012); Tronick and Lester, (2013); Spittle et al. (2016a, 2017).

- *Psychometric properties:* The NNNS has very good reliability, internal and concurrent validity. Normative values are available. Scores on the NNNS improve over time in preterm infants prior to term and in both preterm and term-born infants post term (Provenzi et al. 2018). The NNNS has been shown to have efficacy as an early neurobehavioural assessment for a range of clinical populations including maternal depression, neonatal exposure to methadone, and preterm birth. NNNS is primarily a discriminative tool. Nevertheless, it has been shown to be predictive of a range of neurodevelopmental outcomes. For example, in a study of 41 infants born weighing <15 000g and <34 weeks assessed with the NNNS at term equivalent age, infants who had less regulation and more non-optimal reflexes had lower cognitive scores, whilst infants who had less regulation, more non-optimal reflexes, hypertonicity, and handling had lower motor scores at 18 months on the Bayley-II (El-Dib et al. 2012). Latent profile analysis has demonstrated that different NNNS profiles were correlated to different neurodevelopmental outcomes, for example infants who had a hypotonic profile, that is, infants with signs of hypotonia, along with the highest mean standardized scores for lethargy and non-optimal reflexes, had lower psychomotor scores on the Bayley-II (Sucharew et al. 2012). These profiles are useful for research purposes but can be difficult to translate into clinical practice.
- *Training:* It is more comprehensive than many other neonatal and infant examinations and thus requires the assessor to undertake specific training on the assessment by a qualified NNNS trainer. The training is several days in length and includes the trainer administering the examination and thus involves handling of infants. The high level of training and time to administer and score the NNNS ensures high reliability in the NNNS scores, along with a comprehensive neurobehavioural evaluation but may limits its clinical utility.

The Assessment of Preterm Infants' Behavior (APIB)

The APIB is a comprehensive neurobehavioural examination developed by Heidelise Als. It is based upon the Synactive model and takes into account how the infant is interacting with the environment (Als et al. 1982). It is derived from the NBAS in order to make it applicable for vulnerable infants, such as those born preterm, who are in an environment that is challenging (e.g. neonatal unit rather than in the mother's womb). The APIB takes into account that an infant, from birth, is able to interact, collaborate and communicate with the caregiver when given the appropriate support. The APIB pays particular attention to the infant's body language, signs of stress and stability to assist in providing developmentally appropriate care for the infant. The APIB involves a comprehensive, extended training process, which can be up to 12 months. The assessment also takes time; it can take up to half a day to administer and document. Therefore, the APIB is most suited to health professionals who are working in settings where they are assessing large numbers of at-risk infants in detail. An example consists of neonatal units that implement the Newborn Individualized Developmental Care and Assessment Program (NIDCAP). The properties of the assessment may be summarized as follows (Table 10.6 provides a quick overview):

- *Purpose of the test:* To assess an infant's individual neurobehavioural competence, based on observation of the behavioural subsystems interacting with each other and the environment (Als et al. 2005). The assessment helps to identify which tasks an infant handles with ease, which tasks can be managed with help from the examiner, and which tasks are too difficult for the infant at the time of assessment.
- *Population:* From birth to one month post CA in preterm, at risk and full-term newborns.

Table 10.6   The Assessment of Preterm Infants Behavior (APIB)

Purpose	Systematic identification of an infant's differentiation and modulation of behavioural systems
Age range/population	Preterm, term and at-risk infants from birth to 1-month
Domains	Functional subsystems include autonomic, motor, state organization, attend and self-regulation systems, degree of support needed for reorganization, and balance
Scoring	Six subsystems scored from 1 to 9; lower scores (1–3) indicate well-modulated, organized behaviour, higher scores (7–9) indicate poorer, disorganized behaviour
Format/time needed	Progressive delivery of six packages including: 1. Sleep/Distal Stimulation; 2. Uncover and Supine Positioning; 3. Low Tactile Stimuli; 4. Medium Tactile and Vestibular Stimulation; 5. High Tactile and Vestibular Stimuli; and 6. Attention/Interaction (performed any time). The status of the infant at baseline, during the packaging and post are observed for packages 1 to 5.
Time needed	Assessment takes 30–60 minutes, reporting may take up to 3 hours
Normative sample	Not applicable
Reliability	Excellent test–retest reliability[a]
Validity	*Construct validity:* APIB scores of at-risk preterm infants differ from infants born at term[b] *Concurrent validity:* APIB scores correlate with concurrent MRI and EEG findings in preterm and healthy term-born infants[c]
Training	Health professional needs experience in handling preterm, term and at-risk infants. Training is individualized to experience and takes between 8 and 12 months, with preparatory studies and hands-on training required
Costs	Individualized training costs up to $29 000

[a]Als et al. (1988); [b]Sell et al. (1995); Mouradian et al. (2000); [c]Als et al. (2005).

- *Description of outcome parameters:* Six subsystems of functioning including the autonomic (respiration, digestion, colour), motor (tone, movement, postures), state organization (range, robustness, transition patterns), attention (robustness, transitions), and self-regulation (effort, success), along with the examiner facilitation (amount of support required to balance and reorganize these subsystems) are scored from 1 to 9. Lower scores indicate a well-modulated system and high scores indicated a disorganized, poorly modulated system.
- *Administration:* The APIB uses the manoeuvres of the NBAS, as a graded series of packages, beginning with distal stimulation present during sleep (habituation), then adding in mild tactile stimulation, which gradually increase throughout the examination to high tactile stimulation paired with vestibular input (Als et al. 2005). The social interaction/attention package can be administered at any time during the examination when the infant is in the appropriate state. The autonomic subsystem is as assessed by observation of physiological functions such as respiration, colour changes or visceral functions such as hiccoughing and gagging. The motor subsystem is assessed by observing posture and movement patters. State-organization is assessed by observing the range, transition, and robustness of behavioural states. The attention and interaction is assessed by the ease of the infant being alert and maintaining an alert state in the context of the environment. The system regularly takes into account the strategies to balance all of these subsystems. Finally, the amount of facilitation by the examiner and/or the environment for the infant to balance these systems is observed. The assessment can take up to an hour, whilst the documentation of findings can take up to 3 hours depending on the complexity of the infant.
- *Psychometric properties:* The APIB has excellent test–retest reliability. Its construct validity has been demonstrated by differentiating between populations of at-risk preterm infants from 34 to 40 weeks' gestation and term-born infants (Sell et al. 1995; Mouradian et al. 2000). It has been shown to be effective in documenting the effects of the NIDCAP (Als et al. 2005).
- *Training:* The assessment involves a dialogue between the infant and the examiner, and thus experience in handling infants, along with specific training, is required. The training process is individualized to the experience of the professional and takes between 8 and 12 months including preparatory study and training.

CONCLUDING REMARKS: IMPLEMENTATION IN FAMILY CENTRED CARE

Early developmental assessments provide a unique insight into the developing nervous system and provide useful information for the management of high-risk infants. Different assessment tools are available, and no single assessment tool can be recommended in isolation. Rather, a combination of assessment tools is needed, depending on the clinical history, age of the infant, and purpose of the assessment.

Assessment in early infancy requires the clinician to have skills in a number of areas, not only in handling an infant and understanding infant behavioural cues to ensure that the infant is coping with the examination but also in working with families. As the ultimate goal of the assessment is to guide the management of the infant, the clinician needs to have skills in communicating with the family and other caregivers. Early developmental assessments can be utilized to help caregivers to understand their infant's individual strengths and areas where the infant needs support. For example, showing parents how their baby can orientate to them, if the infant is given the appropriate postural support, may improve parent–infant interactions.

Early developmental assessments should be considered in relation to the clinical history, including medical (e.g. extremely preterm birth), neuroimaging (e.g. magnetic resonance imaging and cranial ultrasound), and social risk factors (e.g. parent education) when used for prognostic or predictive purposes (see Chapter 2). The predictive value of motor, neurological, and neurobehavioural assessment tools is modest to strong – depending on the tool. A consistent finding across the assessment tools is that a typical outcome of the assessment is reassuring, whereas an 'atypical' or 'suboptimal' early examination result may be an early sign for later adverse development or may reflect transient impairment that is followed by recovery. This indicates that assessments at early age often need to be followed by a series of longitudinal assessments.

Clinicians need to understand the psychometric properties of the particular assessment that they are performing, so that they can accurately convey the assessment findings to families. This is particularly important when discussing the risk for developmental impairments, such as cerebral palsy. The importance of family centred care is discussed in further detail in Chapter 12. With respect to the assessments at early age family centred care implies the involvement of the family in the assessment. For the families, this means to get feedback on the infant's strengths and the areas that may be targeted for improvement; to discuss with the professional the predictive value of the assessment; to discuss and understand the importance of assessing the baby's development over time; to get written information and having ample opportunity to ask questions; and – last but not least – obtaining early intervention when appropriate for the infant.

REFERENCES

Allinson LG, Denehy L, Doyle LW, et al. (2017) Physiological stress responses in infants at 29–32 weeks' postmenstrual age during clustered nursing cares and standardised neurobehavioural assessments. *BMJ Paediatr Open* **1**: e000025. doi: 10.1136/bmjpo-2017-000025.

Als H (1982) Toward a synactive theory of development: promise for assessment and support of infant individuality. *Infant Mental Health J* **3**: 234.

Als H, Butler S, Kosta S, McAnulty G (2005) The Assessment of Preterm Infants' Behavior (APIB): furthering the understanding and measurement of neurodevelopmental competence in preterm and full-term infants. *Ment Retard Dev Disabil Res Rev* **11**: 94–102.

Als H, Duffy FH, McAnulty G (1988) THe APIB: an assessment of functional competence in preterm and full-term newborns regardless of gestational age at birth: II. *Infant Behav Dev* **11**: 305–318.

Als H, Lester BM, Tronick EZ, Brazleton T (1982) Manual for the assessment of preterm infants' behaviour (APIB). In FitzGerald HE, Lester BM, Yogman ME, editors, *Theory and Research in Behavioral Pediatrics*. New York: Plenum Press, pp. 65–123.

Amiel-Tison C, Gosselin J (2000) *Neurological Development from Birth to Six Years. Guide for Examination and Evaluation.* Baltimore: The Johns Hopkins University Press.

Barlow J, Herath NI, Bartram Torrance C, Bennett C, Wei Y (2018) The Neonatal Behavioral Assessment Scale (NBAS) and Newborn Behavioral Observations (NBO) system for supporting caregivers and improving outcomes in caregivers and their infants. *Cochrane Database Syst Rev* **3**: CD011754. doi: 10.1002/14651858. CD011754.pub2.

Bosanquet M, Copeland L, Ware R, Boyd R (2013) A systematic review of tests to predict cerebral palsy in young children. *Dev Med Child Neurol* **55**: 418–426. doi: 10.1111/dmcn.12140.

Bouwstra H, Dijk-Stigter GR, Grooten HM, et al. (2009) Prevalence of abnormal general movements in three-month-old infants. *Early Hum Dev* **85**: 399–403. doi: 10.1016/j.earlhumdev.2009.01.003.

Bouwstra H, Dijk-Stigter GR, Grooten HM, et al. (2010) Predictive value of definitely abnormal general movements in the general population. *Dev Med Child Neurol* **52**: 456–461. doi: 10.1111/j.1469-8749.2009.03529.x.

Brazelton TB, Nugent JK (2011) *Neonatal Behavioural Assessment Scale*, 4th edn. London: Mac Keith Press.

Brown N, Spittle A (2014) Neurobehavioral evaluation in the preterm and term infant. *Curr Pediatr Rev* **10**: 65–72.

Brown NC, Doyle LW, Bear MJ, Inder TE (2006) Alterations in neurobehaviour at term reflect differing perinatal exposures in very preterm infants. *Pediatrics* **118**: 2461–2471.

Brown NC, Inder TE, Bear MJ, Hunt RW, Anderson PJ, Doyle LW (2009) Neurobehaviour at term and white and gray matter abnormalities in very preterm infants. *J Pediatr* **155**: 32–38. doi: 10.1016/j.jpeds.2009.01.038.

Campbell SK, Hedeker D (2001) Validity of the Test of Infant Motor Performance for discriminating among infants with varying risk for poor motor outcome. *J Pediatr* **139**: 546–551. doi: 10.1067/mpd.2001.117581.

Campbell SK, Kolobe TH, Osten ET, Lenke M, Girolami GL (1995) Construct validity of the test of infant motor performance. *Phys Ther* **75**: 585–596.

Campbell SK, Kolobe TH, Wright BD, Linacre JM (2002) Validity of the Test of Infant Motor Performance for prediction of 6-, 9- and 12-month scores on the Alberta Infant Motor Scale. *Dev Med Child Neurol* **44**: 263–272.

Campbell SK, Swanlund A, Smith E, Liao PJ, Zawacki L (2008) Validity of the TIMPSI for estimating concurrent performance on the test of infant motor performance. *Pediatr Phys Ther* **20**: 3–10. doi: 10.1097/PEP.0b013e-31815f66a6.

Chin EY, Baral VR, Ereno IL, Allen JC, Yeo CL (2019) Evaluation of neurologcal behaviour in late-preterm newborn infants using the Hammersmith Neurological Examination. *J Paediatr Child Health* **55**, 349–357. doi: 10.1111/jpc.14205.

De Bock F, Will H, Behrenbeck U, Jarczok MN, Hadders-Algra M, Philippi H (2017) Predictive value of General Movement Assessment for preterm infants' development at 2 years – implementation in clinical routine in a non-academic setting. *Res Dev Disabil* **62**: 69–80. doi: 10.1016/j.ridd.2017.01.012.

De Graaf-Peters VB, De Groot-Hornstra AH, Dirks T, Hadders-Algra M (2006) Specific postural support promotes variation in motor behaviour of infants with minor neurological dysfunction. *Dev Med Child Neurol* **48**: 966–972.

Dubowitz L, Dubowitz V, Mercuri E (1999) *The Neurological Assessment of the Preterm and Full Term Infant*, 2nd edn. London: Mac Keith Press.

Dubowitz L, Mercuri E, Dubowitz V (1998) An optimality score for the neurological examination of the term newborn. *Disabil Rehabil* **133**: 406–416.

Dubowitz L, Ricci D, Mercuri E (2005) The Dubowitz Neurological Examination of the full-term newborn. *Ment Retard Dev Disabil Res Rev* **11**: 52–60.

Dusing SC, Murray T, Stern M (2008) Parent preferences for motor development education in the NICU. *Pediatr Phys Ther* **20**: 363–368.

El-Dib M, Massaro AN, Glass P, Aly H (2012) Neurobehavrioual assessment as a predictor of neurodevelopmental outcome in preterm infants. *J Perinatol* **32**: 299–303.

Eeles AL, Olsen JE, Walsh JM, et al. (2017) Reliability of neurobehavioral assessments from brth to term equivalent age in preterm and term born infants. *Phys Occup Ther Pediatr* **37**: 108–119. doi: 10.3109/01942638.2015.1135845.

Einspieler C, Prechtl HF, Bos AF, Ferrari F, Cioni G (2004) *Prechtl's Method on the Qualitative Assessment of General Movements in Preterm, Term and Young Infants*. London: Mac Keith Press.

Fink N, Tronick E, Olson K, Lester B (2012) Healthy newborns' neurobehaviour: norms and relations to medical and demographic factors. *J Pediatr* **161**: 1073–1079. doi: 10.1016/j.jpeds.2012.05.036.

Guzzetta A, Haataja L, Cowan FM, et al. (2005) Neurological examination in health term infants aged 3–10 weeks. *Biol Neonate* **87**: 187–196.

Hadders-Algra M (2001) Evaluation of motor function in young infants by means of the assessment of general movements: a review. *Pediatr Phys Ther* **13**: 27–36.

Hadders-Algra M (2004) General movements: a window for early identification of children at high risk for developmental disorders. *J Pediatr* **145** (2 Suppl): S12–S18.

Hadders-Algra M (2007) Putative neural substrate of normal and abnormal general movements. *Neurosci Biobehav Rev* **31**: 1181–1190.

Hadders-Algra M (2018) Neural substrate and clinical significance of general movements: an update. *Dev Med Child Neurol* **60**: 39–46. doi: 10.1111/dmcn.13540.

Hadders-Algra M, Mavinkurve-Groothuis AM, Groen SE, Stremmelaar EF, Martijn A, Butcher PR (2004) Quality of general movements and the development of minor neurological dysfunction at toddler and school age. *Clin Rehabil* **18**: 287–299.

Heineman KR, Hadders-Algra M (2008) Evaluation of neuromotor function in infancy – a systematic review of available methods. *J Dev Behav Pediatr* **29**: 315–323.

Kim SA, Lee YJ, Lee YG (2011) Predictive value of Test of Infant Motor Performance for infants based on correlation between TIMP and Bayley Scales of Infant Development. *Ann Rehabil Med* **35**: 860–866. doi: 10.5535/arm.2011.35.6.860.

Kolobe TH, Bulanda M, Susman L (2004) Predicting motor outcome at preschool age for infants tested at 7, 30, 60, and 90 days after term age using the Test of Infant Motor Performance. *Phys Ther* **84**: 1144–1156.

Lester BM, Tronick EZ, Brazelton TB (2004) The Neonatal Intensive Care Unit Network Neurobehavioural Scale procedures. *Pediatrics* **113**: 676–678.

Liu J, Bann C, Lester B, et al. (2010) Neonatal neurobehavior predicts medical and behavioral outcome. *Pediatrics* **125**: e90–98. doi: 10.1542/peds.2009-0204.

Majnemer A, Snider L (2005) A comparison of developmental assessments of the newborn and young infant. *Ment Retard Dev Disabil Res Rev* **11**: 68–73. doi: 10.1002/mrdd.20052.

Marcroft C, Khan A, Embleton ND, Trenell M, Plötz T (2015) Movement recognition technology as a method of assessing spontaneous general movements in high risk infants. *Front Neurol* **5**: 284. doi: 10.3389/fneur.2014.00284.

McReady R, Simpson J, Panyavudhikrai S (2000) Neonatal neurological testing in resource-poor settings. *Ann Trop Paediatr* **20**: 323–336.

Mercuri E, Guzzetta A, Haataja L (1999) Neonatal neurological examination in infants with hypoxic ischaemic encephalopathy: correlation with MRI findings. *Neuropediatrics* **30**: 83–89.

Mercuri E, Guzzetta A, Laroche S (2003) Neurological examination of preterm infants at term age: comparison with term infants. *Disabil Rehabil* **142**: 647–655.

Mouradian L, Als H, Coster W (2000) Neurobehavioural functioning of healthy preterm infants of varying gestational ages. *Dev Behav Pediatr* **21**: 408–416.

Noble Y, Boyd R (2012) Neonatal assessments for the preterm infant up to 4 months corrected age: a systematic review. *Dev Med Child Neurol* **54**: 129–139. doi: 10.1111/j.1469-8749.2010.03903.x.

Nijhuis JG, Prechtl HF, Martin CB Jr, Bots RS (1982) Are there behavioural states in the human fetus? *Early Hum Dev* **6**: 177–195.

Novak I, Morgan C, Adde L, et al. (2017) Early, accurate diagnosis and early intervention in cerebral palsy: Advances in diagnosis and treatment. *JAMA Pediatr* **171**: 897–907. doi: 10.1001/jamapediatrics.2017.1689.

Peyton C, Yang E, Msall ME, et al. (2017) White matter injury and general movements in high-risk preterm infants. *AJNR Am J Neuroradiol* **38**: 162–169. doi: 10.3174/ajnr.A4955.

Prechtl HF (1974) The behavioural states of the newborn infant (a review). *Brain Res* **76**: 185–212. doi: 10.1016/0006-8993(74)90454-5.

Prechtl HFR (1977) *The Neurological Examination of the Full Term Newborn*, 2nd edn. London: Spastic Society with Heinemann Medical.

Prechtl HF (1990) Qualitative changes of spontaneous movements in fetus and preterm infant are a marker of neurological dysfunction. *Early Hum Dev* **23**: 151–158.

Provenzi L, Olson K, Giusti L, Montirosso R, DeSantis A, Tronick E (2018) NICU Network Neurobehavioral Scale: 1-month normative data and variation from birth to 1 month. *Pediatr Res* **83**: 1104–1109. doi: 10.1038/pr.2018.25.

Ricci D, Romeo DM, Haataja L (2008) Neurological examination of preterm infants at term equivalent age. *Early Hum Dev* **84**: 751–768.

Salisbury AL, Fallone MD, Lester B (2005) Neurobehavioural assessment from fetus to infant. *Ment Retard Dev Disabil Res Rev* **11**: 14–20.

Schröder SA, Hesse N, Weinberger R, et al. (2020) General Movement Assessment from videos of computed 3D infant body models is equally effective compared to conventional RGB video rating. *Early Hum Dev*, epub ahead of print. doi: 10.1016/j.earlhumdev.2020.104967.

Sell EJ, Figueredo AJ, Wilcox TG (1995) Assessment of preterm infants' behaviour (APIB): confirmatory factor analysis of behaviour constructs. *Infant Behav Dev* **18**: 447–457.

Spittle AJ, Doyle LW, Boyd RN (2008) A systematic review of the clinimetric properties of neuromotor assessments for preterm infants during the first year of life. *Dev Med Child Neurol* **50**: 254–266. doi: 10.1111/j.1469-8749.2008.02025.x.

Spittle AJ, Ferretti C, Anderson PJ, et al. (2009) Improving the outcome of infants born at <30 weeks' gestation – a randomized controlled trial of preventative care at home. *BMC Pediatr* **9**: 73. doi: 10.1186/1471-2431-9-73.

Spittle AJ, Olsen J, Kwong A, et al. (2016a). The Baby Moves prospective cohort study protocol: using a smartphone application with the General Movements Assessment to predict neurodevelopmental outcomes at age 2 years for extremely preterm or extremely low birthweight infants. *BMJ Open* **6**: e013446. doi: 10.1136/bmjopen-2016-013446.

Spittle AJ, Walsh J, Olsen JE, et al. (2016b) Neurobehaviour and neurological development in the first month after birth for infants born between 32–42 weeks' gestation. *Early Hum Dev* **96**: 7–14. doi: 10.1016/j.earlhumdev.2016.02.006.

Spittle AJ, Walsh JM, Potter C, et al. (2017). Neurobehaviour at term-equivalent age and neurodevelopmental outcomes at 2 years in infants born moderate-to-late preterm. *Dev Med Child Neurol* **59**: 207–215. doi: 10.1111/dmcn.13297.

Sucharew H, Khoury JC, Xu Y, Succop P, Yolton K (2012) NICU Network Neurobehavioral Scale profiles predict developmental outcomes in a low-risk sample. *Paediatr Perinat Epidemiol* **26**: 344–352. doi: 10.1111/j.1365-3016.2012.01288.x.

Sweeney JK, Heriza CB, Blanchard Y, Dusing SC (2010) Neonatal physical therapy. Part II: Practice frameworks and evidence-based practice guidelines. *Pediatr Phys Ther* **22**: 2–16. doi: 10.1097/PEP.0b013e3181cdba43.

Tronick E, Lester B (2013) Grandchild of the NBAS: The NICU Network Neurobehavioural Scale (NNNS). *J Child and Adol Psychiatric Nursing* **26**: 193–203.

Ustad T, Helbostad JL, Campbell SK, et al. (2016). Test-retest reliability of the Test of Infant Motor Performance Screening Items in infants at risk for impaired functional motor performance. *Early Hum Dev* **93**: 43–46. doi: 10.1016/j.earlhumdev.2015.12.007.

Van Balen LC, Dijkstra LJ, Bos AF, Van Den Heuvel ER, Hadders-Algra M (2015) Development of postural adjustments during reaching in infants at risk for cerebral palsy from 4 to 18 months. *Dev Med Child Neurol* **57**: 668–676. doi: 10.1111/dmcn.12699.

Assessment of Infants and Toddlers

Annette Majnemer, Laurie Snider, and Mijna Hadders-Algra

SUMMARY POINTS

- This chapter highlights several standardized measures of neurological, sensory, motor, global developmental, and functional domains of infant/toddler development.
- The rapid development during the first 2 years of life necessitates longitudinal assessments of developmental skills.
- The developmental measures continue to be updated to ensure that they are ecologically valid and norm-referenced.
- The proper use of the standardized assessments is stressed.

Assessment of individuals in the earliest stages of growth and development is challenging as the infant is rapidly evolving and changing. This is particularly true in terms of the acquisition of gross and fine motor milestones, but also for the emergence of early expressive and receptive language skills, cognition, and social-emotional development. An infant may appear to be following a typical developmental trajectory; however, they may at some point fall off this trajectory, if the child begins to manifest delays or difficulties in the acquisition of more complex developmental skills in particular domains. For example, motor milestones may be age-appropriate during the first year of life; however, in the second year of life, the infant may exhibit lags in the ability to use words to express his needs. It is therefore important to follow the development of children, particularly those at higher risk (e.g. preterm survivor, sibling of a child with autism), intermittently over the first years of life, across developmental domains (Council on Children with Disabilities 2006).

This chapter focuses on five domains of assessment of infants and toddlers between 3 months and 2 years of age. These include (1) neurological assessment; (2) sensory assessment; (3) motor assessment; (4) general developmental assessment; and (5) assessment of function in daily life. Each domain is briefly defined and two to three measures are described as representative examples of standardized age-appropriate psychometrically sound measures within the domain. Each of these measures are meant to provide detailed information regarding the infant's abilities and challenges in the domain of interest, and can also be used to show progress over time. Of importance, infant assessments are used to indicate a need for services aimed at enhancing the child's development.

SCREENING VERSUS ASSESSMENT

Screening tests are often conducted as part of regular neurodevelopmental surveillance by primary care providers, in order to determine if an infant needs a more comprehensive assessment (Rydz et al. 2005). They may also be used by programs that follow high-risk infants. Screening tools that focus on developmental milestone acquisition are meant to identify potential infants at high risk for developmental delay. Concerns highlighted by parents and those identified following developmental screening and surveillance may warrant referral for comprehensive assessment to promote early identification of developmental disorders. Some examples of screening tools include the Ages and Stages Questionnaire and the Parents' Evaluations of Developmental Status (Glascoe and Marks 2012). There are also more structured screeners that are performed by health professionals, such as the screening versions of two developmental assessments we describe below: Battelle Developmental Inventory Screening Test and the Bayley Infant Neurodevelopmental Screen. A recently developed tool is the Standardized Infant NeuroDevelopmental Assessment (SINDA; Hadders-Algra et al. 2019, 2020). SINDA has been designed for infants aged 6 weeks to 12 months corrected age (CA). (Note that from this point onwards, all ages in this chapter refer to ages corrected for prematurity. This is not further indicated [with the abbreviation CA].) It consists of three scales: a neurological, a developmental, and a socio-emotional scale. The scales have good reliability, proper construct validity, and promising predictive validity (Table 11.1).

NEUROLOGICAL ASSESSMENT

Neurological examinations aim to assess the integrity of the nervous system. Following the pioneering work of Albrecht Peiper (1963), André-Thomas and Saint-Anne Dargassies (1952), standardized neurological assessments for infants emerged. The assessments were developed in a clinical context and relatively little attention was paid to their psychometric properties. Yet, this did not preclude their worldwide application in the care of infants at risk of developmental disorders.

Currently, two methods are commonly used, the Amiel-Tison Neurological Assessment (ATNA) and the Hammersmith Infant Neurological Examination (HINE). These assessments reflect the increasing knowledge about the developing nervous system. Gradually, it became clear that the infant's neurological condition is not only exemplified by muscle tone and reflexes, but also – or even more so – by the quality of the infant's spontaneous motor behaviour (Prechtl 1990; Touwen 1990; Hadders-Algra 2010). These conceptual changes explain why ATNA, the instrument with the oldest roots, focusses on muscle tone and postural reactions, whereas HINE includes also one item on the quality of spontaneous motor behaviour. However, HINE pays considerably less attention to the quality of spontaneous movements than the recently developed neurological scale of the screening instrument SINDA.

Amiel-Tison Neurological Assessment (ATNA)

The ATNA is a standardized neurological assessment for children from birth to 6 years. It is firmly rooted in (a) the neuromaturational theories of neuromotor development and (b) the concept that motor function is governed by two control systems (i.e. the subcorticospinal and the corticospinal system). The properties of the ATNA may be summarized as follows (for details see Gosselin and Amiel-Tison 2011; Table 11.2 provides a quick overview):

- *Purpose of the test:* ATNA primarily aims to describe the child's current neurological condition. Its developers warn against early diagnostic conclusions, as the child's neurological condition frequently changes during infancy.

Table 11.1	**Standardized Infant NeuroDevelopmental Assessment (SINDA)**
Purpose	Screening to detect infants at high risk of developmental disorders (discriminative and evaluative tool)[a,b]
Age range/population	6 weeks–12 months, low and high risk populations[a,b]
Domains	Neurological scale: spontaneous movements; cranial nerve function; motor reactions; muscle tone; reflexes – special attention to quality of spontaneous movements (seven items)[a] Developmental scale: cognition; language; gross motor; fine motor[b] Socio-emotional scale: interaction; emotionality; self-regulation; reactivity[b]
Scoring/description	Neurological and developmental scales: total scores with a cut-off for 'at risk' Socio-emotional scale: four behaviours, scored as typical or atypical All scales: cut-off for 'at risk' independent of infant's age[a,b]
Format	Neurological scale: 28 dichotomous items (1 page form)[a] Developmental scale: 113 dichotomous items (15 /per month; 2 pages form)[b] Socio-emotional scale (six dichotomous items), recorded on developmental form[b]
Time needed	Assessment including scoring takes – neurological scale: 10 minutes[a] – developmental and socio-emotional scales together: at 2–3 months: 5–7 minutes; 4–9 months: 7–10 minutes; 10–12 months: 10–15 minutes (1 page form for 2–6 months; 1 page form for 7–12 months)[b]
Normative sample	n = 1100 infants, 6 weeks–12 months, representative of Dutch population 2017–2019[c]
Reliability	Neurological scale: intrarater reliability: ICC 0.92–0.95; interrater reliability: ICC 0.96.[a] Developmental scale: interrater reliability: $\rho = 0.972$[b] Socio-emotional scale: interrater reliability: $\kappa = 0.783$–0.896[b]
Validity	*Construct validity:* scale scores largely independent of infant's age; developmental scale and socio-emotional scales especially assist caregiver counselling[a,b] *Predictive validity:* (in mixed high risk samples) Neurological scale: prediction of at risk scores (≤21) of atypical outcome at 2 years: sensitivity 83–89%, specificity 94–96%; prediction of CP at 2 years: sensitivity 91–100%, specificity 81–85%[a,b] Developmental scale: prediction of at risk scores (≤7) of intellectual disability at 2 years: sensitivity 77%, specificity 92%[b] Socio-emotional scale: prediction of atypical 'emotionality' and atypical 'self-regulation' of behavioural or emotional disorder at 2 years: sensitivities 32% and 40%, specificities 85% and 98% respectively[b]
Training	Only manual needed: Expected 2nd quarter of 2021 via https://www.kohlhammer.de/go.php?isbn=978-3-17-037922-0; manual accompanied by many videos, no formal training required
Costs	Manual about 70€; scoring sheets: no costs

[a]Hadders-Algra et al. (2019); [b]Hadders-Algra et al. (2020); [c]Hadders-Algra et al. (2021).

- *Population:* ATNA is applicable to children aged 0–6 years. It is mainly applied in high-risk populations. ATNA has three age-bands: 0–9 months, 9–24 months and 2–6 years. Here we focus on the two youngest age bands.
- *Domains:* ATNA is primarily a neurological examination, but it includes also a section on developmental motor milestones (head control, sitting, walking independently, putting a cube into a cup, and grasping a pellet). The neurological scale assesses the skull, cranial nerve function, passive tone, motor activity, reflexes, and postural reactions. The focus is on muscle tone and postural reactions.

Table 11.2 Amiel-Tison Neurological Assessment (ATNA)	
Purpose	To describe neurological condition; to detect infants at risk of developmental disorders (discriminative and evaluative tool)[a]
Age range/population	0–6 years, high risk populations[a]
Domains	Neurological scale: skull; cranial nerve function; passive tone; motor activity; reflexes; postural reactions – focus is on tone and postural reactions Developmental milestones[a] Psychometric properties only available of neurological scale
Scoring/description	<2 years: description of neurological condition, summarizing conclusion not recommended; ≥2 years: five summarizing categories: normal; isolated signs; symptomatic triad; non-disabling CP; disabling CP.[a] First two categories usually considered as typical[b]
Format	Three age categories (0–9 months, 41 items; 9–24 months, 36 items; 2–6 years, 38 items) with four-page chart for each category; trichotomous items[a]
Time needed	Assessment including scoring takes 10–15 minutes[a]
Normative sample	Not available
Reliability	Interrater reliability: κ = 0.92[c]
Validity	*Construct validity:* presence[d] and severity[e] of neonatal brain lesions, degree of perinatal asphyxia,[b] and worse neonatal risk scores[f] associated with worse ATNA outcome classification *Predictive validity:* (in mixed high risk samples) Prediction of disabling impairment at 1 year of disabling impairment at 14–15 years: sensitivity 38%, specificity 98%[g] Worse neurological classification in first 2 years associated with worse IQ and higher risk of special education at school age[h]
Training	Only manual needed. Digital manual available at https://www.editions-chu-sainte-justine.org
Costs	Digital manual $28

[a]Amiel-Tison and Grenier (1986); Gosselin and Amiel-Tison (2011); [b]Hadzimuratovic et al. (2014); [c]Simard et al. (2009); [d]Paro-Panjan et al. (2005); [e]Rose et al. (2009); [f]Zaramella et al. (2008); [g]Roth et al. (2001); [h]Kodric et al. (2014); Harmon et al. (2015).

- *Description of outcome parameters:* Before the age of 2 years, ATNA results in a clinical description of the child's neurological condition. First at the age of 2 years, ATNA provides a classification consisting of five categories: (1) disabling cerebral palsy (CP), implying that the child is not able to walk independently at 2 years of age; (2) non-disabling CP, implying that the child has CP but could walk independently before or at the age of 2 years; (3) symptomatic triad consisting of (a) presence of unilateral or bilateral phasic stretch at rapid extension of the triceps sural muscle; (b) imbalance of the passive tone in the trunk, that is, resistance during passive movements of the trunk extensor muscles exceeds that of the trunk flexor muscles; (c) small, sharp ridges on the squamous (parietotemporal) sutures of the skull, which the test-developers consider a sign of slow brain growth during the first postnatal months (Amiel-Tison et al. 1996); (4) isolated signs, implying the isolated presence of the symptomatic triad; (5) neurologically normal.
- *Administration:* ATNA is a clinical assessment; its results are recorded on age-band specific charts of four pages. It takes 10–15 minutes to complete an ATNA.
- *Psychometric properties:* Simard et al. (2009) reported that the interrater reliability of ATNA's final conclusion was excellent (κ = 0.92). ATNA's construct validity has been demonstrated by studies

indicating that the presence and severity of brain lesions are associated with worse ANTA outcomes. The predictive validity of ATNA assessments during the first year has not been reported, which is presumably related to the test-developers' hesitancy to classify the child's persisting neurological condition at an early age. Some studies addressed the predictive validity of ATNA at 1–2 years of age: worse ATNA categories were associated with worse cognitive outcome at school-age and beyond.

- *Training:* The second edition of the ATNA manual constitutes its basic background information.

Hammersmith Infant Neurological Examination (HINE)

The HINE is a standardized neurological examination for infants aged 2–24 months. The properties of the HINE may be summarized as follows (for details see Mercuri et al. 2007; Romeo et al. 2016; Table 11.3 provides a quick overview).

- *Purpose of the test:* HINE is a neurological examination, especially used to monitor development of infants at risk of neurological sequelae, such as infants born preterm or infants with neonatal encephalopathy (Mercuri et al. 2007). In addition, HINE serves research purposes.
- *Population:* Infants at high risk of developmental disorders, aged 2–3 to 24 months.

Table 11.3 Hammersmith Infant Neurological Examination (HINE)	
Purpose	To describe neurological condition; to detect infants at risk of developmental disorders; optimality score serves research purposes (discriminative and evaluative tool)[a]
Age range/population	2–3 to 24 months, high-risk populations[b,c]
Domains	Neurological scale: cranial nerve function; posture; movements; tone; reflexes[a] Developmental milestones scale; behaviour[a] Psychometric properties only available of neurological scale
Scoring/description	Total scores of items scored as 'optimal'; cut-offs for 'at risk' differ for various ages and various studies; cut-offs only reported for 3, 6, 9, 12, and 18 months[b,c]
Format	Neurological scale, 26 items, scored 1–4 (1 page form)[c]
Time needed	Assessment including scoring takes 5–10 minutes
Normative sample	Not available; only data of low risk term infants available for: n = 74, longitudinal data between 3 and 8 months; n = 92, 12-months-olds, n = 43, 18 months old (all UK)
Reliability	Interrater reliability: ρ = 'close to 1'[a]
Validity	*Construct validity:* Late preterm infants worse HINE scores than term infants;[d] more severe brain lesions associated with lower HINE scores[e] *Predictive validity:* (in mixed high risk samples; samples with n < 20 excluded): Prediction of at risk scores (for which cut-offs varied with age and sample) of CP: sensitivity 90–100%; specificity 85–100%[c] Lower HINE scores associated with lower gross motor abilities in children with CP at 2 years,[f] and in very preterm children with less optimal neurological condition at 11 years[g]
Training	No manual available, but website with instructional videos: http://hammersmith-neuro-exam.com/ No formal training required
Costs	None

[a]Haataja et al. (1999); [b]Mercuri et al. (2007); [c]Romeo et al. (2016); [d]Chatziioannidis et al. (2018); [e]Haataja et al. (2001); [f]Romeo et al. (2008); [g]Setänen et al. (2016).

- *Domains:* HINE is primarily a neurological examination, but it includes also a section on developmental motor milestones (including head control, sitting, crawling, walking, and voluntary grasp) and three behavioural items (state of consciousness, emotional state, and social orientation). The neurological scale assesses cranial nerve function, posture, movements (one item quality, one item quantity), tone, reflexes. As the literature only reports on the properties of the neurological scale, we focus on this scale.
- *Description of outcome parameters:* On the basis of the total number of items scored as 'optimal' a classification of 'non-optimal' or 'at risk' is determined. The cut-offs for 'at risk' vary, however, with the infant's age and across studies (Romeo et al. 2016).
- *Administration:* HINE's neurological scale consists of 26 items, scored 1–4, recorded on a one-page form. Each item is scored as optimal or non-optimal, based on comparison with groups of term-born infants. Addition of the number of items on which the infant scores as optimal generates the total or optimality score (Haataja et al. 1999; Mercuri et al. 2007). The HINE takes about 10 minutes to complete.
- *Psychometric properties:* Haataja et al. (1999) reported that the assessment of the interrater reliability of HINE demonstrated a correlation coefficient close to 1, suggesting excellent interrater reliability (Haataja et al. 1999). HINE's construct was validated with studies demonstrating that preterm birth and infants with more severe brain lesions were associated with worse HINE scores. Multiple studies showed that 'at risk' HINE scores had high sensitivities and specificities to predict CP. However, the studies used varying cut-offs to determine 'at risk', which interferes with the determination of the infant's risk in clinical practice.
- *Training:* No HINE manual is available, but HINE's website supplies background material and demonstration videos.

SENSORY ASSESSMENT

Sensory information plays a pivotal role in motor development. It is required for the sculpturing of the brain, for trial and error learning, for the adaptation of movements to the environment, and for the construction of internal frames of reference (see Chapter 3). Children with developmental motor disorders frequently exhibit additional impairments in the processing of sensory information (Gomez and Sirigu 2015; McClelland 2017).

Sensory processing is a complex phenomenon involving the brain's perception, modulation, and integration of multiple sensory modalities, such as visual, auditory, somatosensory, and vestibular information. The assessment of sensory processing at an early age is difficult as it requires either a direct assessment of brain function with techniques such as evoked potentials or near infrared spectroscopy, or an indirect assessment based on the young child's behaviour. The latter strategy is more feasible in clinical practice, but it should be realized that the infant's behaviour is not only determined by the capacity to process sensory information, but also by the child's motor and cognitive abilities (Eeles et al. 2013a).

Eeles et al. (2013b) reviewed the clinical tests available to evaluate young children's capacities to process sensory information, and found three assessments that may serve this function: the Sensory Rating Scale, the Infant/Toddler Sensory Profile and the Test of Sensory Function in Infants. The authors of the review stressed, however, that the reliability of the three tests varied in the literature from poor to adequate and that limited data on validity were available. Therefore, we refrained from a tabular summary of the three assessments. We restrict ourselves to short descriptions in the text below.

The *Sensory Rating Scale* is a caregiver questionnaire evaluating sensory responsiveness in children aged 0–3 years (Provost and Oetter 1993; see also Eeles et al. 2013b). It has two age bands, 0–8 months

(88 questions) and 9 months to 3 years (136 questions). The questions are rated on a 5-point scale; it is not clear how much time completion of the questionnaire takes. The questionnaire addresses six sections: touch; movement and gravity; hearing; vision; taste and smell; temperament and general sensitivity. The sum of the section scores result in a total score.

The *Infant/Toddler Sensory Profile* is also a caregiver questionnaire assessing sensory processing in children 0–3 years (Dunn 2002; see also Eeles et al. 2013b). It has two age bands, 0–6 months (36 questions) and 7 months to 3 years (48 questions). It primarily addresses sensory processing in terms of neurological threshold and self-regulation. It results in four basic patterns of sensory responsiveness: (1) 'low registration', consisting of the combination of a high neurological threshold and a passive self-regulation strategy; (2) 'sensation seeking', implying a high neurological threshold and an active self-regulation strategy; (3) 'sensory sensitivity', combining a low neurological threshold with a passive self-regulation strategy; (4) 'sensation avoiding', implying the presence of a low neurological threshold and an active self-regulation strategy. The questions are rated on a 5-point scale and take 15–20 minutes to complete. They address the following sensory domains: general processing; auditory processing; visual processing; tactile processing; vestibular processing; and oral sensory processing. The assessment's end-result consists of the child's scores on the four basic patterns of sensory responsiveness.

The *Test of Sensory Function in Infants* is a performance-based assessment for infants aged 4 to 18 months (Degangi and Greenspan 1989; for details see also Eeles et al. 2013b). The test – performed by a health professional – requires interaction with the infant and stimulation with various materials. The test primarily assesses sensory defensive behaviours and focuses on tactile deep pressure, visual tactile integration, vestibular functions, and ocular motor control. The test has 24 items and takes 15–20 minutes. It has a multi-point scoring system. The test generates scores in five domains (reactivity to tactile deep pressure; adaptive motor function; visual-tactile integration; ocular-motor control; reactivity to vestibular stimulation) and a total score.

MOTOR ASSESSMENT

Motor development rapidly unfolds over the first years of life, providing the young child with greater opportunities to explore the environment and to learn. Motor development includes an increase in postural control and a gradual acquisition of gross and fine motor skills (see Chapter 6). Detailed appraisal of the motor behaviours (e.g. quality of posture and movement) that occur between 3 and 24 months of life are provided by motor assessments. Impaired motor behaviours are associated with increased risk for poor neurodevelopmental outcomes. This section focuses on general motor development tests. It does not review the tests available for the assessment of hand function of infants at risk for a unilateral spastic CP, nor those available to assess infant oral motor feeding. The most promising instruments for the evaluation of these properties, the Hand Assessment for Infants (HAI; Krumlinde-Sundholm et al. 2017) and the Neonatal Oral Motor Assessment Scale (NOMAS; Zarem et al. 2013) and the Functional Evaluation of Eating Difficulties Scale (FEEDS; Cavallini et al. 2019), respectively, appear clinically useful, but need additional evaluation of psychometric properties (Krumlinde-Sundholm et al. 2015; Bickell et al. 2018).

Infant Motor Profile (IMP)

The Infant Motor Profile (IMP) is a video-based standardized assessment of motor behaviour in infants aged 3–18 months, or, in the assessment of infants experiencing a developmental delay, until the infant has achieved a few months of experience in independent walking. It focuses on the quality of the infant's movements, but it also provides information on the skills that the infant has obtained (see below).

The IMP is based upon the Neuronal Group Selection Theory (NGST), a theoretical framework that explains motor variation in typical development (see Chapter 3). Within the context of the NGST, movement variation, the infant's ability to select movement strategies, symmetry, and fluency are indicators of neurological integrity. The underlying premise is that, in the first phase of variability, the infant has already a varied repertoire of movements, for instance of reaching and kicking movements, but is not yet able to select the most efficient movement in specific situations. In the second phase of variability, the infant develops the ability to adaptively select behaviours from the available repertoire in response to environmental stimuli. Both properties, the size of the repertoire (variation, or when variation is absent: stereotypy), and the degree to which the infant is able to select efficient strategies (adaptability) are promising markers of current and later neuromotor condition.

The properties of the IMP may be summarized as follows (for details see Hadders-Algra and Heineman 2021; Table 11.4 provides a quick overview).

- *Purpose of the test:* The IMP is a motor assessment with three aims: (1) to counsel caregivers about the strengths and challenges of the infant; (2) to assist professionals, especially paediatric physiotherapists, to offer suggestions and set goals for early intervention; and (3) to detect infants at high risk of developmental disorders.
- *Population:* All infants, but especially infants at high risk of developmental disorders, aged 3–18 months or rather to the age of being able to walk independently for some months. The latter means that the IMP also may be applied in non-ambulant children older than 18 months.
- *Domains:* the IMP has five domains. Four of the five domains assess a qualitative aspect of the infant's movements: variation (evaluating the infant's movement repertoire), adaptability (assessing the infant's ability to select efficient movement strategies from the repertoire), symmetry and fluency. The fifth domain assesses performance (i.e. the skills that the infant is able to achieve).
- *Description of outcome parameters:* The IMP results in five domain scores (in infants ≤6 months: four domain scores as no score on adaptability is generated) and a total score (based on the mean of the domain scores). The raw scores may be converted to percentile scores.
- *Administration:* The IMP is a video-based assessment of the infants spontaneous movement and/or its movements elicited during play; it takes about 15 minutes. The 80 items are recorded off-line on a seven-page form or in the IMP app; this takes another 10 minutes. The IMP app generates the IMP domain and total scores.
- *Psychometric properties:* Studies addressing intra- and interrater reliability showed good to excellent reliability. IMP's construct was validated by demonstrating that IMP scores were lower in infants born preterm, in infants with a brain lesion, and infants of families with a lower socio-economic status. In addition, the total IMP score and the scores of the adaptability, symmetry, and performance domains increase with increasing infant age, whereas the scores of the variation and fluency domains are independent of age (Heineman et al. 2008; Heineman et al. 2010; Hadders-Algra and Heineman 2021). The studies on IMP's predictive validity indicated that lower IMP scores are associated with an increased risk of CP at 18 months and cognitive and behavioural impairment up to and including schoolage (Heineman et al. 2011; Heineman et al. 2018; Wu et al. 2020) In addition, the IMP turned out to be a responsive instrument to measure developmental change, including change associated with specific means of intervention (Akhbari Ziegler et al. 2020; Hielkema et al. 2011; Sgandurra et al. 2016, 2017).
- *Training:* In addition to use of the manual, a 2-day training course is recommended.

Table 11.4 Infant Motor Profile (IMP)	
Purpose	To assess infant motor development with three aims: caregiver counselling; assist professional's suggestions for early intervention strategies; detect infants at risk of developmental disorders (evaluative and discriminative tool)[a]
Age range/population	3–18 months (or being able to walking independently for some months); low and high risk populations[a]
Domains	Five domains: Movement variation (25 items); adaptability (15 items); symmetry (10 items); fluency (7 items); performance (23 items)
Scoring/description	Observational, based on infant's spontaneous motor activity or movements elicited through play in five positions (supine, prone, sitting, standing, walking) and during reaching and grasping (supine, supported sitting) – depending on the age of the child Assessment results in five (in infants ≤6 months: four) domain scores, and a total IMP score; all generated by the IMP app (provided with manual) Raw scores may be converted to percentile scores[a]
Format	Seven-page form (or app) with 80 items; at each age, some items are skipped or have standard scores; item scores vary from dichotomous, trichotomous or multi-point
Time needed	Assessment takes about 15 minutes, scoring an additional 10 minutes[a]
Normative sample	n = 1700 infants, 2–18 months, representative of Dutch population, 2017–2019[a]
Reliability	Intrarater reliability: total score: ρ = 0.9[b], ICC = 0.92–0.98[c]; domain scores: ρ = 0.6–1.0[b], ICC = 0.51–0.99 (median: 0.82)[c] Interrater reliability: total score: ρ = 0.9[b], ICC = 0.91–0.95[c,d]; domain scores: ρ = 0.4–1.0[b], ICC = 0.58–0.99 (median: 0.70)[c], ICC = 0.74–0.99 (median: 0.91)[d]
Validity	*Construct validity:* prematurity, brain lesion, and lower socio-economic class associated with lower total IMP scores.[b,e] Total IMP scores increase with increasing age[a,b,e] *Concurrent validity:* Moderate correlations between total IMP scores and Albert Infant Motor Scale scores and neurological condition.[b,d] *Predictive validity:* Total IMP scores throughout infancy predicted CP well: area under receiver operating characteristic curve 0.89–0.99 (most pronounced for variation and performance domains). [f] IMP scores during infancy associated with cognition and behaviour at 4 and 9 years[g] *Responsiveness to change:* Three early intervention studies indicated that the IMP is a sensitive instrument to measure developmental changes associated with specific forms of intervention[h]
Training	Manual (accompanied by many videos; https://www.tandfonline.com) in combination with 2-day course, see http://www.developmentalneurology.com/website/index.php/en
Costs	Manual (expected early 2021): 70€; scoring sheets: no costs

[a]Hadders-Algra and Heineman (2021); [b]Heineman et al. (2008); [c]Hecker et al. (2016); [d]Heineman et al. (2013); [e]Heineman et al. (2010); [f]Heineman et al. (2011); [g]Heineman et al. (2018); Wu et al. (2020); [h]Hielkema et al. (2011); Sgandurra et al. (2016, 2017); Akhbari Ziegler (2020).

Alberta Infant Motor Scale (AIMS)

The AIMS measures change in an infant's gross motor performance over time and is able to monitor change in infants with delayed/immature motor skills despite the presence of essentially normal patterns of movement. It is *not* appropriate to use the AIMS to measure change over time in infants who are demonstrating atypical patterns of movement (e.g. an infant with a diagnosis of CP). The AIMS is intended to be used as a serial assessment, not as a one-time assessment to determine if a child has

Table 11.5	Alberta Infant Motor Scales (AIMS)
Purpose	To measure gross motor development for infants at risk for motor delay[a]
Age range/ population	Infants 0–18 months (born preterm or at term) or until child is able to independently walk[a]
Domains	Four domains: Supine (9 items); Prone (21 items); Sitting (12 items); Standing (16 items)
Scoring/ description	Observational, not video-based method, scoring of motor performance. Motor behaviours are elicited through play in prone, supine, sitting, and standing. Observed behaviours are credited a point, resulting in four domain subscale scores and total scores. Raw scores are converted to percentile scores[a]
Format	Multipage form with 58 items
Time needed	Assessment including scoring takes 30–45 minutes
Normative sample	n = 2202 infants, 0–18 months, representative of Canadian population, 1990–1992
Reliability	Test–retest reliability; Interrater reliability: high (ICC 0.76–0.99) Intrarater reliability: high: [ICC] > = 0.99)[b]
Validity	*Concurrent validity:* strong associations between low AIMS scores and delayed gross motor development assessed with the Bayley-III, gross motor domain, and between AIMS scores and PDGMS-2 scores.[c] *Predictive validity:* AIMS scores <10th percentile (P10) at 4 months and <P5 at 8 months regarded as indicators of motor developmental delay or abnormality. These points provide the best balance of sensitivity and specificity. For infants >8 months, the P5 is recommended as a cut-off, but has not been formally evaluated. Sensitivity and positive predictive values ranged from 0.33 at 3 months to 0.82 at 12 months. The P5 cut-off correctly classified a higher number of children with or without disabilities than the P10 cut-off[d]
Training	No training session required. Evaluator should be experienced in motor assessment of high-risk infants[e]
Costs	Manual 80€ and package of 50 scoring sheets 25–40€

[a]Piper and Darrah (1994); [b]Almeida et al. (2008); [c]de Albuquerque et al. (2018); Valentini and Saccani (2012); [d]Kolobe and Bulanda (2006); [e]Darrah et al. (1998).

delayed development (Kolobe and Bulanda 2006). It takes into consideration three criteria related to quality of movement: weight distribution, posture, and movement against the force of gravity.

The properties of the AIMS may be summarized as follows (for details see Piper and Darrah 1994; Table 11.5).

- *Purpose of the test:* The AIMS is a gross motor assessment designed to measure the motor development for infants at risk for motor delay, focusing on attaining motor milestones and components necessary to attain them. This scale breaks down the components of infant movement from birth until independent walking is achieved.
- *Population:* Infants aged 0–18 months (born preterm or at term) or until the child is able to independently walk.
- *Domains:* The AIMS has four subscales: (1) supine (lying on back), (2) prone (lying on tummy), (3) sitting, (4) standing.
- *Description of outcome parameters:* the AIMS consists of 58 items, including four positions: prone (21 items), supine (9 items), sitting (12 items), and standing (16 standing). The infant motor abilities

and quality of posture and movement are assessed in four these positions. It is possible to determine a total overall score and subscores for each assessed position.

- *Administration:* Observational, performance-based, norm-referenced. The assessment does not require video-recording; but it may be based on a video of the assessment (Boonzaaijer et al. 2017) Each item is scored as 'observed' or 'not observed'. The scorer identifies the least and most mature item observed. The items between these items represent the 'motor window'. Each item within the 'motor window' is scored as 'observed' or 'not observed'. One point is given for each item prior to the least mature item and one point within the motor window. All points for each subscale are added up, the four subscales are summed for a total score and plotted on the percentile graph. Scores are recorded as a percentile. The level of motor performance is determined as compared to age peers and compared to previous performances. It takes 30–45 minutes to complete the AIMS, including recording of the data.
- *Psychometric properties:* Studies addressing intrarater and interrater reliability showed excellent reliability. Also, internal consistency is excellent (motor development score: α = 0.90; domain scores: α = 0.84–0.92; Valentini and Saccani 2012). The AIMS moderately well predicts later motor developmental delay or abnormality with sensitivities and positive predictive values ranging from 0.33 at 3 months to 0.82 at 12 months when the 5th percentile of the AIMS was used as cut-off.
- *Training:* To be used by health professionals skilled at handling high-risk infants; no specific training is required.

Gross Motor Function Measure (GMFM-66 and GMFM-88), 3rd Edition

The GMFM is a standardized assessment tool designed and validated to assess change in the gross motor abilities of children with CP or to measure change in gross motor function over time. The third edition is due to publish in mid 2021 (Russell et al. 2021). Developed for evaluative purposes, the GMFM-88 is the original version. With Rasch analysis, the GMFM-66 was created (i.e. a subset of 66 items). The GMFM-66 is arranged into a hierarchal structure based on the degree of difficulty of the items and misfitting items have been eliminated. This allows a calculation of a total score when not all items are administered. The GMFM-66 is only valid for use with children with CP. An item set version (GMFM-66-IS) and a basal and ceiling version (GMFM-66-B&C) have been developed. If the primary goal of assessment is to measure change, the full GMFM-66 is still regarded as the criterion standard. The GMFM-66-IS is the preferred shortened measure for children with unilateral CP (Avery et al. 2013). The GMFM-88 and GMFM-66 have been extensively utilized in paediatric rehabilitation settings and translated into many languages. The properties of the GMFM may be summarized as follows (Table 11.6 provides a quick overview):

- *Purpose of the test:* The GMFM is a set of evaluative measures of gross motor function that also can be used to monitor change in gross motor status over time in children with neurologically based conditions (GMFM-88) or CP (GMFM-66).
- *Population:* Children (age: 5 months–16 years) with CP, Down syndrome, other neurologically based conditions.
- *Domains:* Five dimensions: (A) lying and rolling (17 and 4 items for GMFM-88 and GMFM-66, respectively); (B) sitting (20 and 15 items); (C) crawling and kneeling (14 and 10 items); (D) standing (13 items) and (E) walking, running, and jumping (24 items).
- *Description of outcome parameters:* Each item is evaluated on a 4-point scale. The scoring key is based on 0 (does not initiate) to 3 (completes). The GMFM-88 item scores are summed into dimension scores and a total score. The GMFM-66 item scores are converted by the Gross Motor Ability

Table 11.6	Gross Motor Function Measure (GMFM)
Purpose	To evaluate gross motor function and to monitor change in gross motor status over time in children with neurologically based conditions (GMFM-88) or CP (GMFM-66). 'Gold standard' for measuring gross motor function in children with CP[a]
Age range/ population	Children (age: 5 months–16 years) with CP, Down syndrome, other neurologically based conditions
Subscales	Five dimensions: A: Lying and Rolling (17 and 4 items); B: Sitting (20 and 15 items); C: Crawling and Kneeling (14 and 10 items); D: Standing (13 items); E: Walking, Running, and Jumping (24 items) – different number of items refer to GMFM-88 and GMFM-66 respectively[b]
Scoring/ description	Each item is evaluated on a 4-point scale (0: does not initiate, 3: completes). Provides outcome scores that reflect how much of an activity a child can accomplish (function) rather than how well activity is performed
Format	Standardized observational measure
Time needed	Assessment including scoring takes 45–60 minutes
Normative sample	Sample of 170 children (CP: n = 111; traumatic brain injury: n = 25; non-disabled: n = 34)[a]
Reliability	Both versions of GMFM highly reliable: intrarater and interrater ICCs >0.98 (95% confidence interval 0.965–0.994)[b]
Validity	*Construct and concurrent validity:* high correlation with other measures of functional outcome, including Bayley Scales, and Pediatric Evaluation of Disability Inventory[a] GMFM-88 and GMFM-66 useful to detect changes in gross motor function in children with CP undergoing interventions[b,c]
Training	Designed for use by paediatric therapists who are familiar with evaluation of gross motor skills in children with CP. Tools to become an assessor: Training video: one hour training video https://canchild.ca/en/shop/33-gross-motor-function-measure-training-video GMFM User's Manual, 3rd Edition (GMFM-66 and GMFM-88) (Russell et al. 2021) GMFM App+ "https://www.canchild.ca/en/shop/38-the-gross-motor-function-measure-app"CanChild Shop
Costs	Manual: 70-80€; training video $200; GMFM app $100

[a]Brunton and Bartlet (2011); [b]Russell et al. (1989); [c]Alotaibi et al. (2014); Ketelaar et al. (2001).

Estimator program to an interval level summary score provide outcome scores that reflect how much of an activity a child can accomplish (function) rather than how well the activity is performed.

- *Administration:* The GMFM is based on the observation of the child performing the items. It takes 45–60 minutes to perform the GMFM.
- *Psychometric properties:* Reliability: Both versions of GMFM were shown to be highly reliable, with intrarater and interrater ICCs of greater than 0.98 (95% confidence interval 0.965–0.994; Russell et al. 2000). Content validity was confirmed in the comparison between the hierarchy of the motor items and GMFM-66 total scores for differing groups of children (Russell et al. 2000). Construct validity was confirmed by the relationship between the relative difficulty of an item to age, sex, type/distribution of CP and the Gross Motor Functional Classification Scale (Russell et al. 2000). Children with CP over the age of 5 years tended to demonstrate less change than those who were

younger. Responsiveness was observed in the mean changes of GMFM-66 scores for children with CP changed over 12 months. The preponderance of change was observed in children less than 5 years of age and in children with less severe levels of the Gross Motor Function Classification System (GMFCS). The authors suggested that another measure such as the Pediatric Evaluation Disability Index (PEDI) should be used for evaluating change in gross motor function for children over the age of 5 (see Table 11.6).

- *Training:* The GMFM is administered by a paediatric therapist who is skilled at assessing the motor skills of children with cerebral palsy. A self-training CD-ROM is available with the user's manual.

Peabody Developmental Motor Scales – Second Edition (PDMS-2)

Originally published in 1983, the Peabody Developmental Motor Scales was developed as a comprehensive evaluative measure of motor development to be used for assessment and program intervention for young children with disabilities. The hierarchical sequence of component skills for both gross motor and fine motor domains formed a developmental framework for the measure. The motor development assessment scale is accompanied by a series of program activity cards designed for intervention. The properties of the PDMS-2 may be summarized as follows (Table 11.7 provides a quick overview).

- *Purpose of the test:* The PDMS-2 is an evaluative measure of motor development to be used for assessment and program intervention for young children with disabilities.
- *Population:* Can be used in young children from birth to 84 months.
- *Domains:* The PDMS-2 has two scales: (1) Gross Motor Developmental Scale with four subtests: reflexes (to 11 months; 8 items); stationary (30 items); locomotion (89 items); and object manipulation (≥12 months; 24 items); (2) Fine Motor Developmental Scale with two subtests: grasping (26 items) and visual–motor integration (72 items).
- *Description of outcome parameters:* Items are scored 2, 1, and 0 according to established specified criteria for mastery. Item scores are summed; this is used to generate composite quotient scores. These Gross Motor, Fine Motor and Total Motor Quotient standard scores have a mean of 100 and SD of 15 (GMQ, FMQ, TMQ). Percentiles are derived from standard scores. Age equivalent scores are also presented.
- *Administration:* The test takes approximately 20–30 minutes for each subtest or 45–60 minutes for entire assessment; the time to complete depends on the child's age and stage of development.
- *Psychometric properties:* In children with CP the intrarater and interrater for subtests and composite scores are high. Also test–retest reliability is high. The content, criterion, and construct validity are good. The concurrent validity has been assessed to a limited extent only; correlations between PDMS-scores and Bayley-II score were relatively low (Provost et al. 2004). The responsiveness of the PDMS for children with CP is acceptable.
- *Training:* The test may be purchased by individuals with a master's degree in psychology, education, occupational therapy, speech-language pathology, social work, or in a field closely related to the intended use of the assessment, and formal training in the ethical administration, scoring, and interpretation of clinical assessments.

DEVELOPMENTAL ASSESSMENT

Developmental delays refer to a lag in one or more developmental domains, using a cut-off (e.g. typically two standard deviations below the normative mean) on a standardized test (Allen and Lipkin 2005). The International Classification of Functioning, Disability, and Health (World Health Organization

Table 11.7 Peabody Developmental Motor Scales (PDMS-2)	
Purpose	To evaluate motor development and to program intervention for young children with disabilities[a]
Age range/ population	Children with disabilities from birth to 84 months
Domains	Six domains resulting in two scales: (1) Gross Motor Developmental Scale: Reflexes (to 11 months): 8 items; Stationary: 30 items; Locomotion: 89 items; Object Manipulation (from 12 months): 24 items; (2) Fine Motor Developmental Scale: Grasping: 26 items; Visual-motor Integration: 72 items[a]
Scoring/ description	Items are scored on 3-point scale. Item scores are summed and result in Gross Motor (GMQ), Final Motor (FMQ) and Total Motor Quotient (TMQ) standard scores (mean: 100, SD 15). Percentiles may be derived from standard scores. Age equivalent scores are also presented
Format	Standardized tests with specific test items; recorded in booklet
Time needed	Assessment including scoring takes 45–60 minutes (each subtest: 20–30 minutes)
Normative sample	n = 2003 North American children; 10% with disabilities
Reliability	In children with CP: intrarater and interrater reliability high (ICCs of subtests and composite scores 0.98–0.99);[a] test–retest reliability high (ICCs of composite scores 0.88–1.00)[b]
Validity	*Content validity:* theory-based, not validated *Criterion-prediction validity:* high correlations between GMQ and FMQ of PDMS and PDMS-2 (r = 0.84; r = 0.91) and high correlations with Mullen Scales of Early Learning: (r = 0.80–0.91)[b] *Construct validity:* rationale presented in the test manual, not formally evaluated[b] *Concurrent validity:* correlations between PDMS scores and Bayley-II scores low[c] *Responsiveness:* the PDMS-2 is a useful outcome measures to detect changes in motor development[a,d]
Training	Professionals in child development may become an assessor by following the instructions in the manual; see http://www.proedinc.com
Costs	PDMS-2 complete kit: $560

[a]Folio and Fewell (2000); [b]Wang et al. (2006); [c]Provost et al. (2004); [d]Palisano et al. (1995).

2008) interprets developmental delays broadly, with elements fitting within body functions and structures (e.g. eye–hand coordination, balance), and others fitting within activities and participation (stringing beads, holding a cup). Most developmental assessments focus on capacity – what the infant can do. This contrasts with functional assessments that focus on what the infant does do in real life (Mazer et al. 2012). Measures with recent updates to normative sampling were preferentially selected for the description below.

Bayley Scales of Infant and Toddler Development – 3rd Edition

The Bayley Scales of Infant and Toddler Development recently released its fourth edition. Relatively little information is available for the fourth edition. Hence, we focus on the properties of the third edition. The Bayley assessment is widely used, both in clinical practice and as an outcome measure in research to identify delays in early child development (1–42 months). Two additional scales were added to the third edition (five subscales in total) and it was re-normed. When compared to Bayley II, children tested with both measures score higher on the Bayley III (Reuner et al. 2013). Furthermore, Bayley III scores at 2 years have a stronger predictive validity for later motor development than other infant assessments performed at that age (Griffiths et al. 2018). Psychometric properties are strong, and toys are engaging. A variety of scores can be generated, depending on the purpose. As mentioned above, there is also a screening version of this measure. Normative data may vary across countries and should be verified (Hoskens et al. 2018). The properties of the Bayley assessment may be summarized as follows (Table 11.8 provides a quick overview).

- *Purpose of the test:* The Bayley assessment is a measure of development of infants and toddlers, providing a profile of developmental strengths and weaknesses. It is used to identify young children with developmental delays.
- *Population:* Infants from 1 to 42 months of age. Typically it is used for children suspected of having developmental delays.
- *Domains:* The Bayley assessment has five domains: (1) Cognitive (91 items): memory, visual preference and acuity, habituation, concept formation, concept formation, sensorimotor development, exploration and manipulation, object permanence; (2) Gross and fine motor (138 items): prehension,

Table 11.8	Bayley Scales of Infant and Toddler Development – 3rd edition
Purpose	To measure development of infants and toddlers and to identify developmental delays[a]
Age range/ population	Infants and toddlers (1–42 months)
Domains	Five domains: cognitive (91 items); Gross and Fine Motor (138 items); Expressive and Receptive Language (97 items); Socio-Emotional (35 items); Adaptive Behaviour (241 items)[a]
Scoring/ description	Items scored on categorical scale; raw scores converted into subscale scores, standard scores, composite scores with age equivalents and cut-offs
Format	Cognitive, gross and fine motor, and language domains: standardized tests with specific test items recorded on domain specific score sheet. Socio-emotional and adaptive behaviour: caregiver questionnaire
Time needed	Testing of the three domains, including recording: 45–90 minutes (depending on age)[b]
Normative sample	1700 children, representative of the USA 2000 census profile; various country-specific norm samples
Reliability	Internal consistency: high (0.91–0.93) for cognitive, motor, language scales; Test–retest: $r = 0.67–0.94$[a]
Validity	*Criterion:* correlations with Wechsler Intelligence Scale-3 (cognitive $r = 0.72–0.79$; language $r = 0.71–0.83$); with PDMS-2 ($r = 0.49–0.57$); with Vineland Adaptive Behavior ($r = 0.58–0.70$); with AIMS ($0.58–0.98$)[b] *Predictive validity:* Bayley III cognitive and language scores in preterms at 2 years correlated with intelligence scores ($r = 0.81$, $r = 0.78$) at 4 years[c]
Training	Many formats to include DVD training, workshops, prerecorded webinars, independent study. Details: https://www.pearsonclinical.com/childhood/ordering/how-to-order.html; Can be ordered in over a dozen countries with dedicated websites (link to other countries listed on primary website)
Costs	Complete testing kit: $1000–1300; package of 25 test record forms $80–90; package of 25 questionnaires $125; 2-day training $400–650

[a]Bayley (2006); [b]Hoskens et al. (2018); [c]D'Eugenio et al. (2014)

perceptual-motor integration, motor planning and speed, static and dynamic positioning and balance, quality of movement; (3) Expressive and receptive language (97 items): babbling, gesturing, turn taking, joint referencing, vocabulary, morpho-syntactic development, identifying objects; (4) Socio-emotional (35 items): communicating needs, self-regulation using emotional signals; (5) Adaptive behaviour (Adaptive Behaviour Assessment System, 2nd edition; up to 241 items): communication, self-care, self-direction, leisure, pre-academic functions, socialization.

- *Description of outcome parameters:* Items are scored on a categorical scale and then raw scores are converted into subscale scores, standard scores, composite scores with age equivalents and cut-offs.
- *Administration*: The Bayley assessment takes approximately 45–90 minutes to administer (depending on age); the items in cognitive, motor and language domains are administered by an examiner, the items on socio-emotional and adaptive behaviour are assessed in the form of questionnaires that are completed by a caregiver.
- *Psychometric properties:* Internal consistency was found to be high for cognitive, motor, language scales. Test–retest reliability was sufficient (Bayley 2006). Criterion validity was supported by correlations with scores on the Wechsler Intelligence Scale-3, the PDMS-2, the Vineland Adaptive Behavior and with the AIMS. In preterm infants aged 2 years, Bayley III cognitive and language scores correlated with intelligence scores at 4 years, supporting its predictive validity.
- *Training:* In addition to use of the manual, a 2-day training course is recommended.

Battelle Developmental Inventory – 2nd Edition

The Battelle Developmental Inventory (Battelle II) is another measure of developmental performance across domains in children under 8 years of age, that is widely used by clinicians and researchers. It was developed in 1984 and revised in 2005 by Jean Newborg (Newborg 2005). A comprehensive toolkit is provided with child-friendly toys and test items. In addition to structured activities, some items are administered by interviewing the caregiver using a script and some by observation (Mazer et al. 2012). Administration of domains can be done in any order. The standardized version is available in English; however, a Spanish translated version is also available (Cunha et al. 2018). The properties of the Battelle may be summarized as follows (Table 11.9 provides a quick overview).

- *Purpose of the test:* To measure development of young children covering multiple domains. The Battelle is used to identify children with developmental delays and to measure progress. It also screens for school readiness and need for special education services.
- *Population:* Young children between 0 and 7 years, 11 months of age. It can be used with children with disabilities.
- *Domains:* There are five domains, each with subdomains (13 subdomains and 450 items in total). (1) Motor: gross, fine, and perceptual motor; (2) Cognitive: attention and memory, reasoning and academic abilities, perception, and concepts; (3) Communication: expressive, receptive; (4) Adaptive: self-care, personal responsibility; (5) Personal-social: adult interaction, peer interaction, self-concept, and social role.
- *Description of outcome parameters:* There is a 3-point scoring system that generates norm-referenced, raw scores converted to scale scores, percentile ranks and age equivalents. Developmental quotients can be obtained for each subscale. Software is available to facilitate scoring.
- *Administration:* The Battelle takes about 60–90 minutes to administer (depending on age); the screening version can be administered in 10–30 minutes. The assessment uses a structured play-based administration of items plus also includes observation and interview formats. There are both English and Spanish versions.

Table 11.9   Battelle Developmental Inventory – 2nd edition

Purpose	To measure development of young children; to identify children with developmental delays and to screen for school readiness and need for special education services[a]
Age range/population	Young children (0–7 years, 11 months)
Domains	Five domains (with 13 subdomains and 450 items in total); motor; cognitive; communication; adaptive; personal-social[a]
Scoring/description	Norm-referenced, raw scores converted to scale scores, percentile ranks and age equivalents. Developmental quotients for each subscale Software available to facilitate scoring
Format	Structured play-based administration of items plus observation and interview formats; screening version available. English and Spanish versions[a,b]
Time needed	Assessment including scoring takes 60–90 minutes (depending on age); screener: 10–30 minutes[a,b]
Normative sample	2500 children, representative of USA population; norms have been re-weighted based on 2015 census
Reliability	Internal consistency: high (subdomains and quotients: α = 0.85–0.96)[a] Interrater reliability: high: ICC = 0.97–0.99[a] Test–retest: acceptable (subdomains and domains: r = 0.74–0.92)[a]
Validity	*Criterion:* correlations with Bayley II (r = 0.61–0.75); with Denver Developmental Screening test-2 (r = 0.83–0.90); with Preschool Language Scale (r = 0.63–0.73) *Construct:* subdomains scores highly correlated with domain scores and total score (except for motor/total, r = 0.49)[a] *Predictive:* acceptable sensitivity and specificity to developmental delay[c]
Training	No formal training required. Evaluators with expertise in child development can review manual and learnt evaluation components. See: https://www.hmhco.com/search/shop?term=battelle+developmental+inventory
Costs	Complete kit: $1500; Screener kit $450; test record sheets: package of 15 sheets $85; screener record sheets: package of 30 sheets $95

[a]Newborg (2005); [b]Cunha et al. (2018); [c]Elbaum et al. (2010).

- *Psychometric properties:* Internal consistency is high and interrater reliability is excellent. Criterion validity has been established with strong correlations with the Bayley II, the Denver Developmental Screening test-2 and with the Preschool Language Scale (r = 0.63–0.73). The construct validity was confirmed by high correlations between the most subdomain scores and domain scores and total score (Newborg 2005). Acceptable sensitivity and specificity for developmental delay were found, further supporting validity (Elbaum et al. 2010).
- *Training:* No formal training is required, although knowledge of child development is expected for evaluators.

Griffiths Scales of Child Development – 3rd Edition

The Griffiths Scale, first published in 1954 by Ruth Griffiths, was among the first scales designed to assess a child's strengths and weaknesses across developmental domains. A second version was published in 1996 and a third edition in 2016. The latter has a thorough re-standardization by the Association for Research in Infant and Child Development. This new version was considerably redesigned based on feedback from

Table 11.10	Griffiths Scales of Child Development – 3rd edition
Purpose	To measure child development; to identify children with developmental delays and track development over time[a]
Age range/population	Birth to 6 years (72 months)
Domains	Five domains (total 321 items): foundations of learning; language and communication; eye and hand coordination; personal–social–emotional; gross motor[a]
Scoring/description	Developmental ages and quotients for each subscale; total quotients, stanines for all subscales, percentiles
Format	Standardized test with specific test items recorded in booklet
Time needed	Assessment including scoring takes about 60 minutes (depending on age)
Reliability	No data available Griffith-III
Validity	No data available Griffith-III
Training	E-Learning package included in the kit (3–6 hours to complete), 3-day face-to-face workshops available worldwide (https://www.aricd.ac.uk/training-courses/). Additional information: orders@hogrefe.co.uk. Also licensed distributors outside the UK
Costs	Complete kit: 1900€; package of 10 scoring booklets 63€; on-line training, two parts, each part 45–110€; face-to-face course, two parts, each part 550€

[a]Green et al. (2015).
Note: Psychometric properties of this instrument are not yet available (Gee and Gee, https://www.hogrefe.co.uk/shop/griffiths-scales-of-child-development-third-edition.html).
For an overview of the psychometric properties of the 2nd edition see Hadders-Algra et al. (2020).

experts and users. A literature review was also conducted to develop guiding principles for test development. This version is meant to be more user-friendly, with streamlined administration and has washable equipment. The normative sample included 426 children (representative) from the United Kingdom and Republic of Ireland, and was completed in 2015. As yet, there are no published manuscripts with information regarding the psychometric properties or application of this revised assessment. The properties of the Griffiths Scale may be summarized as follows (Table 11.10 provides a quick overview).

- *Purpose of the test:* The Griffiths Scale is a measure of child development that profiles a child's developmental strengths and weaknesses. It is used to identify children with developmental delays and track development over time.
- *Population:* Can be used in young children from birth to 6 years (72 months) of age.
- *Domains:* There are five main domains with in total 321 items: (1) Foundations of learning: cognition (e.g. include attention, processing speed, executive function, dimensions of reasoning, organizing information, concept formation, sequencing), visual and auditory memory, play; (2) Language and communication: expressive and receptive language, syntactic, semantic, and pragmatic language; (3) Eye and hand coordination: fine motor skills, manual dexterity, coordination, visual perception; (4) Personal–social–emotional: self-concept, empathy/perspective-taking, emotional development, moral reasoning; (5) Gross motor: postural control, balance, motor sequencing.
- *Description of outcome parameters:* Developmental ages and quotients can be obtained for each subscale as well as total quotients, stanines for all subscales, percentiles.
- *Administration:* The Griffiths Scale takes approximately 60 minutes to complete; time to complete depends on the child's age and stage of development.

- *Psychometric properties:* No publications as yet.
- *Training:* No formal training is required, although knowledge of child development is expected for evaluators.

FUNCTIONAL ASSESSMENT

Vineland Adaptive Behavior Scale – 3rd Edition (2016)

The Vineland Adaptive Behavior Scale (VABS) was first developed in 1935, and is a measure of adaptive behaviour. It can be used for individuals from birth to 90 years of age. There are five domains, each with two or three subdomains, representing functional abilities across all activity types (Burger-Caplan et al. 2018). The VABS has recently released a third edition. It has maintained three formats of administration: a semi-structured interview, a caregiver self-report questionnaire, and a teacher questionnaire (for children <18 years only), and the same domains exist. However, item content and normative data have been updated to reflect changes in everyday life experiences. There is now a brief form in addition to the comprehensive form. Normative data may vary across countries and should be verified (Pepperdine and McCrimmon 2018). The properties of the VABS may be summarized as follows (for a quick overview see Table 11.11).

Table 11.11	Vineland Adaptive Behavior Scales – 3rd edition
Purpose	To measure of an individual's daily life functional abilities across the lifespan and to identify activity limitations[a]
Age range/population	Birth to 90 years of age
Domains	Five domains: communication; daily living skills; socialization; motor skills (optional); maladaptive behaviour (optional). The number of items is format dependent (149–502 items)[a]
Scoring/description	Based on item scores, resulting in standard scores, confidence intervals, composite scores with age equivalents and percentile ranks
Format	Three formats: (a) semi-structured interview by health professional; (b) self-report questionnaire by caregivers; (c) teacher report (children 3–21 years)[a]
Time needed	Assessment including scoring takes 45–60 minutes (depending on age)
Normative sample	6535 individuals, representative of the USA, 2014–2015
Reliability	Internal consistency: coefficients ranged 0.90–0.98 across five domains[a,b] Test–retest: r = 0.73–0.92 across domains[a,b] Interrater: r = 0.70–0.81 between two reviewers across domains[a]
Validity	*Content validity:* extensively described[a,b] *Construct validity:* raw scores show expected trends with increasing age[a] *Concurrent validity:* significant correlations with Vineland II, Bayley-III, and Adaptive Behavior Assessment System-3[a,b]
Training	The manual provides detailed information to administer and score the assessment. See: https://www.pearsonclinical.ca/en/products/product-master.html/item-541
Costs	Complete kit with three formats and 25 recording sheets per format $450; additional recording sheets: package of 25 sheets $92

Web source: https://downloads.pearsonassessments.com/images/assets/vineland-3/Vineland-Publication-Summary.pdf.
[a]Burger-Caplan et al. (2018); [b]Pepperdine and McCrimmon (2018).

Table 11.12   Pediatric Evaluation of Disability Inventory (PEDI)

Property	PEDI	PEDI-CAT
Purpose	To measure mastery of functional skills in children aged 6 months to 7.5 years	To revise the PEDI into a series of computer-adaptive tests for the age range of 0–21 years
Age range/ population	Children aged 6 months to 7 years 6 months	Children and youth 0–21 years of age
Domains	Self-care, mobility, social function, caregiver assistance, modifications	Self-care, mobility, social function, responsibility, caregiver assistance, modifications
Scoring/ description	Completed by parent/caregiver report. Part I, Functional Skills, completed as checklist or by structured interview (capable/unable). Parts II and II, Caregiver Assistance Scale and the Modification Scale, administered via structured interview of parents/caregivers	Parents/caregivers complete items on a computer or tablet on which the software program is loaded
Format	Parent/caregiver structured interview by health professional	Computer-assisted list of items administered on a computer or a tablet
Time needed	Interview, including recording, takes 45–60 minutes	Speedy-Cat: 5–15 items/domain Content-Balanced CAT: 30 items/domain
Normative sample	Representative sample of 412 children aged 6 months to 7 years 6 months from USA	Parents of typically developing children (n = 2205) and parents of children and adolescents with disabilities (n = 703) between the ages of 0 and 21 years, stratified by age and sex (USA)
Reliability	Internal consistency reliability coefficients high (α = 0.95–0.99); inter-interviewer reliability in a clinical sample high (ICC = 0.84–1.00) and agreement between parent responses and team responses high (ICC = 0.74–0.96)[a]	Test–retest reliability excellent for all domains of the PEDI-CAT (ICC = 0.96–0.99)[d]
Validity	*Content validity:* based on expert panel; scale validation with Rasch modelling[b] *Criterion validity:* with comparable domains of Battelle Developmental Inventory Screening Test and WeeFIM (r = 0.62–0.97)[b] *Construct validity:* established for (1) age-dependency and (2) construct that Functional Skills and Caregiver Assistance scales measure different aspects of function; (3) PEDI summary scores predict the classification of a child between disabled and non-disabled groups[b]	*Concurrent validity:* PEDI-CAT mobility domain associated with PEDI-Functional Skills Mobility Scale (r = 0.82)[c] *Construct validity:* correlation of PEDI-CAT with Pediatric Quality of Life CP [PedsQL-CP] or (Caregiver Priorities and Child Health Index of Life with Disabilities [CPCHILD]): in children who were walking, Daily Activities (PEDI-CAT vs PedsQL-CP: r = 0.85) and Social/Cognitive (PEDI-CAT) and Speech and Communication (PedsQL-CP) (r = 0.42); in children who did not walk, Daily Activities (PEDI-CAT) and Personal Care (CPCHILD): r = 0.44, social/cognitive (PEDI-CAT) and Communication (CPCHILD) (r = 0.64)[d] PEDI-CAT identified lower levels of support needed for children determined clinically to be in need (32%) than Vineland-3 did (40%)[e]
Training	Reading the manual is advised	Reading the manual is advised, see: https://www.pedicat.com/
Costs	Manual $125; package of 25 scoring sheets $45	Manual and app: $500

[a]Haley et al. (1992); [b]Reid et al. (1994); [c]Dumas and Fragala-Pinkham (2012); [d]Shore et al. (2019); [e]Milne (2020).

- *Purpose of the test:* The measure is meant to capture an individual's daily life functional abilities across the lifespan. The VABS is used to identify activity limitations and to assist in diagnosis of developmental disabilities, program planning and progress reporting.
- *Population:* Can be used in all individuals, from birth to 90 years of age.
- *Domains:* There are five domains with varying numbers of items depending on the format (149–502 items): (1) Communication: receptive, expressive, written; (2) Daily living skills: personal, domestic, community; (3) Socialization: interpersonal relationships, play and leisure, coping skills; (4) Motor skills (optional): fine motor, gross motor; (5) Maladaptive behaviour (optional): internalizing, externalizing, critical items.
- *Description of outcome parameters:* Each item is typically scored on a 3-point scale, with score 2 meaning behaviour is usually performed, score 1 behaviour is sometimes performed, and score 0 behaviour is never performed. Other items receive a 2 for 'yes' and 0 for 'no'. Scoring can be done digitally or manually to calculate scores. The evaluator can generate standard scores, confidence intervals, composite scores with age equivalents and percentile ranks.
- *Administration:* It takes 45–60 minutes to administer (depending on age) and can be administered by semi-structured interview (by a health professional with expertise in child development), or can be completed as a self-report questionnaire (typically by a caregiver). There is also a teacher form to gain this perspective for children 3–21 years.
- *Psychometric properties:* Internal consistency is high. Test–retest reliability across domains and inter-rater reliability between two reviewers across domains were good. Content validity was extensively described. Raw scores show expected trends with increasing age supporting construct validity. There are significant correlations with Vineland II, Bayley-III, and Adaptive Behavior Assessment System-3, demonstrating concurrent validity (Burger et al. 2018; Pepperdine and McCrimmon 2018).
- *Training:* No formal training is required, although knowledge of child development is expected for evaluators.

Pediatric Evaluation of Disability Inventory (PEDI)

Developed to measure mastery of functional skills in children aged 6 months to 7.5 years, the Pediatric Evaluation of Disability Inventory (PEDI) assesses three content domains: (1) self-care; (2) mobility; and (3) social function. The scales can be administered separately if the purposes of the assessment do not include all of the domains. Two other contributing perspectives to functional status include the (1) level of independence in performing of functional activities as well as (2) the extent of modifications required to complete them. The PEDI can be completed using a paper and pencil format or by using the PEDI software program.

- *Purpose of the test:* To measure functional skills and independence in children. The PEDI may also be used as a summary report of the multidisciplinary team when the professionals have observed the child's functional performance.
- *Population:* Designed for use with young children with a range of disabling conditions. Can be utilized with children from ages of 6 months to 7.5 years.
- *Domains:* Functional Skills Scales (197 items) with three domains: self-care, mobility, and social function. A Caregiver Assistance Scale (20 items), measuring the extent of assistance required on a daily basis, and a Modification Scale (20 items) describing the extent to which environmental modifications and adapted equipment are used to support daily routines complete the evaluation.

- *Description of outcome parameters:* Part 1, the Functional Skills Scales is scored dichotomously (capable/unable) on items grouped into self-care, mobility, social function. In Part II, the Caregiver Assistance Scale consisting of 20 complex functional activities, items are scored on a 0–5 scale, where 5 is 'Independent' and 0 is 'Total Assistance'. Part III, the Modification Scale, which also consists of 20 complex functional activities, is scored according to a letter key where N means no modifications, C child-oriented (non-specialized modifications), R rehabilitation equipment and E extensive modifications.
- *Administration:* The PEDI is completed by caregiver report. Part I can be completed as a checklist or by a structured interview. Parts II and III, Caregiver Assistance Scale and the Modification Scale, should be administered via a structured interview of the caregivers. Functional Skills and Caregiver Assistance raw scores are converted into normative standard scores using normative tables provided in the manual. Typically, it takes 45–60 minutes to administer the PEDI.
- *Psychometric properties:* Reliability was high for the three forms evaluated: internal consistency, inter-interviewer reliability in a clinical sample, and agreement between parent responses and team responses.
- *Validity:* Content validity was established by a panel of experts and Rasch modelling was used for purposes of scale validation. Criterion validity was established with comparable domains of the Battelle Developmental Inventory Screening Test and the WeeFIM. Construct validity for the underlying assumptions that (1) function is developmental and therefore age-related and (2) the Functional Skills and Caregiver Assistance scales measure different aspects of the construct of function was supported by developmental data. PEDI summary scores accurately predict the classification of a child between disabled and non-disabled groups.
- *Training:* The professional administering the PEDI should have a background in developmental paediatrics as well as experience in childhood disability. The new interviewer should observe an experienced examiner administer the test and then be observed by the experienced examiner. Importance is placed on learning the structured interview in Part II.

The Pediatric Evaluation of Disability Inventory-Computer Adaptive Test (PEDI-CAT) was developed on the basis of the original PEDI whose limitations included a small age range (6 months to 7.5 years) and a lengthy administration time. Each of the PEDI-CAT scales can be used alone or in conjunction with the others. Statistical modelling is used to estimate the child's performance beginning with an item in the mid-range of difficulty in each domain. The child's response to that first item will determine which test item from the domain item bank is presented next (more or less difficult). Computer algorithms direct the presentation of subsequent test items until stopping criteria are met. The program then presents the results in terms of item map, scaled score, age percentile (Dumas and Fragala-Pinkham 2012). The PEDI-CAT is valid for use up in those up to 20 years of age. Currently, the PEDI-CAT is available in two versions: (1) the 'Speedy CAT', that gives an estimated score while administering 15 or fewer items per domain, and (2) the 'Content-Balanced CAT', where 30 items per domain are administered. A summary (scaled) score and a normative score in percentiles are generated (Haley and Coster 2010). The PEDI-CAT evaluates function in three domains: (1) Daily activities (2) Mobility; (3) Social/Cognitive. Function is measured using a 4-point response scale (easy, a little hard, hard, and unable). Photographs are presented for each item to demonstrate the activity being assessed. A fourth functional domain, PEDI-CAT Responsibility, measures the extent to which the caregiver or child takes responsibility for managing complex, multistep life tasks. Haley et al. (2011) reported on the change of the PEDI into a series of computer-adaptive tests (CATs) covering the 0–21-year age range.

Test–retest reliability was found to be excellent. A study of the concurrent validity of the PEDI-CAT mobility domain with the PEDI-Functional Skills Mobility Scale showed that they were strongly associated. Construct validity of the PEDI-CAT for children who were walking was established with the Pediatric Quality of Life CP. In children who did not walk, PEDI-CAT scores were moderately associated with scores on the CPCHILD measure. A comparison with the Vineland Adaptive Behavior Scales (Vineland-3) showed that the PEDI-CAT identified lower levels of support needed for children determined clinically to be in need (32%) versus the Vineland-3 (40%) (Milne 2020).

CONCLUDING REMARKS

A wide range of psychometrically sound and age appropriate measures exist to assess neurological, sensory, motor, developmental, and functional outcomes of infants and toddlers with or at risk for disability. This chapter highlights several assessment tools in each of these domains of potential interest. These tools continue to be updated and renormed, to reflect ecological and cultural changes that potentially influence infant behaviour and development. Selection of the most appropriate measure, whether for clinical practice or for research, will depend on the purpose of measurement and the construct(s) of interest. It is important that the evaluator is familiar in the appropriate use of the measure and some may require specific training. Nonetheless, these measures are readily available and applicable for use by health professionals with expertise in child development. Unfortunately, a longstanding issue is that many frontline clinicians do not adequately utilize outcome measures to inform clinical decision-making (e.g. to identify impairments, to prioritize goals of intervention based on performance) or to quantify changes and responsiveness to treatment (Majnemer and Mazer 2004; Gmmash and Effgan 2019). We therefore urge rehabilitation and other developmental specialists to carefully consider the measures described in this chapter, in terms of their potential utility in informing best practice.

REFERENCES

Akhbari Ziegler S, von Rhein M, Meichtry A, et al. (2020) The coping with and caring for infant with special needs intervention was associated with improved motor development in preterm infants. *Acta Paediatr.* epub ahead of print. doi: 10.1111/apa.15619.

Allen MC, Lipkin PH (2005) Introduction: developmental assessment of the fetus and young infant. *Ment Retard Dev Disabil Res Rev* **11**: 1–2.

Almeida KM, Dutra MV, Mello RR, Reis AB, Martins PS (2008). Concurrent validity and reliability of the Alberta Infant Motor Scale in premature infants. *J Pediatr (Rio J)* **84**: 442–448. doi: 10.2223/JPED.1836.

Alotaibi M, Long T, Kennedy E, Bavishi S (2014) The efficacy of GMFM-88 and GMFM-66 to detect changes in gross motor function in children with cerebral palsy (CP): A literature review. *Disabil Rehabil* **36**: 617–627. doi: 10.3109/09638288.2013.805820.

Amiel-Tison C, Grenier A (1986) *Neurological Assessment During the First Year of Life*. Oxford: Oxford University Press.

Amiel-Tison C, Njiokiktjien C, Vaivre-Douret L, Verschoor CA, Chavanne E, Garel M (1996) Relation of early neuromotor and cranial signs with neuropsychological outcome at 4 years. *Brain Dev* **18**: 280–286. doi: 10.1016/0387-7604(96)00016-2.

André-Thomas, Saint-Anne Dargassies A (1952) *Études neurologiques sur le nouveau-né et le jeune nourrisson*. Paris: Masson.

Avery LM, Russell DJ, Rosenbaum PL (2013) Criterion validity of the GMFM-66 item set and the GMFM-66 basal and ceiling approaches for estimating GMFM-66 scores. *Dev Med Child Neurol* **55**: 534–538. doi: 10.1111/dmcn.12120.

Bayley N (2006) *Bayley Scales of Infant and Toddler Development, Third edition: Administration Manual and Technical Manual*. San Antonio Texas: Harcourt Assessment.

Bickell M, Barton C, Dow K, Fucile S (2018) A systematic review of clinical and psychometric properties of infant oral motor feeding assessments. *Dev Neurorehabil* **21**: 351–361. doi: 10.1080/17518423.

Boonzaaijer M, van Dam E, van Haastert IC, Nuysink J (2017) Concurrent validity between live and home video observations using the Alberta Infant Motor Scale. *Pediatr Phys Ther* **29**: 146–151. doi: 10.1097/PEP.0000000000000363.

Brunton LK, Bartlett DJ (2011) Validity and reliability of two abbreviated versions of the Gross Motor Function Measure. *Phys Ther* **91**: 577–588. doi: 10.2522/ptj.20100279.

Burger-Caplan R, Saulnier CA, Sparrow SS (2018) Vineland Adaptive Behavior Scales. In: Kreutzer J, DeLuca J, Caplan B, editors, *Encyclopedia of Clinical Neuropsychology*. Cham: Springer International Publishing, pp. 3597–3601.

Cavallini A, Provenzi L, Scotto Di Minico G, et al. (2019) Functional Evaluation of Eating Difficulties Scale to predict oral motor skills in infants with neurodevelopmental disorders: a longitudinal study. *Dev Med Child Neurol* **61**: 813–819. doi: 10.1111/dmcn.14154.

Chatziioannidis I, Kyriakidou M, Exadaktylou S, Antoniou E, Zafeiriou D, Nikolaidis N (2018) Neurological outcome at 6 and 12 months corrected age in hospitalised late preterm infants – a prospective study. *Eur J Paediatr Neurol* **22**: 602–609. doi: 10.1016/j.ejpn.2018.02.013.

Council on Children With Disabilities, Section on Developmental Behavioral Pediatrics, Bright Futures Steering Committee and Medical Home Initiatives for Children With Special Needs Project Advisory Committee (2006) Identifying infants and young children with developmental disorders in the medical home: an algorithm for developmental surveillance and screening. *Pediatrics* **118**: 405–420. https://doi.org/10.1542/peds.2006-1231.

Cunha AC, Berkovits MD, Albuquerque KA (2018) Developmental assessment with young children: A systematic review of Battelle studies. *Infant Young Child* **31**: 69–90. doi: 10.1097/IYC.0000000000000106.

Darrah J, Piper M, Watt MJ (1998) Assessment of gross motor skills of at-risk infants: Predictive validity of the Alberta Infant Motor Scale. *Dev Med Child Neurol* **40**: 485–491.

de Albuquerque PL, de Farias Guerra MQ, de Carvalho Lima M, Eickmann SH (2018) Concurrent validity of the Alberta Infant Motor Scale to detect delayed gross motor development in preterm infants: A comparative study with the Bayley III. *Dev Neurorehabil* **21**: 408–414. doi: 10.1080/17518423.2017.1323974.

Degangi G, Greenspan SI (1989). *Test of Sensory Functions in Infants (TSFI) Manual*. Los Angeles, CA: Western Psychological Services.

D'Eugenio DB, Mettelman BB, Gorss SJ (2014). Predictive validity of the Bayley, Third Edition at 2 years for intelligence quotient at 4 years in preterm infants. *J Dev Behav Pediatr* **35**: 570–575. doi: 10.1097/DBP.0000000000000110.

Dumas HM, Fragala-Pinkham MA (2012) Concurrent validity and reliability of the Pediatric Evaluation of Disability Inventory-Computer Adaptive Test Mobility Domain. *Pediatr Phys Ther* **24**: 171–196. doi: 10.1097/PEP.0b013e31824c94ca.

Dumas HM, Fragala-Pinkham MA, Rosen EL, Lombard KA, Farrell C (2015). Pediatric Evaluation of Disability Inventory Computer Adaptive Test (PEDI-CAT) and Alberta Infant Motor Scale (AIMS): Validity and Responsiveness. *Phys Ther* **95**: 1559–1568. doi.org/10.2522/ptj.20140339.

Dunn W (2002) *Infant/Toddler Sensory Profile. User's Manual*. San Antonio, TX: The Psychological Corporation.

Eeles AL, Anderson PJ, Brown NC, et al. (2013b) Sensory profiles obtained from parental reports correlate with independent assessments of development in very preterm children at 2 years of age. *Early Hum Dev* **89**: 1075–1080. doi: 10.1016/j.earlhumdev.2013.07.027.

Eeles AL, Spittle AJ, Anderson PJ, et al. (2013a) Assessments of sensory processing in infants: a systematic review. *Dev Med Child Neurol* **55**: 314–326. doi: 10.1111/j.1469-8749.2012.04434.x.

Elbaum B, Gattamorta K, Penfield R (2010) Evaluation of the Battelle Developmental Inventory, 2nd Edition, screening test for use in states' child outcomes measurement systems under the Individuals with Disabilities Education Act. *J Early Intervention* **32**: 255–273. doi: 10.1177/1053815110384723.

Folio MK, Fewell R (2000) *Peabody Developmental Motor Scales: Examiner's Manual*, 2nd edn. Austin, TX: PRO-ED, Inc.

Glascoe FP, Marks KP (2012) Screening for developmental and behavioral problems. In: Majnemer A, editor, *Measures for Children with Developmental Disabilities. An ICF-CY approach*. London: Mac Keith Press, pp. 233–248.

Gmmash AS, Effgen SK (2019) Early intervention therapy services for infants with or at risk for cerebral palsy. *Pediatr Phys Ther* **31**: 242–249. doi: 10.1097/PEP.0000000000000619.

Gomez A, Sirigu A (2015) Developmental coordination disorder: core sensori-motor deficits, neurobiology and etiology. *Neuropsychologia* **79**: 272–287. doi: 10.1016/j.neuropsychologia.2015.09.032.

Gosselin J, Amiel-Tison (2011) *Neurological Assessment from Birth to 6*, 2nd edn. Montreal: Éditions du CHU Sainte-Justine.

Green E, Stroud L, Bloomfield S, et al. (2015) *Griffiths Scales of Child Development*, 3rd edn. Amsterdam: Hogrefe.

Griffiths A, Toovey R, Morgan PE, Spittle AJ (2018). Psychometric properties of gross motor assessment tools for children: A systematic review. *BMJ Open* **8**(10). doi: 10.1136/bmjopen-2018-021734.

Haataja L, Mercuri E, Regev R, et al. (1999) Optimality score for the neurologic examination of the infant at 12 and 18 months of age. *J Pediatr* **135**: 153–161.

Haataja L, Mercuri E, Guzzetta A, et al. (2001) Neurologic examination in infants with hypoxic-ischemic encephalopathy at age 9 to 14 months: use of optimality scores and correlation with magnetic resonance imaging findings. *J Pediatr* **138**: 332–337.

Hadders-Algra M (2010) Variation and variability: key words in human motor development. *Phys Ther* **90**: 1823–1837. doi: 10.2522/ptj.20100006.

Hadders-Algra M, Heineman KR (2021) *The Infant Motor Profile.* Abingdon, Oxon: Routledge.

Hadders-Algra M, Tacke U, Pietz J, Philippi H (2021) *SINDA – Standardized Infant NeuroDevelopmental Assessment.* Stuttgart: Kohlhammer.

Hadders-Algra M, Tacke U, Pietz J, Rupp A, Philippi H (2019) Reliability and validity of the Standardized Infant NeuroDevelopmental Assessment neurological scale. *Dev Med Child Neurol* **61**: 654–660. doi: 10.1111/dmcn.14045.

Hadders-Algra M, Tacke U, Pietz J, Rupp A, Philippi H (2020) Standardized Infant NeuroDevelopmental Assessment developmental and socio-emotional scales: reliability and predictive value in an at-risk population. *Dev Med Child Neurol*, **62**: 845–853. doi: 10.1111/dmcn.14423.

Hadzimuratovic E, Skrablin S, Hadzimuratovic A, Dinarevic SM (2014) Postasphyxial renal injury in newborns as a prognostic factor of neurological outcome. *J Matern Fetal Neonatal Med* **27**: 407–410. doi: 10.3109/14767058.2013.818646.

Haley SM, Coster WJ, Dumas HM, et al. (2011) Accuracy and precision of the Pediatric Evaluation of Disability Inventory computer-adaptive tests (PEDI-CAT). *Dev Med Child Neurol* **53**: 1100–1106. doi: 10.1111/j.1469-8749.2011.04107.x.

Haley S, Coster W (2010) *PEDI-CAT: Development, Standardization and Administration Manual.* Boston, MA: CRECare LLC.

Harmon HM, Taylor HG, Minich N, Wilson-Costello D, Hack M (2015) Early school outcomes for extremely preterm infants with transient neurological abnormalities. *Dev Med Child Neurol* **57**: 865–871. doi: 10.1111/dmcn.12811.

Hecker E, Baer GD, Stark C, Herkenrath P, Hadders-Algra M (2016). Inter-and intra-rater reliability of the Infant Motor Profile in 3–18-month-old infants. *Pediatr Phys Ther* **28**: 217–222. doi: 10.1097/PEP. 0000000000000244.

Heineman KR, Bos AF, Hadders-Algra M (2008) The Infant Motor Profile: a standardized and qualitative method to assess motor behaviour in infancy. *Dev Med Child Neurol* **50**: 275–282. doi: 10.1111/j.1469-8749.2008.02035.x.

Heineman KR, La Bastide-Van Gemert S, Fidler V, Middelburg KJ, Bos AF, Hadders-Algra M (2010) Construct validity of the Infant Motor Profile: relation with prenatal, perinatal, and neonatal risk factors. *Dev Med Child Neurol* **52**: e209–215. doi: 10.1111/j.1469-8749.2010.03667.x.

Heineman KR, Bos AF, Hadders-Algra M (2011) Infant Motor Profile and cerebral palsy: promising associations. *Dev Med Child Neurol* **53** (Suppl 4): 40–45. doi: 10.1111/j.1469-8749.2011.04063.x.

Heineman KR, Middelburg KJ, Bos AF, et al. (2013) Reliability and concurrent validity of the Infant Motor Profile. *Dev Med Child Neurol* **55**: 539–545. doi: 10.1111/dmcn.12100.

Heineman KR, Schendelaar P, Van den Heuvel ER, Hadders-Algra M (2018) Motor development in infancy is related to cognitive function at 4 years of age. *Dev Med Child Neurol* **60**: 1149–1155. doi: 10.1111/dmcn.13761.

Hielkema T, Blauw-Hospers CH, Dirks T, Drijver-Messelink M, Bos AF, Hadders-Algra M (2011) Does physiotherapeutic intervention affect motor outcome in high-risk infants? An approach combining a randomized controlled trial and process evaluation. *Dev Med Child Neurol* **53**: e8–15. doi: 10.1111/j.1469-8749.2010.03876.x.

Hoskens J, Klingels K, Smits-Engelsman B (2018). Validity and cross-cultural differences of the Bayley Scales of Infant and Toddler Development, Third Edition in typically developing infants. *Early Hum Dev* **125**: 17–25. doi: 10.1016/j.earlhumdev.2018.07.002.

Ketelaar M, Vermeer A, Hart H, et al. (2001) Effects of a functional therapy program on motor abilities of children with cerebral palsy. *Phys Ther* **9**: 1534–1545.

Krumlinde-Sundholm L, Ek L, Eliasson AC (2015) What assessments evaluate use of hands in infants? A literature review. *Dev Med Child Neurol* **57** (Suppl 2): 37–41. doi: 10.1111/dmcn.12684.

Krumlinde-Sundholm L, Ek L, Sicola E, et al. (2017) Development of the Hand Assessment for Infants: evidence of internal scale validity. *Dev Med Child Neurol* **59**: 1276–1283. doi: 10.1111/dmcn.13585.

Kodric J, Sustersic B, Paro-Panjan D (2014) Relationship between neurological assessments of preterm infants in the first 2 years and cognitive outcome at school age. *Pediatr Neurol* **51**: 681–687. doi: 10.1016/j.pediatrneurol.2014.07.024.

Kolobe TA, Bulanda M (2006) Diagnostic accuracy and consistency of the Alberta Infant Motor Scale in a longitudinal sample. *Pediatr Phys Ther* **18**: 76–77.

Majnemer A, Mazer B (2004) New directions in outcome evaluation of children with cerebral palsy. *Semin Pediatr Neurol* **11**: 11–17.

Mazer B, Majnemer A, Dahan-Oliel N, Sebesteyn I (2012) Global developmental assessments. In: Majnemer A, editor, *Measures for Children with Developmental Disabilities. An ICF-CY Approach.* London: Mac Keith Press, pp. 249–264.

McClelland VM (2017) The neurophysiology of paediatric movement disorders. *Curr Opin Pediatr* **29**: 683–690. doi: 10.1097/MOP.0000000000000547.

Mercuri E, Haataja L, Dubowitz L (2007) Neurological assessment in normal young infants. In: Cioni G, Mercuri E, editors, *Neurological Assessment in the First Two Years of Life.* London: Mac Keith Press, pp. 24–37.

Mercuri E, Haataja L, Ricci D, Cowan F, Dubowitz L (2007) Classical neurological examination in young infants with neonatal brain lesions. In: Cioni G, Mercuri E, editors, *Neurological Assessment in the First Two Years of Life.* London: Mac Keith Press, pp. 38–48.

Milne S, Campbell L, Cottier C (2020) Accurate assessment of functional abilities in pre-schoolers for diagnostic and funding purposes: a comparison of the Vineland-3 and the PEDI-CAT. *Aust Occup Ther J* **67**: 31–38. doi: 10.1111/1440-1630.12619.

Newborg J (2005) *Battelle Developmental Inventory,* 2nd edn. Itasca, IL: Riverside Publishing.

Palisano RJ, Kolobe TH, Haley SM, et al. (1995) Validity of the Peabody Developmental Gross Motor Scale as an evaluative measure of infants receiving physical therapy. *Phys Ther* **75**: 939–951.

Paro-Panjan D, Neubauer D, Kodric J, Bratanic B (2005) Amiel-Tison Neurological Assessment at term age: clinical application, correlation with other methods, and outcome at 12 to 15 months. *Dev Med Child Neurol* **47**: 19–26.

Piper MC, Darrah J (1994) *Motor Assessment of the Developing Infant.* Pennsylvania: W.B. Saunders Company.

Peiper A (1963) *Cerebral Function in Infancy and Childhood.* New York: Consultants Bureau.

Pepperdine CR, McCrimmon AW (2018) Test review: Vineland Adaptive Behavior Scales, Third Edition (Vineland-3) by Sparrow SS, Cicchetti DV & Saulnier CA. *Can J School Psychol* **33**: 157–163. doi: 10.1177/0829573517733845.

Prechtl HFR (1990) Qualitative changes of spontaneous movements in fetus and preterm infant are a marker of neurological dysfunction. *Early Hum Dev* **23**: 151–158.

Provost B, Heimerl S, McClain C, Kim NH, Lopez BR, Kodituwakku P (2004) Concurrent validity of the Bayley Scales of Infant Development II Motor Scale and the Peabody Developmental Motor Scales-2 in children with developmental delays. *Pediatr Phys Ther* **16**: 149–156.

Provost B, Oetter P (1993) The sensory rating scale for infants and young children: development and reliability. *Phys Occup Ther Pediatr* **13**: 15–35.

Reuner G, Fields AC, Wittke A, Loepprich M, Pietz J (2013). Comparison of the developmental testes Bayley-III and Bayley-II in 7-month-old infants born preterm. *Eur J Pediatr* **172**: 393–400. doi: 10.1007/s00431-012-1902-6.

Russell DJ, Avery LM, Rosenbaum PL, Raina PS, Walter SD, Palisano RJ (2000) Improved scaling of the gross motor function measure for children with cerebral palsy: evidence of reliability and validity. *Phys Ther* **80**: 873–885. doi: 10.1093/ptj/80.9.873.

Russell DJ, Rosenbaum PL, Cadman DT, Gowland C, Hardy S, Jarvis S (1989) The Gross Motor Function Measure: means to evaluate the effects of physical therapy. *Dev Med Child Neurol* **31**: 341–352. doi.org/10.1111/j.1469-8749.1989.tb04003.x.

Russell DJ, Rosenbaum PL, Wright M, Avery LM (2021) *Gross Motor Function Measure (GMFM-66 & GMFM-88) User's Manual*, 3rd Edition. London: Mac Keith Press. (In Press)

Romeo DM, Cioni M, Scoto M, Mazzone L, Palermo F, Romeo MG (2008) Neuromotor development in infants with cerebral palsy investigated by the Hammersmith Infant Neurological Examination during the first year of age. *Eur J Paediatr Neurol* **12**: 24–31.

Romeo DM, Ricci D, Brogna C, Mercuri E (2016) Use of the Hammersmith Infant Neurological Examination in infants with cerebral palsy: a critical review of the literature. *Dev Med Child Neurol* **58**: 240–245. doi: 10.1111/dmcn.12876.

Rose J, Butler EE, Lamont LE, Barnes PD, Atlas SW, Stevenson DK (2009) Neonatal brain structure on MRI and diffusion tensor imaging, sex, and neurodevelopment in very-low-birthweight preterm children. *Dev Med Child Neurol* **51**: 526–535. doi: 10.1111/j.1469-8749.2008.03231.x.

Roth S, Wyatt J, Baudin J, et al. (2001) Neurodevelopmental status at 1 year predicts neuropsychiatric outcome at 14–15 years of age in very preterm infants. *Early Hum Dev* **65**: 81–89.

Rydz D, Shevell MI, Majnemer A, Oskoui M (2005) Developmental screening. *J Child Neurol* **20**: 4–21.

Setänen S, Lehtonen L, Parkkola R, Aho K, Haataja L; PIPARI Study Group (2016) Prediction of neuromotor outcome in infants born preterm at 11 years of age using volumetric neonatal magnetic resonance imaging and neurological examinations. *Dev Med Child Neurol* **58**: 721–727. doi: 10.1111/dmcn.13030.

Sgandurra G, Bartalena L, Cecchi F, et al. (2016) A pilot study on early home-based intervention through an intelligent baby gym (CareToy) in preterm infants. *Res Dev Disabil* **53–54**: 32–42. doi: 10.1016/j.ridd.2016.01.013.

Sgandurra G, Lorentzen J, Inguaggiato E, et al. (2017) A randomized clinical trial in preterm infants on the effects of a home-based early intervention with the 'Care-Toy System'. *PLoS One* **12**: e0173521. doi: 10.1371/journal.pone.0173521.

Simard MN, Lambert J, Lachance C, Audibert F, Gosselin J (2009) Interexaminer reliability of Amiel-Tison neurological assessments. *Pediatr Neurol* **41**: 347–352. doi: 10.1016/j.pediatrneurol.2009.05.010.

Touwen BCL (1990) Variability and stereotypy of spontaneous motility as a predictor of neurological development of preterm infants. *Dev Med Child Neurol* **32**: 501–508.

Valentini, NC, Saccani R (2012) Brazilian validation of the Alberta Infant Motor Scale. *Phys Ther* **92**: 440–447. doi: 10.2522/ptj.20110036.

Wang HH, Liao HF, Hsieh CL (2006) Reliability, sensitivity to change, and responsiveness of the Peabody Developmental Motor Scales – Second Edition for children with cerebral palsy. *Phys Ther* **86**: 1351–1359. doi: 10.2522/ptj.20050259.

World Health Organization (2008) *International Classification of Functioning, Disability, and Health: Children & Youth Version (ICF-CY)*. Geneva: World Health Organization.

Wu Y-C, Heineman KR, la Bastide-van Gemert S, Kuiper D, Drenth Olivares M, Hadders-Algra M (2020) Motor behaviour in infancy is associated with cognitive, neurological and behavioural function in 9-year-old children born to parents with reduced fertility. *Dev Med Child Neurol,* epub ahead of print. doi: 10.1111/dmcn.14520.

Zaramella P, Freato F, Milan A, Grisafi D, Vianello A, Chiandetti L (2008) Comparison between the perinatal risk inventory and the nursery neurobiological risk score for predicting development in high-risk newborn infants. *Early Hum Dev* **84**: 311–317.

Zarem C, Kidokoro H, Neil J, Wallendorf M, Inder T, Pineda R (2013) Psychometrics of the neonatal oral motor assessment scale. *Dev Med Child Neurol* **55**: 1115–1120. doi: 10.1111/dmcn.12202.

SUGGESTIONS FOR FURTHER READING

Ages and Stages Questionnaire: www.agesandstages.
Parents' Evaluations of Developmental Status: www.PEDSTest.com.
Vineland-3: https://downloads.pearsonassessments.com/images/assets/vineland-3/Vineland-Publication-Summary.pdf.

PART VI
Early Intervention

Early Intervention: What About the Family?

Peter Rosenbaum, Monika Novak-Pavlic, Schirin Akhbari Ziegler, and Mijna Hadders-Algra

SUMMARY POINTS

- Early intervention services for children at risk for, or with, neurodevelopmental impairments are strongly grounded on principles of neuroplasticity and neuromotor learning. However, the scope of neurodevelopment goes beyond structured early intervention therapies for children that are offered in controlled clinical settings. Child development involves a constant interplay of the external stimuli and neural processes that occur in all life situations and settings.
- Children with developmental challenges might react and respond to those stimuli differently than their typically developing peers. These situations impact family functioning and can be a source of significant family stress, particularly for parents. It is, therefore, essential to make ourselves available not only to support families making medical decisions about their child's developmental needs, but also to support parent and family needs and well-being.
- There are many ways to support parents on their journey of parenting a child with developmental delay or disability. In this chapter, we present the broad case for caring about the family as well as the child. We also introduce two innovative early intervention programs that aim to promote family involvement and well-being: 'COPing with and CAring for infants with special needs' (COPCA) and ENabling VISion and Growing Expectations (ENVISAGE).

INTRODUCTION AND BACKGROUND

For many years, discussions about 'early intervention' (EI) for children with, or at risk of, developmental challenges have focused on the impact of these activities on the development of the infant and young child. This interest is grounded in the strong belief in concepts such as 'neuroplasticity' (discussed in detail in Chapter 3), coupled with ample evidence from animal research that changes in brain structure and function are associated with EI (Kolb et al. 2017). It is very important to provide young children with as much appropriate stimulation, and as many learning opportunities, as possible at a time when the brain is most receptive to those inputs and experiences.

Ideas about, and approaches to, the delivery of services to enhance neuroplasticity, remain essential. Clinical studies indicate that early intervention, aiming to tap into the infant's neuroplasticity, is associated with improved developmental outcome, in particular improved cognitive development (Spittle et al. 2015; Hadders-Algra et al. 2017; see Chapter 14).

Another perspective on how to think about the importance of early experience, and what kinds of 'interventions' to provide, is to recognize that any child, with any neurodevelopmental impairment, is likely to be at high risk of experiencing 'deprivation'. The term 'deprivation' is usually used to refer to caregiver neglect; however, what is meant by the use of this term in this context is a different dimension of 'deprivation' – namely deprivation of life experiences secondary to functional limitations associated with the underlying impairment.

As described in Part III of this book, typical development is an interactive ('transactional') process. That is, a child's emerging skills provide the raw material for experimentation, exploration, learning and development. It is easy to take much of that typical development for granted when it seems to emerge easily and without apparent effort. We can thus miss the incredible subtlety of what is happening *between* child and environment – especially the human environment around the child. The many environments to which a child is exposed every day may facilitate (or perhaps interfere with) the child's relentless efforts to exploit their developing capacities; for this reason, the role of 'environments' (human, physical, social, cultural, experiential) should be a major focus of much of our thinking in EI.

Consider an example. Imagine identical 24-month-old twins, one developing typically and the other with an impairment of mobility (and/or vision, or auditory capacity, or communication). How different are their day-to-day life experiences? How different are the challenges of parenting these otherwise identical children? The child with the impairments will be at considerable risk of being 'deprived' of some of the kinds of experience that the typical twin absorbs, apparently effortlessly. Insofar as 'parenting is a dance led by the child', raising a child with, or at risk of, an impairment is considerably more complex, because the child does not 'dance' (i.e. develop) easily, or perhaps dances to a rhythm that caregivers do not easily perceive. As a consequence, caregivers often don't know how best to exploit what the child *can* do, in whatever ways are easiest for them.

Many professionals believe that families have a difficult job when raising a child with a developmental disorder. It should be recognized that caregivers receive considerable, sometimes conflicting, information about their child's situation, and advice about interventions; they are expected to follow all that advice; and in at least some circumstances both professionals and the caregivers themselves may believe that a child's slow developmental progress is 'caused by' inadequate implementation of intervention at home. This idea is inappropriate, and casts parents in a poor light! It likely reflects clinicians' lack of experience with, and understanding about, how children with challenges in early life, or those with identifiable impairments, may follow a different developmental path, and how different the parenting experiences might be when the child is developing along their own path.

In reality, many factors affect this developmental journey, but are at times not taken into account. These include the well-being of families with whom we work, and their experiences of professionals. Many professionals are aware of the importance of family's circumstances, but despite a considerable body of work on Family-Centred Service (FCS) and evidence of its value to families (King et al. 1997, 1998, 1999, 2004; Rosenbaum et al. 1998; Rosenbaum 2011; Law et al. 2003, 2005; Akhbari Ziegler et al. 2019), it is often challenging for professionals to feel comfortable in knowing how to address and accommodate family realities. Professionals have a responsibility to engage with families on their own terms. That includes sharing knowledge about the child's condition, and especially about how that condition is affecting this specific child (as opposed to what we know about 'the condition' itself). We also need to give the family information about management options that are relevant to their individual reality. There is an increasing expectation that professionals include family members as equal partners in the intervention process and use the goals of the family as a starting point of the intervention. If EI is offered in such a way that family members have the possibility to explore their own goals and capacity to support the child's development within daily routines, intervention may be accommodated best to the family's life circumstances.

The literature on EI for infants and children is extensive, as discussed and reviewed elsewhere in this book. On the other hand, the impact of EI on caregiver and family well-being has received less attention, and generally focuses on caregivers dealing with the situation of a young infant 'at risk' of developmental challenges (Benzies et al. 2013; Van Wassenaer-Leemhuis et al. 2016). The rest of this chapter explores how EI can be used to address the challenges and dilemmas of *parents*, and to consider ways of assessing the benefits of this aspect of professional services for caregivers and families as well as children. These perspectives are seen to be complementary to our interest in promoting a child's best development. They simply focus on the other partner in the parent–child dyad and on parent–child interaction, to reflect on how our advice and services can be made as specific for parents' growth and development as for the child's.

This chapter next explores 'EI' from a caregiver perspective. This is followed by considerations on how professionals can identify ways to be helpful to and supportive of caregivers. The authors outline current work underway to explore these ideas with research to evaluate the impact of these new developments. Finally, the chapter concludes with recommendations for further research.

PERSPECTIVES ON EARLY INTERVENTION FOR PARENTS

Parents as the Focus of Our Work

Professionals who work in the field of child development, and particularly those whose focus is children with or at risk of developmental challenges, easily understand the rationale for EI and the techniques to be applied to try to enhance children's development. Parents, on the other hand, usually know considerably less about the nuances of child development, especially in the context of impairments that interfere with a child's typical development (as described above). However, parents are the experts on their own child's abilities and needs – something that professionals need to recognize and take into account by listening to parents' observations of their child under the myriad of circumstances in which they see them every day. For this reason, it is important to begin our relationship with a family with a consideration of the needs, desires, visions, and goals of parents whose children are the usual target of our EI services.

The most obvious reality – perhaps *so* obvious that it is simply assumed and taken for granted – is that we work with *parents in their roles as caregivers*, and it is their 'predicaments' (that is, their child's impairments, or risk thereof) that we need to understand. However skilled we are as professionals, it is the caregivers who are expected to incorporate our recommended EI activities as part of their child's and family's daily life. This implies, as noted earlier, that professionals understand the principles and practices of FCS in order to be able, optimally, to integrate parents as active partners in the intervention process. In addition, it implies that the focus of our guidance is the family as a unit and not only the child. Thus, we first need to know what the family members have been told, and what they understand, about the developmental situation that led to their child's referral to our services. We may also need to apply principles of 'coaching' to help parents understand how best to build our ideas into their roles as parents.

Sharing Diagnostic and Prognostic Information

It is usually the legal responsibility of doctors and licenced psychologists to convey diagnoses or even concerns about 'risk for' something, and to explain the language and labels we use about children's developmental impairments and their prognosis (see Chapter 14). It should be realized that the issue of 'truth disclosure' – often colloquially referred to as 'telling bad news' – is an area of training that is not done nearly as well as it could be for many professionals. Families often report how our failures to offer honest and open communication create extra worries for them. There is a considerable literature about both the content and the processes of this activity as done by professionals (two powerful essays are those of Siegler [1975] and Cassel [1982]; see also Chapter 2). Thus, if caregivers have been given a bleak prognosis about their child's future – what people sometimes refer to as a 'catalogue of doom' about all the things their child is unlikely to be able to accomplish – they can be forgiven for lacking enthusiasm to apply the best of our ideas about EI.

EI as Part of a Process

We believe that everyone working with a child and family has a responsibility to be involved in these processes as they concern and involve parents. There is, in particular, a special opportunity for allied health and social services professionals to be helpful, at least in part because their engagement with families is usually longer and deeper than that of doctors. These professionals can both listen for, and ask about, how parents are understanding their child's situation, and share this understanding (and, sadly, often misunderstanding) with the child and family's team. However, it should be realized that active listening, asking questions, and provision of relevant information are coaching strategies that have to be learned and practised by the health professionals, as many current curricula of health professionals' basic education do not include these skills. Helping caregivers to be on the same (hopefully realistically optimistic) page as the EI team must be an early and ongoing goal if we expect caregivers to follow through with and apply the EI activities and tools that are known, at their best, to contribute to children's development.

Promoting EI requires professionals to recognize that parents face an impossible challenge: knowing how much EI is 'enough'? Service providers should consider that EI can be both time-consuming and stressful for parents. It is therefore essential to communicate with parents what EI realistically can and cannot be expected to do. For example, will it 'fix' the child? Is doing more going to yield better results? The belief that 'more is better' can be extremely stressful and, in fact, detrimental to families if it entails investing all of family life in EI and potentially depriving parents and children of meaningful and fun family time.

Do We Need a Diagnosis to Start EI?

An issue that often leads to much discussion among professionals is whether there needs to be a formal 'diagnosis' before starting EI. For the authors of this chapter, the answer is: 'absolutely not' (Rosenbaum 2019). If a young child and the family have experienced challenges in the pregnancy, delivery, or early postnatal period, parents will be well aware of 'risks' – and even without a specific diagnosis, the family is likely to be very responsive to input that supports them and their child's development. Similarly, if an infant is already demonstrating some atypical patterns of development or behaviours, parents are often aware of that fact and want support – again, even without a formal diagnosis. Many developmental paths in childhood lead to adulthood (including the considerable variation in 'quantity' (milestones) and 'quality' (style) of development). When offering guidance to families, there is a shared understanding that we are observing and assessing the child's development, but not waiting for 'something to be wrong' with a formal diagnosis. Furthermore, with a few exceptions (such as constraint-induced movement therapy), most of our developmental interventions are not condition- or diagnosis-specific. Rather, what we are offering with EI is based on principles such as family support, 'child development', and 'neurological plasticity', and not on the diagnostic label.

At the same time, health professionals must be attuned to the reality that the absence of a specific diagnosis can create tensions for parents and families. In this situation of uncertainty, parents are sailing between hope and anxiety. Parents want to have a diagnosis, a number, a code, or some other clear indication of the issues their child faces – something that will give them an 'explanation' for the situation they are in, and an idea of what specific issues to consider with that condition. For many people, the uncertainly associated with 'not knowing' is a huge source of stress. Parents have said 'It is worse to not know than to know the worst'. This may be true even in cases when the diagnosis is a serious condition with a poor prognosis. Receiving a specific diagnosis may, for many people, provide a guidepost that reveals to them what to do and where to go.

Communication Skills Are an Essential Element of All EI

Because of the challenges outlined above, we must pay special attention to the communication and rapport-building between parents and clinicians at this time of uncertainty. Without sensitive awareness of the impact of lack of diagnosis, parents may have doubts about the clinicians' competencies, the validity and effectiveness of proposed interventions, clinicians' reasoning, and so on. Among the many strategies in our communication should be to remind families that we are continuing to seek clear and precise answers by watching the child's progress and pursuing appropriate clinical tests; and that, regardless of the diagnosis, we are always following principles of child development. These concepts, which we may or may not share with families, include the neuromotor principles derived from the Neuronal Group Selection Theory (NGST) like variation, exploration, and trial-and-error experiences (see Chapter 3) and the Concept Grounded Cognition (Lobo et al. 2013) that underlines the importance of object interaction, sitting and locomotion for cognitive development – our guides in the advice we offer.

Assessment and Communication as Ongoing Processes

Caregivers' understanding of their child's development, and ours, evolves with time, development, learning, etc. This leads us to ask: How do we counsel and advise as time passes, and things change in this 'moving target' that includes the developing child and their increasingly informed caregivers? Given a relationship-directed form of intervention, based on principles of family-centred service, we may assume that the caregivers are active partners in the intervention process and that they are able to make informed decisions. They are able to formulate their needs, and health professionals are able to coach them to find adaptive solutions for these needs. It is worth noting that professionals (and extended family members) who see the child episodically may have an odd advantage: they may recognize change and development of which the parents, who are there all the time, are less aware! This insight may also be turned into a recommendation to caregivers, that is, to advise them to use their cell phones to record their child's performance from time to time, and then to review these recordings to see how far they and their child have come.

OPPORTUNITIES TO BE HELPFUL TO THE FAMILY

Let Parents Be Parents, and Don't Make Them Therapists

Parents often express concerns about feeling as though they are being expected, by professionals, to be their child's *therapist*, when what they want is to be *parents*. It is likely that, in the past, in our enthusiasm to encourage the application of 'therapies', we have conveyed this expectation of 'parent-as-therapist' too eagerly. One hopes that 20 years into the 21st century, with so much emphasis on FCS (Rosenbaum et al. 1998) and relationship-directed forms of intervention, contemporary clinicians are more sensitive to these perceptions by parents, and more able to engage with them in equal partnerships. We believe that continuing professional development is needed to achieve a full implementation, into daily health care, of relationship-directed forms of EI based on the principles of family-centred practice. The goal is to enhance the family's capacity to participate as an equal and active partner in the intervention process of their child with special needs. This may be achieved by the health professional taking on the role of coach: the professional does not tell the family members what they have to do best, but creates explorative situations, so that the family members may discover for themselves how best to implement principles of developmental stimulation in daily life (Akhbari Ziegler et al. 2019; Akhbari Ziegler and Hadders-Algra 2020).

Remember the Extended Family – Especially the Grandparents

It is important to remind ourselves that very few families live in a vacuum, and that every family belongs to one or more social circles that are fundamentally important to them. People who are most likely to be involved in the family's life are extended family members. This raises the question: how do – how should – professionals be involved with a child's extended family?

Grandparents, in particular, should be recognized for their potential involvement with and influence on the child and caregivers (Novak-Pavlic et al. 2020). They have a unique position with respect to the nuclear family, insofar as they are both the grandparents to the infant or child receiving EI, and the parent to one of their grandchild's caregivers! This dynamic has led to the concept that grandparents may experience 'double grief' (Rush and Shelden 2011), and feel distress about both the infant or child and their own (adult) child's predicament. Given the complexity of these interconnections – and, of course, depending on the nature of pre-existing family dynamics – grandparents may play essential roles with the nuclear family. Therefore, their involvement, perspectives, beliefs, and resources can have a powerful impact on the caregivers and, in turn, on the child. Consider a few possible scenarios in which the grandparents' influence can play out.

At the positive end of the continuum, with warm family relationships, supportive grandparents may provide resources of time, money, experience, wisdom, and engagement with their adult child, grandchild, and family. They may be in a position to offer comfort, material resources, perspectives on life in general, and parenting. On the other side of the ledger, grandparents and their adult children may be estranged; in this circumstance, none of the supports outlined above will be available to the nuclear family.

Even more complex are those situations in which the child's caregivers and grandparents are connected in some ways, perhaps enmeshed, but where there are important differences of opinion and tensions about the child's situation. Caregivers might find themselves caught in a vice between professionals' perspectives and advice and their own parents' or in-laws' views that are substantially different. In this kind of scenario grandparents might, for example, have worries far beyond objective reality; on the other hand, they may deny or try to minimize the reality of a complex situation, and in so doing, challenge the professionals' advice and counsel. More importantly, this kind of situation can create confusion for the caregivers by undermining what they are wanting to do. A further potential complexity, regardless of the pre-existing family dynamics, is that grandparents' perceptions and experiences of 'disability' may be out of date with respect to current concepts and thinking about these same issues (such as those presented in this book).

This dynamic may work the other way around as well. Caregivers who are trying to navigate the family relationships often struggle with how to share the news about their child's condition and health with their own parents and families. They are often emotionally and mentally torn between clinicians' and their own parents' opinions and suggestions.

As professionals, how can we be helpful? We need to listen carefully to caregivers, including how they talk about their supports. In a situation in which caregivers are dealing with and adapting to their child's developmental challenges, the additional burden of managing family relationships can be easily pre-vented by encouraging – welcoming, with caregivers' permission – the involvement of significant family members at clinical appointments or home visits. This idea may provide a win-win situation for both the families and clinicians. In situations where extended family members are highly involved and accompany the family, clinicians are more likely to hear multiple perspectives on the child's development and family functioning. At the same time, the extended family members are given the opportunity to address their concerns and receive relevant information they need. With the clinicians' knowledge and authority, caregivers do not have to take the (sometimes burdensome) responsibility for conveying and 'tailoring' the information to grandparents.

Collaborative Identification of Issues and Goal-setting

One implication of embracing a family-centred philosophy is the importance of joint goal-setting with parents. As expert clinicians, we can often see 'problems' and 'issues' right from the start and begin to formulate an approach to intervention for those issues. Before we do that, however, we need to ask about, and understand, the caregivers' overall concerns about their child's predicament, and their own immediate goals. For example, a child may have a challenge with mobility, for which a range of appropriate inter-ventions is available. If, however, the caregivers are currently most concerned about feeding, that must be our first target for intervention. Gaining a family's trust is essential, and forms a platform on which to build a working relationship. Also, as noted above, we need to help caregivers be creative in how they interweave what we might think of as 'therapies' into their 'parenting', play and daily life with their child and family. This implies that the focus of the intervention has to be on the family as a unit and especially on the caregiver–infant interaction during daily care-giving activities of the family members, including siblings, in naturally occurring caregiving situations (Dirks and Hadders-Algra 2011). Furthermore, supporting caregiver–infant interaction in daily life in an enriched real-life environment may help to minimize social deprivation of young children with special needs. In fact, an important aim of EI is to enhance caregivers' joy in interacting, communicating and playing with the child.

In addition, health professionals should not hesitate to identify the benefits of assistive devices, including power mobility and augmentative communication, both of which may, in the right circum-stances, help to reduce the risk of 'deprivation' discussed earlier in this chapter. We can discuss with family members the idea that a major goal could be 'promoting development and supporting the growth of independence'. Doing so provides a narrative that differs from – and may well be more palatable than – expecting parents to provide 'therapies' that are aimed at 'fixing' an impairment or promoting 'normal' development (Rosenbaum and Gorter 2012).

Current Approaches to Family-based Interventions: The Example of COPCA

'COPing with and CAring for infants with special needs' (COPCA) is an innovative family-centred early intervention program based on principles of family-centred care (Dirks et al. 2011) and the NGST (Chapter 3). COPCA has two objectives: (1) to empower the individual family in processes of decision-making regarding participation in daily life, and (2) to promote activities and partici-pation of the infant with special needs. The latter also includes optimizing the motor capacities of the infant as a means for the child to explore interactions with persons and objects (i.e. social and cognitive development) (Akhbari Ziegler et al. 2019; see also Chapters 6 and 14). The key elements of COPCA's family component are family autonomy, family responsibility, and family-specific par-enting. COPCA aims to encourage the family's own capacities to stimulate the infant's development during daily care in naturally occurring parenting situations (Dirks et al. 2011). In the COPCA approach, caregivers remain caregivers and do not become therapists. COPCA's main intervention strategy involves coaching family members (Dirks et al. 2011; Dirks and Hadders-Algra 2011; Akhbari Ziegler et al. 2019). The coach aims at understanding parental needs. This forms the basis for providing the family with information required to make informed decisions. In this way, families develop new skills that may enhance well-being and participation of the whole family, including the child with, or at risk of, a disability. COPCA uses the principles of the NGST to inform the families about the needs of the infant with atypical motor development for ample opportunities for self-produced motor behaviour, variation, and trial-and-error experiences to promote motor, cognitive, and social development (Chapters 3 and 6). During coaching sessions at home using shared observation, family members may explore and develop their own strategies to cope in daily life with the situation of having an infant with special needs. These strategies offer the possibility for the parents to explore what their young child can do and how they can best support the development of their young child (see Text Box 12.1).

The communication between family members and coach is open, and relationships are based on equal partnership and confidence. The coach listens, asks reflective questions, and provides suggestions to challenge the infant. Positive feedback is used to confirm, clarify, and explore any needs to attain a goal. The caregivers are informed that development proceeds by means of trial-and-error and self-produced activity requiring ample time and practice. Studies on the effectiveness of COPCA in infants at high risk of developmental disorders showed that elements of the COPCA approach, in particular caregiver coaching and challenging the infant to perform motor actions himself or herself, were associated with a better cognitive and functional outcome at 18 months (Blauw-Hospers et al. 2011; Hielkema et al. 2011) and with enhanced family empowerment (Hielkema et al. 2019).

Text Box 12.1 An Example of COPCA Intervention

COPCA coach Jane is introduced to Peter and his family. Peter is 12 months old, and a friendly boy with general developmental delay due to an unidentified genetic syndrome. Apart from Peter, Peter's family consists of mother, father, and Susan, Peter's 4-year-old sister. The family lives on the third floor of an apartment building. Both parents have a part-time job; they share caregiving activities. They have a supportive bond with their own living parents, father's father and mother's mother. However, the grandparents are not able to participate in caregiving activities on a regular basis as they live at a distance of 70 to 100 kilometres.

Peter's mother tells Jane that she would like to participate with both children in the activities on the playground near the apartment building. However, she admits, she has no idea how to tackle this problem, as Peter cannot sit independently and expresses his wishes and discomfort by just a few simple sounds. Therefore, the mother and the COPCA coach decide to go with Peter and Susan to the sandbox on the playground. There, guided by tips and hints of the COPCA coach, the mother explores how Peter may sit in the sand by building a sand chair for him with Susan's help. The COPCA coach also informs the mother how they can experiment with the amount of postural support the sand chair provides. The mother, Peter, and Susan discover what they can do together in the sandbox, and how the joint handling of the sand is fun for all. Their joyful sounds soon attract other children, who also join the building and playing activities in the sand.

After half an hour, the family members and the coach return to the family's apartment. Peter's mother happily tells the coach that she has now discovered how – as a family – they can explore these kinds of activities and how easily and nicely other children respond to Peter and Susan.

The COPCA session shows how the family was empowered in participation and the infant was offered opportunities to practise motor, cognitive, and social skills.

Current Work in Progress with Parents: ENabling VISion and Growing Expectations (ENVISAGE)

The issues outlined in this chapter to this point are based on decades of clinical experience and recent research with families at the beginning of their journey raising a child with any neurodisability. They form part of the foundation of a research program ('ENVISAGE') that has been co-created by the first author's CanChild research group and Australian colleagues, and includes parents as co-developers and co-researchers. The program involves five weekly on-line 'virtual' interactive workshops with five to seven parents working with a researcher and a parent facilitator. As this chapter is being prepared, the ENVISAGE program is under evaluation with parents in both Canada and Australia.

The premise behind ENVISAGE is the belief that parents will be better able to navigate their journey in the choppy waters of 'childhood disability' if they can experience that journey more clearly with the guidance of modern ideas about health, child development and family well-being. From our work to date with Envisage, it is our impression that parents find it helpful when service providers validate their views, experiences, and goals, and give them a language to articulate these (as in the case with the 'F-words' in childhood disability – function, family, fitness, fun, friendships, and future [Rosenbaum and Gorter 2012]).

The themes of the ENVISAGE program include the following ideas, (and the thinking behind them):

(i)   Session 1 provides an introduction to the WHO's framework for health (the International Classification of Functioning, Disability and Health [the ICF]) and the operationalization of these ideas with the 'F-words in child development' (Rosenbaum and Gorter 2012). There is considerable evidence that these ideas resonate with families and service providers, and that they provide ways of contextualizing what we are recommending and why.

(ii)   Session 2 promotes the importance of 'development' (of child and family) as a focus for all our interventions. This theme is based on the idea that we work in the field of 'developmental disability' – and too easily forget the essential first word, despite the fact that development is, or is very likely to be, compromised because of the 'disability'.

(iii)   Session 3 presents a discussion of parenting, especially in the context of developmental differences. The point of this session is to talk about parenting a child with an impairment, whose developmental 'dance' may be compromised by impairment in *any* aspect of development (sensory, motor, cognitive, etc.) and thus make the child a harder child for parents to 'parent'.

(iv)   Session 4 addresses the importance of caregivers taking care of their own health. This session is designed to give caregivers 'permission' to be aware of, and care for, their own physical, mental, marital, family, and spiritual needs, because parenting a child with an impairment is a marathon and not a sprint.

(v)   In Session 5, caregivers are offered ideas about communication, collaboration and connections with others. This final session is designed to empower caregivers to acquiring the skills and strategies that are essential when families need to work with people and systems (e.g. education, recreation, community organizations, government agencies, etc.) because of their child's and family's special issues.

The outcomes being evaluated in the ENVISAGE study are all caregiver-reported accounts of their mental health, their experience of services and their self-perceptions of their approaches to parenting. It is important to state that there is no assumption or expectation that the ENVISAGE program should replace EI for infants and young children, as discussed and promoted in this book. Rather, we see an important complementarity between this proposed approach to 'early intervention for caregivers' and the advice we have to offer to families about their infant or young child with, or at risk of, impaired development. The elements of Envisage (i) focus on the well-being of parents (since the child is always part of a larger family unit), and (ii) focus on the importance of meaningful activities/opportunities to explore their world (through the F-words/ICF framework).

Once a proof of concept of the ENVISAGE program has been established, future studies are planned to explore the impact of this parent-directed program on children's development by assessing a host of child-specific functions before and after caregivers undertake ENVISAGE. If, in fact, engagement with ENVISAGE provides additional evidence of value to 'early intervention', we may be in a position to recommend that we try to influence child development using this two-pronged approach to both child development and family wellbeing.

CONCLUDING REMARKS

It is a statement of the obvious, but 'EI' is an 'intervention'. This chapter identifies, for professionals, a number of issues about the family of the child receiving EI, and how consideration of these dimensions of the child and family's life can be helpful to everyone involved. Also, once again, it is important to stress that attention to the family dimensions of the EI story in no way diminishes the role of EI to enhance child development. Rather, this chapter focuses on the reality that any intervention offered to a child with an impairment must always be considered with an eye to its impact on the child *and* family.

REFERENCES

Akhbari Ziegler S, Dirks T, Hadders-Algra M (2019) Coaching in early physical therapy intervention: the COPCA program as an example of translation of theory into practice. *Disabil Rehabil* **41**: 1846–1854. doi: 10.1080/09638288.2018.1448468.

Akhbari Ziegler S, Hadders-Algra M (2020) Coaching approaches in early intervention and paediatric rehabilitation. *Dev Med Child Neurol* **62**: 569–574. doi: 10.1111/dmcn.14493.

Benzies KM, Magill-Evans JE, Hayden KA, Ballantyne M (2013) Key components of early intervention programs for preterm infants and their parents: a systematic review and meta-analysis. *BMC Pregnancy Childbirth* **13** (Suppl 1): S10. doi: 10.1186/1471-2393-13-S1-S10.

Blauw-Hospers CH, Dirks T, Hulshof LJ, Bos AF, Hadders-Algra M (2011) Pediatric physical therapy in infancy: from nightmare to dream? A two-arm randomized trial. *Phys Ther* **91**: 1323–1338. doi: 10.2522/ptj.20100205.

Cassel EJ (1982) The nature of suffering and the goals of medicine. *N Engl J Med* **306**: 129–142.

Dirks T, Hadders-Algra M (2011) The role of the family in intervention of infants at high risk of cerebral palsy: a systematic analysis. *Dev Med Child Neurol* **53**: 62–67. doi: 10.1111/j.1469-8749.2011.04067.x.

Dirks T, Blauw-Hospers CH, Hulshof LJ, Hadders-Algra M (2011) Differences between the family-centered 'COPCA' program and traditional infant physical therapy based on neurodevelopmental treatment principles. *Phys Ther* **91**: 1303–1322. doi: 10.2522/ptj.20100207.

Hadders-Algra M, Boxum AG, Hielkema T, Hamer EG (2017) Effect of early intervention in infants at very high risk of cerebral palsy – a systematic review. *Dev Med Child Neurol* **59**: 246–258. doi: 10.1111/dmcn.13331.

Hielkema T, Blauw-Hospers CH, Dirks T, Drijver-Messelink M, Bos AF, Hadders-Algra M (2011) Does physiotherapeutic intervention affect motor outcome in high-risk infants? An approach combining a randomized controlled trial and process evaluation. *Dev Med Child Neurol* **53**: e8–15. doi: 10.1111/j.1469-8749.2010.03876.x.

Hielkema T, Boxum AG, Hamer EG, et al. (2019) LEARN2MOVE 0–2 years, a randomized early intervention trial for infants at very high risk of cerebral palsy: family outcome and infant's functional outcome. *Disabil Rehabil*, epub ahead of print. doi: 10.1080/09638288.2019.1610509.

King G, King S, Rosenbaum P, Goffin R (1999) Family-centred caregiving and well-being of parents of children with disabilities: linking process with outcome. *J Pediatr Psychol* **24**: 41–52.

King G, Law M, King S, Rosenbaum P (1998) Parents' and service providers' perceptions of the family-centredness of children's rehabilitation services in Ontario. *Phys Occup Ther Pediatr* **18**: 21–40.

King G, Rosenbaum P, King S (1997) Evaluating family-centred service using a measure of parents' perceptions. *Child Care Hlth Dev* **23**: 47–62.

King S, Teplicky R, King G, Rosenbaum P (2004) Family-centered service for children with cerebral palsy and their families: a review of the literature. *Semin Pediatr Neurol* **11**: 78–86.

Kolb B, Harker A, Gibb R (2017) Principles of plasticity in the developing brain. *Dev Med Child Neurol* **59**: 1218–1223. doi: 10.1111/dmcn.13546.

Law M, Hanna S, King G, et al. (2003) Factors affecting family-centred service delivery for children with disabilities. *Child Care Hlth Dev* **29**: 357–366.

Law M, Teplicky R, King S, et al. (2005) Family-Centred Service: Moving Ideas into Practice. *Child: Care Hlth Dev* **31**: 633–642.

Lobo MA, Harbourne RT, Dusing SC, McCoy SW (2013) Grounding early intervention: physical therapy cannot just be about motor skills anymore. *Phys Ther* **93**: 94–103. doi: 10.2522/ptj.20120158.

Novak-Pavlic M, Abdel Malek S, Rosenbaum P, Macedo LG, Di Rezze B (2021) A scoping review of the literature on grandparents of children with disabilities. Disabil Rehabil, epub ahead of print. doi: 10.1080/09638288.2020.1857850.

Rosenbaum PL (2011) Family-centred research: what does it mean and can we do it? *Dev Med Child Neurol* **53**: 99–100. doi: 10.1111/j.1469-8749.2010.03871.x.

Rosenbaum PL (2019) Diagnosis in developmental disability: a perennial challenge, and a proposed middle ground. *Dev Med Child Neurol* **61**: 620. doi: 10.1111/dmcn.14216.

Rosenbaum PL, Gorter JW (2012) The 'F-words' in childhood disability: I swear this is how we should think! *Child Care Hlth Dev* **38**: 457–463. doi: 10.1111/j.1365-2214.2011.01338.x.

Rosenbaum P, King S, Law M, King G, Evans J (1998) Family-centred services: a conceptual framework and research review. *Phys Occup Ther Pediatr* **18**: 1–20.

Rush D, Shelden M (2011) Coaching families. In: Rush D, Shelden M, editors, *The Early Childhood Coaching Handbook*. Baltimore: Brookes Publishing Company, pp. 123–162.

Siegler M (1975) Pascal's wager and the hanging of crepe. *N Engl J Med* **293**: 853–857. doi: 10.1056/NEJM197510232931705.

Spittle A, Orton J, Anderson PJ, Boyd R, Doyle LW (2015). *Cochrane Database Syst Rev* **24**: 11. doi: 10.1002/14651858.CD005495.pub4.

van Wassenaer-Leemhuis AG, Jeukens-Visser M, van Hus JW et al. (2016) Rethinking preventive post-discharge intervention programmes for very preterm infants and their parents. *Dev Med Child Neurol* **58** (Suppl 4): 67–73. doi: 10.1111/dmcn.13049.

SUGGESTIONS FOR FURTHER READING

Akhbari Ziegler S, Mitteregger E, Hadders-Algra M (2020). Caregivers' experiences with the new family-centred paediatric physiotherapy programme COPCA: a qualitative study. *Child Care Hlth Dev* **46**: 28–36. doi: 10.1111/cch.12722.

Akhbari Ziegler S, Hadders-Algra M (2020). Akhbari Ziegler S, Hadders-Algra M (2020) Coaching approaches in early intervention and paediatric rehabilitation. *Dev Med Child Neurol* **62**: 569–574. doi: 10.1111/dmcn.14493.

Bamm EL, Rosenbaum P (2008) Family-centered theory: origins, development, barriers, and supports to implementation in rehabilitation medicine. *Arch Phys Med Rehabil* **89**: 1618–1624. doi: 10.1016/j.apmr.2007.12.034.

Dunst CJ, Boyd K, Trivette CM, Hamby DW (2002) Family-orientated program models and professional helpgiving practices. *Fam Relat* **51**: 221–229. doi: 10.1111/j.1741-3729.20002.00221.x.

Dunst C, Trivette C, Deal A (1988) *Enabling and Empowering Families – Principles and Guidelines for Practice*. Cambridge, MA: Brookline Books, Inc.

Dunst CJ, Trivette CM, Hamby DW (2007) Meta-analysis of family-centered helpgiving practices research. *Ment Retard Dev Disabil Res Rev* **13**: 370–378. doi: 10.1002/mrdd.20176.

Kemp P, Turnbull AP (2014) Coaching with parents in early intervention: an interdisciplinary research synthesis. *Infant Young Child* **27**: 305–324. doi: 10.1097/IYC.0000000000000018.

King G, Williams L, Hahn Goldberg S (2017) Family-oriented services in pediatric rehabilitation: a scoping review and framework to promote parent and family wellness. *Child Care Hlth Dev* **43**: 334–347. doi.org/10.1111/cch.12435.

Kokorelias KM, Gignac MAM, Naglie G, Cameron JI (2019) Towards a universal model of family centered care: a scoping review. *BMC Health Serv Res* **19**: 564. https://doi.org/10.1186/s12913-019-4394-5.

Kuo DZ, Houtrow AJ, Arango P, Kuhlthau KA, Simmons JM, Neff JM (2012) Family-centered care: current applications and future directions in pediatric health care. *Matern Child Health J.* **16**: 297–305. doi: 10.1007/s10995-011-0751-7.

Kruijsen-Terpstra AJA, Ketelaar M, Boeije H, et al. (2014) Parents' experiences with physical and occupational therapy for their young child with cerebral palsy: a mixed studies review. *Child Care Health Dev* **40**: 787–796. doi: 10.1111/cch.12097

MacKean GL, Thurston WE, Scott CM (2005) Bridging the divide between families and health professionals' perspectives on family-centred care. Health Expectations **8**: 74–85. https://doi.org/10.1111/j.1369-7625.2005.00319.x.

Rosenbaum P (2016) Developmental disability: shouldn't grandparents have a place at the table? *Dev Med Child Neurol* **58**: 5280528. doi.org/10.1111/dmcn.13125.

Rush D, Shelden M (2011) *The Early Childhood Coaching Handbook*. Baltimore: Brookes Publishing Company.

Terwiel M, Alsem MW, Siebes RC, Bieleman K, Verhoef M, Ketelaar M (2017) Family-centred service: differences in what parents of children with cerebral palsy rate important. *Child Care Health Dev* **43**: 663–669. doi: 10.1111/cch.12460.

Early Intervention in the Neonatal Period

Mijna Hadders-Algra

SUMMARY POINTS

- Medically fragile infants, such as infants born preterm or infants with a complex congenital heart disease, are at high risk of neurodevelopmental disorders. Their parents experience high rates of anxiety, stress, and depression.
- Major approaches in the neonatal intensive care unit to promote infant and family outcome consist of family involvement and developmental care.
- Family involvement in the care of medically fragile infants gradually evolves from family-centred care, in which parents mainly have a supportive role and professionals provide most care, to family-integrated care in which parents provide all except the most advanced medical care for their infants. More parental involvement is associated with better family and infant outcome.
- Developmental care primarily aims at promoting parent–infant interaction and stress reduction. It may be applied as the comprehensive model of Neonatal Individualized Developmental Care and Assessment Programme (NIDCAP) or by means of a selection of its components, such as coaching of parent–infant interaction and encouragement of skin-to-skin contact, breastfeeding, nesting, and swaddling.
- Developmental care has a positive effect on the young infant's brain and development. However, no evidence is available that it promotes development beyond the age of 4 months post-term.
- Specific infant directed interventions, such as infant massage, multisensory stimulation, or developmental physiotherapy, may have a minor beneficial effect on the infant's neurodevelopmental condition up to and including term age, but most likely not on the infant's development post-term.
- Research demonstrated that the use of helmet therapy for plagiocephaly does not improve developmental outcome. As application of helmets is associated with side effects, their use is not recommended.

Neonatal care for premature or critically ill newborns, including infants with hypoxic-ischaemic encephalopathy, has dramatically improved since the introduction of assisted ventilation in the seventies of last century (Owen et al. 2017). But not only the infant's medical care made giant leaps, also a major shift occurred in the role of the family. It changed from parents visiting their infant in the neonatal intensive care unit (NICU) only twice a week to the family's daily presence near the infant and involvement in the infant's daily care, extending at many places to an round-the-clock presence (Harrison 1993; Gooding et al. 2011; White 2011; Griffiths et al. 2019).

Notwithstanding the major improvements in perinatal and neonatal care, premature infants and critically ill newborns are at high risk of neurodevelopmental disorders (Allotey et al. 2018; Huisenga et al. 2020). Their parents are prone to stress and anxiety (Mackay et al. 2020). This chapter reviews the strategies used during the infant's stay in the NICU to improve the outcome of the infant and family. The first part addresses developmental care in general, the second part discusses the role of the family, whereas the third part reviews interventional elements that focus especially on infant development. The following section addresses interventions to prevent and to manage plagiocephaly. The chapter ends with concluding remarks.

It should be realized that virtually all intervention studies carried out in the NICU have been performed in preterm infants. Most likely, most intervention strategies that are favourable for preterm newborns will also be beneficial for other medically fragile infants, such as term newborns with hypoxic-ischaemic encephalopathy or complex congenital heart disease. However, this may not always be the case, as the study of Puumala et al. (2020) illustrated: preterm infants fared clinically better in a single family room than in an open-bay NICU, but a similar profit was absent in critically ill term and post-term infants.

DEVELOPMENTAL CARE

Strategies of Developmental Care

Developmental care was introduced in the NICU in the 1980s, a development that was largely facilitated by the work of Heidelise Als (Als et al. 1986, 1994; Als and Gilkerson 1997). She understood that the preterm infant and his parents face a multitude of problems (Fig. 13.1). Being born preterm implies that many organ systems are not yet prepared to cope with extrauterine life. Examples are the preterm's immature lungs, their immature blood pressure regulation and their immature vascular autoregulation in the brain (Gardner et al. 2015; Volpe et al. 2017). In response to this situation, the infant receives life-support assistance in the highly medicalised and technological environment of the NICU. Both the infant's physiological instability caused by the immature organ systems and the technical NICU environment are sources of stress for the infant. The physiological instability, the stress, and their combination may result in major or minor alterations of the brain. The NICU situation is not only stressful for the infant, but also for the parents. The stress starts at the unexpected and untimely birth of the infant, and continues in the medical environment of the NICU (Fig. 13.1).

A major contribution of Als was her introduction in the NICU of standardized behavioural observations of the preterm infant. The behavioural observations allow parents and caregivers to understand the infant's cues, including his signs of stress, and to appreciate the infant's competencies to deal with various caregiving situations, such as feeding, changing a diaper, and feeding.

Current developmental care basically aims at (1) improved parent–infant interaction and bonding, (2) stress reduction, and (3) provision of a supportive environment. To this end, a mix of strategies is used, which vary from involvement of parents as primary caregivers and education of parents and professionals about preterm behaviour, to noise reduction, cycled lightning, skin-to-skin care, swaddling, cue-based care, and clustering of care activities to protect sleep, reduce painful procedures, and promote breastfeeding (Table 13.1; see also Sweeney et al. 2010). Als and colleagues designed a general programme of developmental care, the Neonatal Individualized Developmental Care and Assessment Programme (NIDCAP; Als and Gilkerson 1997), whereas others apply various combinations of the components of developmental care.

The developmental care components summarized in Table 13.1 have been associated with better short-term clinical outcomes of the infant, such as shorter stay in the hospital and improved weight

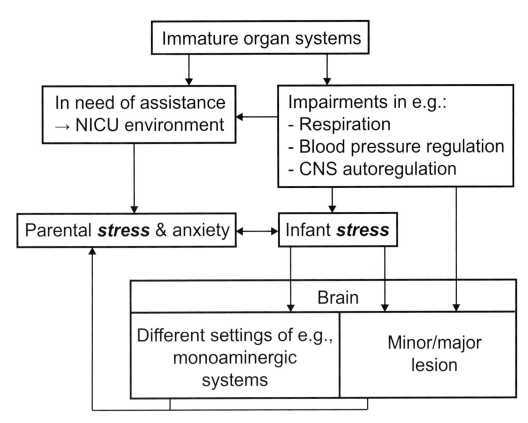

Figure 13.1   Diagram illustrating the pathways of stress and stressful events occurring after preterm birth. The monoaminergic systems (e.g. the dopaminergic, noradrenergic, and serotonergic system) are characterized by their widespread projections to the spinal cord and the cortex.

gain (Griffiths et al. 2019). Also NIDCAP – as a comprehensive program – reduces hospital length of stay and increases daily weight gain (Ohlsson and Jacobs 2013). However, NIDCAP has not been associated with a reduction of chronic lung disease, intraventricular haemorrhage, retinopathy of prematurity, and necrotizing enterocolitis, nor with weight at term age and beyond (Ohlsson and Jacobs 2013).

Effects of Developmental Care on Neurodevelopment

The data on the effects of developmental care on the infant's neurodevelopmental outcome are heterogeneous, which makes it hard to obtain evidence on the effectiveness of strategies.

NIDCAP applied in low-risk preterm infants has been associated with beneficial effects on electroencephalographic and magnetic resonance imaging parameters of brain development at term age (Buehler et al. 1995; Als et al. 2004). Yet, the systematic review and meta-analyses of Ohlsson and Jacobs (2013) demonstrated that the effect of NIDCAP on developmental outcome was limited to a minimal and transient positive effect on motor and cognitive outcome at 9 months. (Recall that ages in this book always refer to corrected ages (unless otherwise indicated).) NIDCAP was not associated with a consistent beneficial effect on developmental outcome at later ages (Ohlsson and Jacobs 2013).

Table 13.1   Developmental care in the NICU: strategies with strong recommendations

Domains	Specific examples
Parent–infant closeness and interaction	– 24hr per day parental access – Early and continuous skin-to-skin contact with parents (kangaroo care); also during painful procedures – Family-centred care – (Single) family rooms – Support of parents to observe and interpret their infant's behaviour – Involve parents as primary caregivers – Provision of parents with education and support to improve parent–infant interactions through, for example, play or reading – Shared decision-making – Availability of parental psychological support
Sensory environment, including pain and stress	– Protection from deleterious stimuli: reduction of ambient noise; single family rooms; minimization of procedural exposures to pain and/or stress – Use of positive sensory stimulation: use of the human voice, during interaction and, for example, during painful procedures; reading to the infant – Procedures that have protective and stimulating components: swaddling to reduce stress and promote self-regulation; provision of postural support; use of slow and gentle movements during caregiving activities
Sleep	– Promotion and protection of sleep (postponement of elective procedures during sleep; appropriate timing of caregiving activities)
Feeding	– Breast is best; first suck feed is preferably a breastfeed – Counselling of mothers on the importance of human milk

See https://newborn-health-standards.org and the best practice guidelines of Griffiths et al. (2019).

Of the single strategies, the effect of skin-to-skin contact on child development has been investigated best. Skin-to-skin contact has been associated with more mature electrophysiological parameters of brain maturation at term age. The meta-analysis of Akbari et al. (2018) indicated that Kangaroo care – often used as a synonym of skin-to-skin care – was associated with better infant self-regulation during the first four months after term age. However, Kangaroo care was not associated with improved neurodevelopment during the rest of the first year. On the other hand, Pineda et al. (2018) reported that increased duration of skin-to-skin care was associated with better scores on gross motor development at 4–5 years. Yet, similar associations with scores on other developmental domains were absent.

Reduction of stress is one of the main principles of developmental care. However, few studies addressed whether interventions aimed at stress reduction for the infant are associated with better developmental outcome. The PremieStart Program evaluated whether training parents to be sensitive to infant stress and to adapt their own interactional behaviour accordingly was associated with a better outcome. The study showed that the intervention resulted in a better microstructure of the brain's white matter at term age (Milgrom et al. 2010). However, when the children were re-assessed at 2 and 4.5 years of age the PremieStart Program was not associated with better cognitive or behavioural outcome (Milgrom et al. 2019). Most studies on neonatal stress and neurodevelopment evaluated associations between the two. It has been shown that nurse handling activities are associated with increased levels of infant physiological stress (Zeiner et al. 2016) and that higher degrees of stress exposure are associated with less mature electrophysiological parameters of brain development at term age (Smith et al. 2011). However, it should be kept in mind that the most severely ill infants also experience the most stress-inducing events. The long-term follow-up studies reported below adjusted as well as possible for this potential confounding.

They quantified neonatal stress by calculating the number of skin-breaking procedures (e.g. heel lance, peripheral intravenous or central line insertion, chest-tube insertion, tape removal, and nasogastric tube insertion). Increased levels of these skin-breaking procedures were associated with reduced cortical thickness (in particular, frontally and parietally), reduced cerebellar volumes in specific subregions, and an altered microstructure of the white matter (Ranger et al. 2013, 2015; Vinall et al. 2014). The latter two abnormalities were associated with lower intelligence quotient scores at school age (Vinall et al. 2014; Ranger et al. 2015), and the reduced cerebellar volumes also with impaired visuomotor integration (Ranger et al. 2015). In addition, the number of skin-breaking procedures was associated with reduced volumes of the thalamus, amygdala, and hippocampus. These reduced volumes were associated with poorer cognitive, visual-motor, and behavioural performances at school age (Chau et al. 2019).

The systematic reviews by Morag and Ohlsson (2016) and Almadhoob and Ohlsson (2016) indicated that cycled lighting and noise reduction had an unclear effect on infants' well-being and development.

Finally, some studies addressed the effect of nesting and swaddling. Maguire et al. (2009) reported that nesting and positioning had no significant effect on growth and development at 1 and 2 years of age. More recent studies focussed on the application of alternative positioning aids ('sleeping bag devices') made of stretchable cotton designed to provide containment while allowing the infant to move freely, similar to the uterine situation. The first studies suggested that the application of such stretchable positioning aids may be associated with a slightly better neuromotor outcome at term age (Madlinger-Lewis et al. 2014; Kitase et al. 2017). However, no long-term outcome data are available.

THE FAMILY AND DEVELOPMENTAL CARE

Parents of medically fragile infants, including infants born preterm and infants with complex congenital heart disease, perceive feelings of guilt, loss, helplessness, and stress that may affect bonding and attachment. The stress, the technological NICU environment, and the fragile infant's behaviour interfere with a proper development of the parental role and may result in parental posttraumatic stress (Brett et al. 2011; Benzies et al. 2013; Mackay et al. 2020).

Gradually, as the evidence was accumulating that increased parental engagement is associated with improved parent-infant interaction and a reduction of parental stress and anxiety (Brett et al. 2011; Benzies et al. 2013; Mackay et al. 2020), families were increasingly involved in the care of the medically fragile infants. Over time, three approaches to family involvement were developed – in general, designed for the care of very preterm infants, that is, infants before 32 weeks of gestation (see Table 13.2 for details):

- *Family-centred care:* parents are encouraged to participate in the care of their infant, especially by providing skin-to-skin contact and breastfeeding; parents are taught about principles of developmental care and parent–infant interaction; parent-to-parent contact is promoted and educational seminars provided (Gooding et al. 2011).
- *Family centred developmental care:* this approach takes the family-centred care principles one step further by involving family members as important persons in providing developmental care of the infant (Craig et al. 2015).
- *Family integrated care:* parents are encouraged to provide all care for their fragile infant, except for the most advanced medical care, such as adjustment of the continuous positive airway pressure or oxygen levels; this contrasts with the other forms of family centred care in which the health professionals provide most of the infant's care; parents take their role of primary caregiver and are coached and mentored by the NICU staff when needed (O'Brien et al. 2015).

Table 13.2   Three approaches to involvement of the family in developmental care in the NICU

Strategy	Family-centred care	Family-centred developmental care	Family integrated care
Family and the NICU caregiving team			
Role of parents			
– Parents are participants in care	✓	✓	✓
– Parents have mainly supportive role in care, professionals provide most of care	✓	✓	
– Parents incorporated as full participatory partners			✓
– Parents provide all except the most advanced medical care for their infants with support from the medical teams			✓
Parental participation in rounds			
– Parents present during rounds	✓	✓	✓
– Parents participate in medical rounds and nursing shift reports		✓	✓
– Parents encouraged to actively participate on ward round, chart their infant's growth and progress			✓
Parental role in decision-making			
– Parents participate in decision-making	✓	✓	✓
– Parents have full access and input to both paper and electronic medical records		✓	✓
– Parents participate in medical decisions			✓
Family support from staff			
– Support of family members, e.g. siblings, grandparents, and parents' friends	✓	✓	✓
– Family support of transition from NICU to home	✓	✓	✓
Parents and the infant			
Parental presence in NICU			
– Unlimited presence in the NICU	✓	✓	✓
– Explicit encouragement of prolonged presence			✓
Encouragement of parental role			
– Promotion of skin-to-skin contact and breastfeeding	✓	✓	✓
– Explicit encouragement of parent–infant interaction		✓	✓

Table 13.2 Three approaches to involvement of the family in developmental care in the NICU (Continued)

– Parental support to understand infant's behaviour, developmental progress and means to reduce infant stress during caregiving activities	✓		
– Parents are in charge of the infant's care, including bathing, feeding, dressing, diaper changing, administering oral medication, taking temperature; access to coaching by staff	✓		
Educational strategies to communicate developmental care			
– Teaching parents principles of developmental care	✓	✓	
– Coaching of parents during caregiving activities	✓		
Parent support and education			
– Parents receive in particular emotional support and are coached in coping strategies and stress reducing activities	✓	✓	✓
– Parent to parent support	✓	✓	
– Parent to parent support, including veteran parents	✓	✓	
– Parent education seminars	✓	✓	✓
– Palliative care and bereavement support	✓	✓	✓
NICU care organization			
– NICU staff well trained in emotional support and family centred care	✓	✓	✓
– Integrated team approach	✓	✓	
– Staff focuses on importance of parental involvement in infant care; staff particularly trained in emotional support and support of parent-interaction	✓		
– Tools for staff to mentor, coach, and support parents	✓		
– Parents as faculty and in advisory councils	?*	✓	

Based on Gooding et al. (2011), Craig et al. (2015), O'Brien et al. (2015, 2018), https://newborn-health-standards.org/.
*Not explicitly mentioned in publications.

It is clear that skin-to-skin contact is included in all approaches. It matches the evidence that skin-to-skin contact is clearly associated with stress alleviation and reduction of depression in the parents (Puthussery et al. 2018). Nonetheless, according to a recent study in six European countries, the extent to which the other above mentioned ideas are implemented in neonatal care shows striking variation (Raiskila et al. 2017). For instance, parental presence in the NICU varied between 3 to 22 hours per day. This suggests that families often encounter barriers when trying to fulfil their parental role in the NICU, such as the lack of an opportunity to stay overnight in the NICU (Raiskila et al. 2017).

In parallel to the developmental changes in the approaches of family involvement in the care of medically fragile infants, the use of single-family rooms has been advocated, as it promotes parent–infant interaction, skin-to-skin contact, breastfeeding, and parental well-being (Lester et al. 2016; Tandberg et al. 2019). Whether single-family rooms are associated with better developmental outcomes of the infant is currently not clear: the first study suggested that motor performance and language development at 2 years of age of infants cared for in a private ward was worse than that of infants cared for in the open ward (Pineda et al. 2014). In contrast, Lester and colleagues reported that infants having been nursed in a single-family room had a better neurobehavioural condition at term age than the infants of the open-bay NICU; yet, at 18 months neurodevelopmental outcome of the two groups was similar (Lester et al. 2014, 2016). However, in the subgroup of infants with a birthweight below 1250 grams, the single-family room was associated with an advantage in cognitive, language and fine motor abilities at 18–24 months of age (Vohr et al. 2017).

INTERVENTIONS FOCUSING ON INFANT STIMULATION

In the preterm period various forms of infant stimulation are applied. The most frequently applied interventions are summarized:

- *Infant massage:* This intervention mostly consists of a combination of tactile and kinaesthetic stimulation, often following the protocol of Field et al. (1986). According to this protocol, the parent first gently strokes the infant placed in prone position for 5 minutes. Next, the infant is placed in supine position and the parent gently moves the limbs of the infant for 5 minutes. The intervention ends with a repetition of the first sequence of 5 minutes of tactile stimulation in prone position. Infant massage is associated with improved weight gain, a shorter hospital stay (Vickers et al. 2004; Wang et al. 2013), and a beneficial effect on parent–infant interaction (Brett et al. 2011). However, the effects on neurodevelopment are inconsistent. Guzzetta et al. (2011) reported a positive effect on maturational parameters of EEG during the preterm period and Abdallah and colleagues (Abdallah et al. 2013) found that infant massage in preterm infants was associated with a better cognitive outcome at the age of 1 year. Nonetheless, the meta-analysis of Wang and colleagues (Wang et al. 2013) suggested that massage was not associated with better neurobehavioural performance at term age.
- *Multisensory stimulation:* This intervention uses the combined application of an appropriate amount of auditory, tactile, visual, and vestibular stimulation. The auditory stimulation is provided by means of the voice of the parent, who talks or sings to the infant; the tactile stimulation consists of gentle stroking; visual stimulation involves eye-to-eye contact, and vestibular stimulation consists of rhythmic rocking (Nelson et al. 2001). The few studies available on this intervention report that it may have a positive effect on the early development of sucking (Medoff-Cooper et al. 2015). However, multisensory stimulation has not been associated with better infant behaviour or parent–infant interaction in the first months post-term (Nelson et al. 2001).

- *Developmental physiotherapy:* This description covers physiotherapeutic interventions that consist of actions promoting postural control and midline orientation, generally in combination with education to parents on how to interact with the infant. In this way also a head preference posture and plagiocephaly may be prevented. Available evidence suggests that developmental physiotherapy during the preterm period has a minor, temporary beneficial effect on neuromotor development: it has been associated with better neuromotor performance at 37 weeks gestational age (Ustad et al. 2016), but not with improved neuromotor outcome at 3–4 months post-term (Cameron et al. 2005; Fjørtoft et al. 2017). Øberg et al. (2020) suggested that a higher dosage of developmental physiotherapy was associated with better neuromotor outcome at 3 months post-term; however, not accounted for in the analyses was the fact that more seriously ill infants received less intervention.

INTERVENTIONS TO PREVENT OR MANAGE POSITIONAL HEAD PREFERENCE AND PLAGIOCEPHALY

Both preterm and term-born infants easily develop a positional head preference: at the age of 2 months about half of the infants in the general Dutch population have a positional head preference (Straathof et al. 2020). The head preference may result in a deformational plagiocephaly, but most often head preferences spontaneously resolve (Straathof et al. 2020; see Chapter 7).

The study of Aarnivala and colleagues (2015) showed that positional head preference may be prevented by parent guidance during the infant's newborn period. Their randomized controlled trial (RCT), that started in the neonatal period, showed that parent guidance compared to standard care was associated with a substantial reduction of deformational plagiocephaly at 3 months. The parent guidance consisted of detailed information about the infant's environment (taking care that the interesting environment, e.g. light, colourful objects, does not always come from the same side), about positioning the infant (creating variation in infant position during, for example, feeding and carrying), and promoting tummy time when the infant is awake.

The RCT of Van Vlimmeren et al. (2008) showed that in infants with positional head preference at the age of 7 weeks a period of 4 months of paediatric physiotherapy was associated with a significantly stronger reduction in the prevalence of severe deformational plagiocephaly than usual care (Van Vlimmeren et al. 2008). Yet, motor development in both groups was similar. The paediatric physiotherapy consisted of exercises to reduce positional preference and to stimulate motor development. In addition, parents were informed how they could promote the infant's symmetry during daily life activities, similar to the parent guidance of the above mentioned study of Aarnivala et al. (2015).

The RCT of Van Wijk et al. (2014) demonstrated that 6 months of helmet therapy in infants with deformational plagiocephaly had a comparable effect on head form and motor development at 2 years as no therapy (i.e. allowing the infant to follow its natural developmental course). Many of the parents reported side effects of helmet therapy, including skin irritation, augmented sweating, pain due to the helmet, and an unpleasant smell of the helmet. Parents also felt hindered in cuddling their baby. This implies that helmet therapy is not recommended for the treatment of deformational plagiocephaly in infancy.

Infants with positional head preference and deformational plagiocephaly are often treated by osteopathic manual therapy. However, no evidence is available that this therapy has a beneficial effect on the infant's head form or motor development, as only few studies of low methodological quality are available (Posadzki et al. 2013; Lanaro et al. 2017). As long as no evidence on the effectiveness of osteopathic manual therapy is provided, I would suggest not to use osteopathic manual therapy for positional head preference or deformational plagiocephaly but rather to apply paediatric physiotherapy using recommended approaches (see also Chapter 14).

CONCLUDING REMARKS

The care of medically fragile infants has changed dramatically over the last decades. The changes consisted in particular of the introduction of developmental care and family involvement. The latter gradually develops into family integrated care in which parents adopt the primary care giving role for their infant.

Developmental care primarily aims at promoting parent–infant interaction, stress reduction, and providing a supportive environment. It may be applied as the comprehensive model of NIDCAP or by means of a selection of its components, such as coaching of parent–infant interaction and encouragement of skin-to-skin contact, breastfeeding, nesting, and swaddling. Developmental care has a positive effect on the young infant's brain and development. However, no evidence is available that it promotes development beyond the age of 4 months (i.e. development after the major phase of transition in brain development occurring around 3–4 months) (see Chapters 3 and 5).

Specific infant directed interventions, such as infant massage, multisensory stimulation, and developmental physiotherapy, may have a minor beneficial effect on the infant's neurodevelopmental condition up to and including term age, but most likely not on the infant's development post-term.

REFERENCES

Aarnivala H, Vuollo V, Harila V, Heikkinen T, Pirttiniemi P, Valkama AM (2015) Preventing deformational plagiocephaly through parent guidance: a randomized, controlled trial. *Eur J Pediatr* **174**: 1197–1208. doi: 10.1007/s00431-015-2520-x.

Abdallah B, Badr LK, Hawwari M (2013) The efficacy of massage on short and long term outcomes in preterm infants. *Infant Behav Dev* **36**: 662–669. doi: 10.1016/j.infbeh.2013.06.009.

Akbari E, Binnoon-Erez N, Rodrigues M, et al. (2018) Kangaroo mother care and infant biopsychosocial outcomes in the first year: a meta-analysis. *Early Hum Dev* **122**: 22–31. doi: 10.1016/j.earlhumdev.2018.05.004.

Allotey J, Zamora J, Cheong-See F, et al. (2018) Cognitive, motor, behavioural and academic performances of children born preterm: a meta-analysis and systematic review involving 64 061 children. *BJOG* **125**: 16–25. doi: 10.1111/1471-0528.14832.

Almadhoob A, Ohlsson A (2020) Sound reduction management in the neonatal intensive care unit for preterm or very low birth weight infants. *Cochrane Database Syst Rev* **1**: CD010333. doi: 10.1002/14651858.CD010333.pub3.

Als H, Gilkerson L (1997) The role of relationship-based developmentally supportive newborn intensive care in strengthening outcome of preterm infants. *Semin Perinatol* **21**: 178–189.

Als H, Duffy FH, McAnulty GB, et al. (2004) Early experience alters brain function and structure. *Pediatrics* **113**: 846–857.

Als H, Lawhon G, Brown E, et al. (1986) Individualized behavioral and environmental care for the very low birth weight preterm infant at high risk for bronchopulmonary dysplasia: neonatal intensive care unit and developmental outcome. *Pediatrics* **113**: 1123–1132.

Als H, Lawhon G, Duffy FH, McAnulty GB, Gibes-Grossman R, Blickman JG (1994) Individualized developmental care for the very low-birth-weight preterm infant. Medical and neurofunctional effects. *JAMA* **272**: 853–858.

Benzies KM, Magill-Evans JE, Hayden KA, Ballantyne M (2013) Key components of early intervention programs for preterm infants and their parents: a systematic review and meta-analysis. *BMC Pregnancy Childbirth* **13** (Suppl 1): S10. doi: 10.1186/1471-2393-13-S1-S10.

Brett J, Staniszewska S, Newburn M, Jones N, Taylor L (2011) A systematic mapping review of effective interventions for communicating with, supporting and providing information to parents of preterm infants. *BMJ Open* **1**: e000023. doi: 10.1136/bmjopen-2010-000023.

Buehler DM, Als H, Duffy FH, McAnulty GB, Liederman J (1995) Effectiveness of individualized developmental care for low-risk preterm infants: behavioral and electrophysiologic evidence. *Pediatrics* **96**: 923–932.

Cameron EC, Maehle V, Reid J (2005) The effects of an early physical therapy intervention for very preterm, very low birth weight infants: a randomized controlled clinical trial. *Pediatr Phys Ther* **17**: 107–119.

Chau CMY, Ranger M, Bichin M, et al. (2019) Hippocampus, amydala, and thalamus volumes in very preterm children a 8 years: neonatal pain and genetic variation. *Front Behav Neurosci* **13**: 51. doi: 10.3389/fnbeh.2019.00051.

Craig JW, Glick C, Phillips R, Hall SL, Smith J, Browne J (2015) Recommendations for involving the family in developmental care of the NICU baby. *J Perinatol* **35** (Suppl 1): S5–8. doi: 10.1038/jp.2015.142.

Field TM, Schanberg SM, Scafidi F, et al. (1986) Tactile/kinesthetic stimulation effects on preterm neonates. *Pediatrics* **77**: 654–658.

Fjørtoft T, Ustad T, Follestad T, Kaaresen PI, Øberg GK (2017) Does a parent-administered early motor intervention influence general movements and movement character at 3 months of age in infants born preterm? *Early Hum Dev* **112**: 20–24. doi: 10.1016/j.earlhumdev.2017.06.008.

Gardner SL, Carter BS, Enzman-Hines MI, Hernandez JA (2015) *Merenstein & Gardner's Handbook of Neonatal Intensive Care*, 8th edn. Amsterdam: Elsevier.

Gooding JS, Cooper LG, Blaine AI, Franck LS, Howse JL, Berns SD (2011) Family support and family-centered care in the neonatal intensive care unit: origins, advances, impact. *Semin Perinatol* **35**: 20–28. doi: 10.1053/j.semperi.2010.10.004.

Griffiths N, Spence K, Loughran-Fowlds A, Westrup B (2019) Individualised developmental care for babies and parents in the NICU: evidence-based best practice guideline recommendations. *Early Hum Dev* **139**: 104840. doi: 10.1016/j.earlhumdev.2019.104840.

Guzzetta A, D'Acunto MG, Carotenuto M, et al. (2011) The effects of preterm infant massage on brain electrical activity. *Dev Med Child Neurol* **53** (Suppl 4): 46–51. doi: 10.1111/j.1469-8749.2011.04065.x.

Harrison H (1993) The principles for family-centered neonatal care. *Pediatrics* **92**: 643–650.

Huisenga D, La Bastide-Van Gemert S, Van Bergen A, Sweeney J, Hadders-Algra M (2020) Developmental outcomes after early surgery for complex congenital heart disease: a systematic review and meta-analysis. *Dev Med Child Neurol*, Epub ahead of print. doi: 10.1111/dmcn.14512.

Kitase Y, Sato Y, Takahashi H, et al. (2017) A new type of swaddling clothing improved development of preterm infants in neonatal intensive care units. *Early Hum Dev* **112**: 25–28. doi: 10.1016/j.earlhumdev.2017.06.005.

Lanaro D, Ruffini N, Manzotti A, Lista G (2017) Osteopathic manipulative treatment showed reduction of length of stay and costs in preterm infants: a systematic review and meta-analysis. *Medicine (Baltimore)* **96**: e6408. doi: 10.1097/MD.0000000000006408.

Lester BM, Hawes K, Abar B, et al. (2014) Single-family room care and neurobehavioral and medical outcomes in preterm infants. *Pediatrics* **134**: 754–760. doi: 10.1542/peds.2013-4252.

Lester BM, Salisbury AL, Hawes K, et al. (2016) 18-month follow-up of infants cared for in a single-family room neonatal intensive care unit. *J Pediatr* **177**: 84–89. doi: 10.1016/j.jpeds.2016.06.069.

Mackay LJ, Benzies KM, Barnard C, Hayden KA (2020) A scoping review of parental experiences caring for their hospitalized medically fragile infants. *Acta Paediatr* **109**: 266–275. doi: 10.1111/apa.14950.

Madlinger-Lewis L, Reynolds L, Zarem C, Crapnell T, Inder T, Pineda R (2014). The effects of alternative positioning on preterm infants in the neonatal intensive care unit: a randomized clinical trial. *Res Dev Disabil* **35**: 490–497. doi: 10.1016/j.ridd.2013.11.019.

Maguire CM, Walther FJ, Van Zwieten PH, et al. (2009) No change in developmental outcome with incubator covers and nesting for very preterm infants in a randomised controlled trial. *Arch Dis Child Fetal Neonatal Ed* **94**: F92–F97.

Medoff-Cooper B, Rankin K, Li Z, Liu L, White-Traut R (2015) Multisensory intervention for preterm infants improves sucking organization. *Adv Neonatal Care* **15**: 142–149. doi: 10.1097/ANC.0000000000000166.

Milgrom J, Martin PR, Newnham C, et al. (2019) Behavioural and cognitive outcomes following an early stress-reduction intervention for very preterm and extremely preterm infants. *Pediatr Res* **86**: 92–99. doi: 10.1038/s41390-019-0385-9.

Milgrom J, Newnham C, Anderson PJ, et al. (2010) Early sensitivity training for parents of preterm infants: impact on the developing brain. *Pediatr Res* **67**: 330–335. doi: 10.1203/PDR.0b013e3181cb8e2f.

Morag I, Ohlsson A (2016) Cycled light in the intensive care unit for preterm and low birth weight infants. *Cochrane Database Syst Rev* **8**: CD006982. doi: 10.1002/14651858.CD006982.pub4.

Nelson MN, White-Traut RC, Vasan U, et al. (2001) One-year outcome of auditory-tactile-visual-vestibular intervention in the neonatal intensive care unit: effects of severe prematurity and central nervous system injury. *J Child Neurol* **16**: 493–498.

Øberg GK, Girolami GL, Campbell SK, et al. (2020) Effects of a patient-administered exercise program in the neonatal intensive care unit: dose does matter – a randomized controlled trial. *Phys Ther* **100**: 860–869. doi: 10.1093/ptj/pzaa014.

O'Brien K, Bracht M, Robson K, et al. (2015) Evaluation of the Family Integrated Care model of neonatal intensive care: a cluster randomized controlled trial in Canada and Australia. *BMC Pediatr* **15**: 210. doi: 10.1186/s12887-015-0527-0.

O'Brien K, Robson K, Bracht M, et al. (2018) Effectiveness of Family Integrated Care in neonatal intensive care units on infant and parent outcomes: a multicentre, multinational, cluster-randomised controlled trial. *Lancet Child Adolesc Health* **2**: 245–254. doi: 10.1016/S2352-4642(18)30039-7.

Ohlsson A, Jacobs SE (2013) NIDCAP: a systematic review and meta-analyses of randomized controlled trials. *Pediatrics* **131**: e881–893. doi: 10.1542/peds.2012-2121.

Owen LS, Manley BJ, Davis PG, Doyle LW (2017) The evolution of modern respiratory care for preterm infants. *Lancet* **389**: 1649–1659. doi: 10.1016/S0140-6736(17)30312-4.

Pineda RG, Neil J, Dierker D, et al. (2014) Alterations in brain structure and neurodevelopmental outcome in preterm infants hospitalized in different neonatal intensive care unit environments. *J Pediatr* **164**: 52–60.e2. doi: 10.1016/j.jpeds.2013.08.047.

Pineda R, Bender J, Hall B, Shabosky L, Anncca A, Smith J (2018) Parent participation in the neonatal intensive care unit: Predictors and relationships to neurobehavior and developmental outcomes. *Early Hum Dev* **117**: 32–38. doi: 10.1016/j.earlhumdev.2017.12.008.

Posadzki P, Lee MS, Ernst E (2013) Osteopathic manipulative treatment for pediatric conditions: a systematic review. *Pediatrics* **132**: 140–152. doi: 10.1542/peds.2012-3959.

Puthussery S, Chutiyami M, Tseng PC, Kilby L, Kapadia J (2018) Effectiveness of early intervention programs for parents of preterm infants: a meta-review of systematic reviews. *BMC Pediatr* **18**: 223. doi: 10.1186/s12887-018-1205-9.

Puumala SE, Rich RK, Roy L, et al. (2020) Single-family room neonatal intensive care unit design: do patient outcomes actually change? *J Perinatol* **40**: 867–874. doi: 10.1038/s41372-019-0584-6.

Raiskila S, Axelin A, Toome L, et al. (2017) Parents' presence and parent-infant closeness in 11 neonatal intensive care units in six European countries vary between and within the countries. *Acta Paediatr* **106**: 878–888. doi: 10.1111/apa.13798.

Ranger M, Chau CM, Garg A, et al. (2013) Neonatal pain-related stress predicts cortical thickness at age 7 years in children born very preterm. *PLoS One* **8**: e76702. doi: 10.1371/journal.pone.0076702.

Ranger M, Zwicker JG, Chau CM, et al. (2015) Neonatal pain and infection relate to smaller cerebellum in very preterm children at school age. *J Pediatr* **167**: 292–298.e1. doi: 10.1016/j.jpeds.2015.04.055.

Smith GC, Gutovich J, Smyser C, et al. (2011) Neonatal intensive care unit stress is associated with brain development in preterm infants. *Ann Neurol* **70**: 541–549. doi: 10.1002/ana.22545.

Straathof EJM, Heineman KR, Hamer EG, Hadders-Algra M (2020) Prevailing head position to one side in early infancy – a population-based study. *Acta Paediatr* **109**: 1423–1429. doi: 10.1111/apa.15112.

Sweeney JK, Heriza CB, Blanchard Y, Dusing SC (2010) Neonatal physical therapy. Part II: Practice frameworks and evidence-based practice guidelines. *Pediatr Phys Ther* **22**: 2–16. doi: 10.1097/PEP.0b013e3181cdba43.

Tandberg BS, Flacking R, Markestad T, Grundt H, Moen A (2019) Parent psychological wellbeing in a single-family room versus an open bay neonatal intensive care unit. *PLoS One* **14**: e0224488. doi: 10.1371/journal.pone.0224488.

Ustad T, Evensen KA, Campbell SK, et al. (2016) Early parent-administered physical therapy for preterm infants: a randomized controlled trial. *Pediatrics* **138**, pii: e20160271. doi: 10.1542/peds.2016-0271.

Van Wijk RM, Van Vlimmeren LA, Groothuis-Oudshoorn CG, Van der Ploeg CP, IJzerman MJ, Boere-Boonekamp MM (2014) Helmet therapy in infants with positional skull deformation: randomised controlled trial. *BMJ* **348**: g2741. doi: 10.1136/bmj.g2741.

Van Vlimmeren LA, Van der Graaf Y, Boere-Boonekamp MM, L'Hoir MP, Helders PJ, Engelbert RH (2008) Effect of pediatric physical therapy on deformational plagiocephaly in children with positional preference: a randomized controlled trial. *Arch Pediatr Adolesc Med* **162**: 712–718. doi: 10.1001/archpedi.162.8.712.

Vickers A, Ohlsson A, Lacy JB, Horsley A (2004) Massage for promoting growth and development of preterm and/or low birth-weight infants. *Cochrane Database Syst Rev* **2**: CD000390.

Vinall J, Miller SP, Bjornson BH, et al. (2014) Invasive procedures in preterm children: brain and cognitive development at school age. *Pediatrics* **133**: 412–421. doi: 10.1542/peds.2013-1863.

Vohr B, McGowan E, McKinley L, Tucker R, Keszler L, Alksninis B (2017) Differential effects of the single-family room neonatal intensive care unit on 18- to 24-month Bayley scores of preterm infants. *J Pediatr* **185**: 42–48. e1. doi: 10.1016/j.jpeds.2017.01.056.

Volpe J, Inder T, Darras B, et al. (2017) *Volpe's Neurology of the Newborn*, 6th edn. Amsterdam: Elsevier.

Wang L, He JL, Zhang XH (2013) The efficacy of massage on preterm infants: a meta-analysis. *Am J Perinatol* **30**: 731–738. doi: 10.1055/s-0032-1332801.

White RD (2011) The newborn intensive care unit environment of care: how we got here, where we're headed, and why. *Semin Perinatol* **35**: 2–7. doi: 10.1053/j.semperi.2010.10.002.

Zeiner V, Storm H, Doheny KK (2016) Preterm infants' behaviors and skin conductance responses to nurse handling in the NICU. *J Matern Fetal Neonatal Med* **29**: 2531–2536. doi: 10.3109/14767058.2015.1092959.

FURTHER READING

De Vries LS, Van Haastert IC (2013) *Beyond the Neonatal Intensive Care Unit*. Utrecht: Video Atlas, University Utrecht.

Lagercrantz H, Hanson MA, Ment L, Peebles DM (2010) *The Newborn Brain – Neuroscience and Clinical Applications*, 2nd edn. Cambridge: Cambridge University Press.

Early Intervention in the First Two Years Post-Term

Mijna Hadders-Algra

SUMMARY POINTS

- Early intervention programs are family centred.
- Infants who were critically ill in the neonatal period without acquiring a significant brain lesion are infants at low to moderate risk of developmental motor disorders. Early intervention programs designed for these infants focus on support and education of the caregivers, support of sensitive and responsive parent–infant interaction, and infant stimulation.
- For infants at low to moderate risk, many intervention programmes are available. The programs are associated with improved infant cognitive development and better maternal well-being. Only three intervention programmes have been associated with improved infant motor development (IBAIP, CareToy and COPCA).
- Families of infants at very high risk of developmental motor disorders deal with prolonged periods of stress and uncertainty. This is true for the period before disclosure of the diagnosis and the period thereafter. Early intervention has to take this into account and provide family support.
- Two family approaches are available for early intervention in infants with or at very high risk of developmental motor disorders: one advocating a combination of training and coaching, and the other applying only coaching.
- The term coaching in early intervention is used heterogeneously. It is often used for parent education that uses a combination of training, instruction, and teaching. Yet, the concepts of training, instruction, and teaching are incompatible with coaching as they are based on different attitudes and tune into different goals. Therefore, it is recommended to reserve the term coaching for relationship-directed family-centred interventions and to label intervention forms that primarily use training, instruction and teaching as parent training.
- Early intervention in infants with or at very high risk of a developmental motor disorder:
  - does not only address mobility, but also learning and applying knowledge and communication;
  - primarily addresses activities, not impairments such as deviant muscle tone or abnormal reflexes;
  - has as important ingredients self-generated movements, challenging the infant with activities at the limit of his abilities, and trial and error;
  - restricts hands-on techniques to minimal postural support in the initial phases of learning a new activity by trial and error;
  - supports the use of assistive devices in infants with severe impairments.
- NeuroDevelopmental Treatment (NDT) is frequently applied in early intervention with an astounding diversity. It is not recommended in infants with low to moderate risk. Its effect on developmental outcome in infants with or at very high risk of a developmental motor disorder is not clear.

Therapeutic intervention in children with developmental motor disorders got a boost in the 1950s and 1960s. Before that time, therapeutic intervention focussed on the medical issues of children with cerebral palsy (CP; Mantovani and Scrutton 2014). But in the beginning of the second half of the 20th century, various intervention programmes for children with CP emerged. Examples are the programs of Karel and Berta Bobath (Bobath and Bobath 1950), András Petö (1955), Jean Ayres (1966), and Václav Vojta (1968). In the following decades, many professionals followed courses in which they learned how to apply these programs, also in infants with or at risk of a developmental motor disorder. As a result, the programs were implemented across the world. Also in recent versions of early intervention applied by paediatric physiotherapists in the Netherlands and Switzerland elements of the programmes, especially those of the Bobaths, are variably present (Dirks et al. 2011; Akhbari et al. 2018; Hielkema et al. 2018).

This chapter first discusses the paradigm shifts in the last decades that underlie the concepts applied in early intervention of infants with or at risk of developmental motor disorders. It will address changing insights in motor development and the role of the family, and changes in the perspectives on disability. The discussions focus on the current situation. The second section shortly reviews the early intervention programs that were developed in the second half of last century. The third section discusses currently used early interventions. Finally, the chapter completes with concluding remarks.

PARADIGM SHIFTS IN CONCEPTS UNDERLYING EARLY INTERVENTION

Changes in Theoretical Concepts of Motor Development

Over the years, the possibility of studying details of typical and atypical motor development increased exponentially. For instance, the ubiquity of video equipment allowed for manifold in-depth longitudinal descriptions of the development of motor skills. Also, kinematic, kinetic, electrophysiological, and neuro-imaging technologies, which grew increasingly accurate, facilitated the understanding of the relationships between the developing brain and motor behaviour. The accumulating knowledge induced a shift in the theoretical concepts of motor development (see Chapter 3). The changes in concepts and their putative consequences for early intervention are presented below.

CONTINUOUS INTERACTION BETWEEN GENES, BRAIN, BODY, AND ENVIRONMENT

For a large part of the 20th century, motor development was considered to be an innate process following preprogrammed pathways of developmental milestones. Nowadays, these neuromaturationist theories have been discarded. Motor development is regarded as the net result of a continuous interaction between genetic information (the basic structure of the neural networks), the body and the environment (Edelman 1989; Hadders-Algra 2018a). The interaction results in experiential selection of movement strategies that are best adapted to the environment. Selection is based on trial and error experience and its associated sensory information. This means that selection is promoted by an environment that invites the infant to explore and try out. This is often referred to as an enriched environment (Kolb et al. 2017).

The dynamic, interactional development induces a large variation in the moment at which infants achieve specific milestones (Chapter 6). This includes variation in the order in which the milestones are acquired. The variation between infants increases with increasing age, due to the individual trajectories of interaction between genetic information, brain, body, and environment. This implies that motor development does not demand a strict order in the achievement of milestones, as previously was thought (Vojta 1976; Bobath 1980).

SPONTANEOUS ACTIVITY IS MORE IMPORTANT THAN REFLEXES AND MUSCLE TONE

In the first two thirds of the 20th century, motor behaviour was thought to be mainly organized in terms of reflexes and muscle tone (Bobath 1980). Yet, during the last four decades, it became clear that motor behaviour is primarily based on spontaneous, patterned activity of the nervous system. From early foetal life onwards, cortical networks participate in the spontaneous activity (Hadders-Algra 2018a). This contrasts with earlier ideas that assumed that the neocortex only gradually became functional in the first year of life and did not function at term age (Peiper 1963). The paradigm shift in neural control of motor behaviour implies that early intervention should primarily address the child's self-generated movements rather than focusing on normalization of muscle tone and reflex inhibition.

BRAIN LESION AND REPERTOIRE REDUCTION

It became increasingly clear that an early lesion of the brain is not only expressed in atypical muscle tone regulation and a slower acquisition of mile stones, but also, and even more so, in a reduction of the child's movement repertoire. This is, for instance, prominently expressed in the general movements of young infants with a brain lesion (Prechtl 1990; Hadders-Algra 2018b). Animal research (Kolb et al. 2017) and available human studies suggest that early intervention is well able to improve cognitive development, but that it generally does not result in an enlargement of the movement repertoire (Hielkema et al. 2011, 2020a; Spittle et al. 2015). However, there are exceptions: in some children, part of the repertoire reduction is not only the direct effect of the brain lesion but also that of disuse. A point in case are children with a unilateral spastic CP: the asymmetry in upper limb use induced by the brain lesion is aggravated by disuse, as it is for the child more convenient to use the least affected limb than the most affected one (Gordon 2011; Eliasson et al. 2014a). In these children, intervention may result in some restoration of the repertoire (i.e. it may eliminate the reduction caused by disuse) (Eliasson et al. 2018).

Nonetheless, in general a major part of the repertoire reduction induced by an early lesion of the brain is an impairment that (nowadays) cannot be fixed. As the brain always searches for its own best functional solutions, the brain of a child with CP will find alternative solutions when the typical ones are lacking. This suggests that it is not a good idea to aim for typical movement sequences in children with CP. The better aim is to help the child in finding his own best functional movement strategies and stop worrying about their appearance.

Importantly, the story is not black or white. In children with a severe reduction of the repertoire, the resulting stereotyped movements and postures will induce contractures and deformities. When this is a potential threat, an important goal of intervention is to prevent these secondary sequelae of repertoire reduction. This cannot be achieved by imposing typical movement sequences, but only by means of external help (i.e. by providing the child with assistive devices, such as orthoses, lying-, seating-, and standing-equipment) (see Chapter 15).

DISUSE AND REPERTOIRE REDUCTION

Infants who are critically ill in early life without having acquired a lesion of the brain, such as many of the infants having been born very preterm or many of the infants with complex congenital heart disease, often experience a situation that hampers the typical exploration of the own body and environment. The limited opportunities for exploration may be brought about by the infant's illness – as systemic illness reduces the infant's drive to explore the available movement repertoire (Bos et al. 1997) – and by the hospital environment during the first weeks of postnatal life. The net effect may induce a mild reduction of the movement repertoire. This is, for instance, often observed in preterm infants (Hadders-Algra 2007; Heineman et al. 2008). Recent studies showed that the mild reductions in the movement repertoire of medically fragile infants without a lesion of the brain are sensitive to early intervention. Early intervention in preterm infants without a lesion of the brain – interventions during which the infants were challenged to explore their own body and the environment – were associated with an enlargement of the infant's movement repertoire (Sgandurra et al. 2016, 2017; Akhbari Ziegler et al. 2020). This underlines the notion that repertoire reduction due to disuse based on a lack of internal motivation or unfavourable environmental conditions may be counteracted by early intervention.

NEED OF EXTRA TRIAL AND ERROR EXPERIENCE

Virtually all children with developmental motor disorders (i.e. children with CP and children with developmental coordination disorder [DCD]) have impairments in the processing of sensory information (Odding et al. 2006; Bleyenheuft and Gordon 2013; Wilson et al. 2017). These impairments interfere with the selection of the most efficient movement strategies. It has been estimated that children with developmental motor disorders need about 10 times more trial and error experience than typically developing children (Gordon 2011; Akhbari Ziegler et al. 2019). Knowing that typically developing infants easily produce 10 000 movements per day (Adolph et al. 2012; Smith et al. 2015; Trujillo-Priego et al. 2017; see Chapter 6), this means that infants with or at risk of a developmental motor disorder would require some 100 000 movements per day to keep up with typical developmental progress. This is an extremely challenging requirement and – I think – not compatible with typical family life. In order to cope with this challenge the following may be considered. First, families of infants with or at risk of developmental motor disorders need to be informed that their infant needs more trial and error practice and more time to achieve mobility goals than their typically developing peers. In addition, it should be realized that the drive to explore own movements, the body and the environment may be reduced in children with a lesion of the brain, in particular in children with severe impairments (Festante et al. 2019). This means that these children depend more than typically developing infants on a stimulating and challenging environment. Families need to be informed about these characteristics of their infant. Such information is not easily digested. Therefore, families deserve coaching support and time to cope with the new prospects and to transform the information into ideas for novel routines in daily life. It may be helpful to share the notions that trying out and producing errors is an excellent form of learning. Also, that being slow is not necessarily worse than being fast (cf. slow and fast cooking). Second, an ample amount of self-produced movements with trial and error experiences is more easily achieved when the infant's activities are integrated in daily care giving routines than by practising activities once a week for half an hour in a clinical physiotherapy setting.

The Role of the Family

During the last decades, the orientation in early intervention and paediatric rehabilitation moved from the medical modal with its child focus to the biopsychosocial model with a family focus. This does not mean that in the earlier decades parents were ignored. They did participate, but their role was mainly restricted to acting as their infant's therapist (Köng 1966; Vojta 1976).

Gradually, it dawned upon health professionals that the infant with or at risk of a developmental disorder is inextricably bound up with his family and that early intervention primarily needs to focus on the family and not primarily on the child. The development of the World Health Organization's framework of the International Classification of Functioning, Disability and Health (ICF) in 2001 and its Children and Youth version (ICF-CY) in 2007 largely facilitated this change in focus. The ICF-CY highlights that the child's health condition is significantly affected by environmental context. Beyond doubt, the family is for infants the most important environment (Lach et al. 2014). Nevertheless, it is good to realize that the framework of the ICF-CY takes the child as the starting point, not the family. Nonetheless, it is the family that is primarily affected by the infant's developmental motor disorder and it is the family that is in charge of raising the child, especially when the child is young.

Over the years, the complexity of the needs of families with an infant with special needs grew increasingly clear (see Chapter 12). Important components deserving consideration are discussed below.

BECOMING AWARE OF AND COPING WITH THE INFANT'S SPECIAL NEEDS: A LONG-LASTING PROCESS

The pathways to awareness that the infant has a developmental motor disorder vary. In some infants (e.g. infants born very preterm or with hypoxic-ischaemic encephalopathy or a complex congenital heart disease), parents are soon aware that the infant is at increased risk of developmental disorders. These parents immediately experience the shock, stress, anxiety, depression, and uncertainty associated with the infant's fragile condition in the neonatal intensive care unit (see Chapter 13). In other infants, the perinatal and neonatal period is uneventful. Only gradually, the picture emerges that the infant develops differently from other infants. Either the parents themselves become aware of the atypical development, or relatives (e.g. grandparents), friends, or professionals during standardized health checks alert the parents. In both situations (i.e. the situations with or without a history of medical complications), it takes time before a final diagnosis can be established (see Chapter 2). This is due to the developmental processes in the brain; the brain needs developmental time to express the clinical picture of CP (Chapter 3; see also Hamer et al. 2018; Van Balen et al. 2018). Of course, in some infants the high likelihood of CP can be determined before the age of 6 months. (Recall that all ages mentioned are corrected ages, unless otherwise specified.) This is especially true for infants with neonatal complications in whom this high likelihood can be ascertained with the combination of general movements assessment around 3 months corrected age and neonatal magnetic resonance imaging of the brain (Novak et al. 2017). The epidemiological study of Granild-Jensen et al. (2015) revealed that in about a quarter of the children with CP the diagnosis had been made before the age of 6 months. At the age of 12 months about half of the children had obtained their diagnosis, but in about 5% the diagnosis was first made after the age of 4 years. This observation corresponds to that of the registries of cerebral palsy (Smithers-Sheedy et al. 2014). Another study assessed the age at diagnosis in a cohort of graduates of a neonatal intensive care unit with CP (Guttmann et al. 2018). The parents reported that about 40% of the children had received the diagnosis at the age of 1 year and about two-thirds at 2 years. The figures of both studies indicate that a substantial proportion of families with infants at risk of a developmental motor disorder have to deal with prolonged times of uncertainty about their child's developmental outcome and diagnosis. They sway back and forth between fear and hope (Guttmann et al. 2020). This emotional turmoil is energy demanding. Moreover, the emotional phases of both parents, and also those of grandparents, often are not synchronized, as each caregiver follows his or her own trajectory to cope with the uncertain situation.

It is important that health professionals explain why a diagnosis often cannot be ascertained at early age, as caregivers otherwise may think 'He/she does know the outcome, but he/she does not dare to disclose it'. Crucially, the absence of a diagnosis does not mean that 'nothing can be done'. The presence of high risk of a developmental diagnosis warrants early intervention. The intervention serves two goals: (1) the family learns to cope with the situation of having an infant 'at risk' and eventually with having an infant with a developmental motor disorder, and (2) the infant achieves his optimal level of participation.

At a certain point, the developmental diagnosis is provided, the 'truth is told' or the 'bad news is delivered'. The various expressions reflect the dramatic effect of the diagnosis. It is therefore quintessential that the diagnosis is communicated carefully (for details see the best practice guidelines of Novak et al. 2019). Caregivers generally experience mixed feelings when the diagnosis is disclosed. It is perceived as positive that the uncertainty about a diagnosis is replaced by the certainty of the specific diagnosis, such as CP. But the diagnosis itself evokes grief – the dreamt future of the typically developing child is lost – stress and new uncertainty (Marvin and Pianta 1996; Rentinck et al. 2007). The latter is understandable, as CP manifests itself in largely different clinical pictures. Parents frequently ask the question 'Will my child be able to walk?' In infants with severe impairments, the question usually can be answered relatively early, providing the family with a sad certainty. Yet, in many infants, the question about walking is not easily answered as early functional skills only moderately well predict later mobility. This is illustrated by the study of Gorter et al. (2009) on the significance of the classification according to the Gross Motor Function Classification System (GMFCS) in children younger than 2 years. In many children, the GMFCS level they had been assigned to before the age of 2 changed into another one at a later age.

Both before and after disclosure of the diagnosis, families with an infant with a developmental motor disorder often perceive stress. Actually, receiving the diagnosis is not an event, it is a long-lasting process (Lach et al. 2014). The process does not stop, as caregivers realize in each new phase of the child's life that their child differs from typically developing children, and that all family members have to cope with the challenges associated with the child's different abilities. The implication for early intervention is that health professionals need to be aware of the psychological stress of caregivers. It is well known that stress interferes with memory and the control of emotion due to its impact on the function of the amygdala, the hippocampus, and the prefrontal cortex (Bremner 2013). As a result, stress affects the caregivers' ability to cope with life in general, to interact with the infant and with the health professional. This implies that caregiver support, patient listening, repetition of information, and the promotion of responsive parenting are essential ingredients of early intervention (Hutchon et al. 2019).

ROLE OF THE FAMILY

In contrast to practices in a major part of the previous century, it is nowadays generally acknowledged that early intervention should focus on the family as a unit and not only on the child (Rosenbaum 2011; Akhbari Ziegler et al. 2019). It is recognized that each family is unique and that caregivers are the experts on the child's abilities and the child's life (King et al. 2004). However, the extent to which family-centred early intervention is implemented in daily practice varies. For instance, consensus exists that family-centred intervention includes an emphasis on the strengths of the family and infant and enabling family choice and control (King and Chiarello 2014). The latter is achieved by shared decision-making, implying that both family members and health professionals have access to relevant information, get the opportunity to ask questions and time to consider, and may propose alternative options (Hubner et al. 2016). However, evaluation of the contents of physiotherapeutic early intervention sessions revealed that therapists often do not act according to the principles of family-centred care, even though they assume they do. Often, the therapist sets the goal, designs the intervention plan, and informs the family (Dirks et al. 2011). It is often overlooked that the shift from the child-focussed medical model, in which the health professional decides, informs, and sets the goals, to proper family-centred care aiming at family empowerment, parental engagement, and equal partnership requires a fundamental change in attitude and habits (King and Chiarello, 2014). Such a change requires education, practice, and time (Akhbari Ziegler and Hadders-Algra, 2020).

The change from child-focused to family-focused early intervention also necessitates a different way to approach and communicate with families (Fig. 14.1). In the early days of intervention, therapists treated the infants and parents were trained to perform therapeutic actions with their infants in the home setting (Köng 1966; Vojta 1976). As the unidirectional approach of caregiver training does not

MODEL

INTERVENTION APPROACH

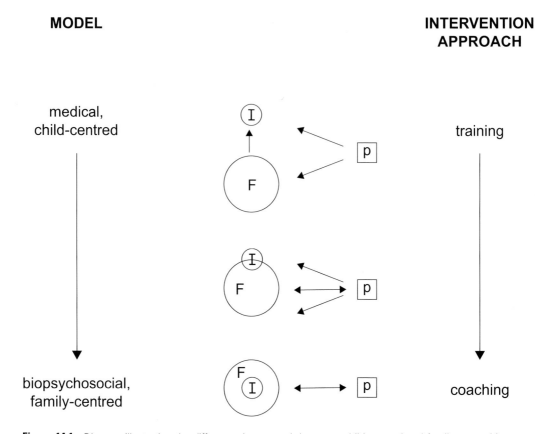

medical,
child-centred

training

biopsychosocial,
family-centred

coaching

Figure 14.1 Diagram illustrating the difference in approach between child-centred and family-centred intervention. The upper row represents the child-focused approach of the medical model that was most prevalent during the last century. The professional (P) treated the infant (I) and instructed the family (F) how to continue therapeutic actions in the home setting. The bottom row depicts the family-centred approach of the biopsychosocial model. The professional coaches the family in a bidirectional dialogue; the infant is an integral part of the family. The middle row illustrates the situation that is most commonly practised currently.

match up with the concept of family-centred services, the tool of caregiver coaching was introduced in early intervention. Coaching has been embraced by many therapists, but with large heterogeneity (Morgan et al. 2014; Eliasson et al. 2016; Akhbari Ziegler et al. 2019). The diversity can be attributed mostly to the ambiguity with which coaching is defined in the literature. Actually, the literature does not well differentiate between coaching and training of families. We therefore recently suggested labelling intervener-directed forms of intervention that use teaching, instruction, and training as 'parent training' and to reserve the term 'coaching' in early intervention for relationship-directed family-centred interventions. This also implies that it is impossible to combine parent training and parent coaching defined in this way, as these practices are based on mutually exclusive attitudes (Akhbari Ziegler and Hadders-Algra 2020).

One of the challenges that accompanied the shift from child-focused to family-focused intervention is that caregivers may perceive that it is entirely their responsibility how well the infant develops, especially as a mantra of early intervention seems to be 'more is better'. Caregivers may struggle to find the right balance between paying attention to the infant with special needs and the other demands of daily life (Lach et al. 2014; Kruijsen-Terpstra et al. 2014; Basu et al. 2015). It is conceivable that this conflict more easily arises when intervention consists of a predetermined set of therapy actions than when intervention consists of coaching how the child's development can be promoted while interaction with the child during daily caregiving routines (Akhbari Ziegler et al. 2019; Stewart and Applequist 2019).

Changes in the Perspectives on Disability

The implementation of the ICF and ICF-CY in the beginning of this century illustrates the shift in thinking about disability. Previously, disability was mainly considered in terms of the medical model. Intervention primarily focused on the impairments of children with developmental motor disorders and particularly addressed management of impaired muscle tone and the normalization of posture and movements (Vojta 1976; Bobath 1980). Again, as often is the case in developmental paediatrics, the story is not black or white. The Bobath program also paid attention to the child's activities and participation (Mayston 2016) and Pető's conductive education entirely focused on participation (Hari and Tillemans 1984).

The ICF and ICF-CY facilitated the transition from thinking about disability in terms of impairments and limitations to functional strengths and modifications of the environment (Buntinx 2013). The new conceptual framework is really out in the world. However, societies across the world still need to make large steps to achieve its full implementation. Currently, young and older people with a visible disability are still often primarily perceived as beings 'with whom something essentially is wrong' and beings 'who need to be pitied' instead of as individuals with specific strengths and weaknesses just as anybody else. I know this from personal experience, rolling around in a manually driven wheelchair. Also, health professionals often radiate – unconsciously – this attitude while offering with totally good intentions their help to families and children. As health professionals we really have to come to terms with how we view disability. See also Text Box 1.3 for some considerations.

EARLY INTERVENTION PROGRAMMES DEVELOPED IN THE SECOND HALF OF THE 20TH CENTURY

In this section four early intervention methods are described that were developed in the second half of the 20th century: the methods of Vojta, Ayres, Pető, and the Bobaths. The latter, known as well as NeuroDevelopmental Treatment (NDT), receives most attention as it is also nowadays frequently used across the world (Zanon et al. 2018).

Treatment According to Vojta

Vojta's treatment is based on the concept of 'reflex locomotion'. With the latter term Vojta described total movement patterns that are not spontaneously generated, but only can be elicited by stimulation of specific body parts (the 'trigger zones'). He distinguished reflex crawling and reflex rolling. Vojta assumed that these reflex patterns, which can be evoked in newborn infants, were based on subcortical activity. He proposed that infants at high risk of cerebral palsy should receive a frequent application of the patterns of reflex locomotion in order to prevent the development of CP or to improve the motor skills of children with CP. The application of the therapy is mainly the task of the caregivers (Vojta 1976, 1984). The treatment is a challenge for caregivers and infants, as the treatment, that should be applied multiple times per day frequently, makes the infant cry.

Vojta therapy is also nowadays applied, even though little information is available on its effect. In more than 50 years only three studies have been published that evaluated the effect of Vojta therapy in young children. Two of them evaluated the effect of Vojta in infants at high risk of CP (d'Avignon et al. 1981; Kanda et al. 2004). Both studies evaluated small groups and suffered from weak methodological quality (Blauw-Hospers and Hadders-Algra 2005). The third study compared the effect of 8 weeks of Vojta therapy with that of a similar period of NDT in young infants with postural asymmetry (Jung et al. 2017). The postural asymmetry diminished in both groups, but significantly more in the group with Vojta treatment. The effect on the infants' activities and participations was not assessed.

Overall, I would not recommend Vojta treatment for infants with or at high risk of developmental motor disorders, as (1) the evidence of effectiveness in these infants is lacking; (2) the underlying neurophysiological hypothesis does not correspond to current developmental neuroscience; and (3) the treatment by the parents often makes the infant cry, which interferes with the establishment of responsive parent–infant interaction.

Sensory Integration Therapy According to Jean Ayres

Jean Ayres primarily developed her therapeutic approaches for older children with developmental disorders, in particular children with learning disorders and/or DCD. Her therapeutic approach also became integrated in early intervention. Ayres postulated that children with or at risk of developmental motor disorders have impairments in the processing of sensory information (i.e. to organize sensory input for use) (Ayres 1966). She assumed that the sensory impairments hamper the inhibition of 'primitive reflexes' and interfere with the development of righting and equilibrium reactions and the typical sequence of motor milestones (White 1984). Central in Ayres' observation and treatment are the postural and behavioural responses in reaction to changing vestibular, proprioceptive, and tactile stimulation. Treatment basically consists of providing sensory stimulation: vestibular and proprioceptive stimulation by means of, for example, swings, hammocks, or large balls to sit or stand on, and tactile stimulation by letting the child experience a large variety of textures, including soft, hard, prickly or slimy surfaces (White 1984). Treatment is mainly performed by a therapist in a therapy setting; parents do not have a specific role.

Most studies addressing the effect of sensory integration therapy have been performed on older children with CP or DCD. Current guidelines recommend that sensory integration therapy should not be used in the guidance of these children (Blank et al. 2019; Novak et al. 2020). Only a few studies addressed the effectiveness of sensory integration therapy in young children with or at risk of a developmental motor disorder. The studies reported a positive effect of sensory integration therapy. However, the studies suffered from methodological flaws, such as the lack of a control group (Blanche et al. 2016; Pekçetin et al. 2016), the presence of co-intervention (optimizing the infant's self-regulation) and insufficient statistical analysis (Lecuona et al. 2017).

In conclusion, evidence that sensory integration therapy as developed by Ayres is effective in enhancing developmental outcome in infants with or at risk of a developmental motor disorder is lacking. Nonetheless, Ayres' idea that impaired sensory processing contributes to the motor deficits of at risk infants is correct. This especially happens in infants with a reduced motor repertoire, where stereotyped movements will generate stereotyped sensory input (Shafer et al. 2017). Conceivably, this means that not the application of passive sensory stimuli, as proposed by Ayres, is effective in enhancing the development of motor skills but rather the generation of varied sensory input through self-generated movements when being exposed to a variety of challenges – as was demonstrated in the studies of Sgandurra et al. (2016, 2017) and Akhbari Ziegler et al. (2020).

Petö's Conductive Education

Petö's conductive education is a holistic educational programme that aims at optimal participation of the child in society. The goals to be achieved are discussed with the parents. Conductive education focuses on learning in its broadest sense (i.e. it does not only include the learning of motor skills but also that of cognitive and social abilities). It is a group-based programme, with the group being led by a conductor. The conductor is a teacher with specific training in conductive education. The conductor guides the group activities through specific teaching strategies that include task series and 'rhythmic intention' (i.e. the use of rhythmical singing, counting, and speech). Specific attention is paid to the child's motivation and self-efficacy. During the group activities specific equipment is used, such as slatted wooden tables and ladder-back chairs. Postural support and assistive devices are used as little as possible (Hari and Tillemans 1984; Bourke-Taylor et al. 2007).

Conductive education has been studied infrequently in a systematic way. The studies available showed that functional outcome after conductive education did not differ from equally intensive, goal-oriented typical physiotherapy, also in the youngest children studied (1–3 years of age; Reddihough et al. 1998). It means that we need more studies to assess which children and which families would benefit in particular from conductive education. For the time being, we may perhaps give conductive education the benefit of the doubt (Myrhaug et al. 2018; Myrhaug et al. 2019). In particular, I would not – as Novak et al. (2020) – discourage families to participate with their young child in conductive education.

Bobath Therapy or NeuroDevelopmental Treatment

Originally, treatment according to the Bobaths was guided by two principles: (1) the inhibition of atypical reflex patterns that were responsible for hypertonia, and (2) the facilitation of 'higher integrated' typical postural reactions (Bobath and Bobath 1950; Bobath 1980). The Bobaths also assumed that motor milestones should be achieved in typical order. Already in the 1960s, Bobath therapy was not only applied in older children but also in infants (Köng 1966). Over the years, the Bobaths learned what worked well and what did not; they gradually changed their approach (Bobath and Bobath 1984). The focus on 'reflex inhibition' diminished and the goals of therapy changed from improvement of impairments into optimizing activities and participation (Bobath and Bobath 1984; Butler and Darrah 2001; Mayston 2016). In addition, the Bobaths realized that it was not necessary that motor development follows a typical sequence. Moreover, they allowed the presence of atypical movement patterns when they assisted participation – even though their treatment continued to aim at the suppression of these patterns (Mayston 2008). As a result, Bobath treatment became a 'living concept' (Howle 2002). Nonetheless, the normalization of muscle tone through facilitation as the basis to learn typical movement sequences remained a key theme of treatment. The facilitation is achieved by hands-on techniques of therapists and parents (Mayston 2004). According to the Bobaths, this should be done as little as possible. It should only be performed when the child is actively involved in the motor action and only during the first phases of the acquisition of a motor skill. The hands-on facilitation is only meant to enable the development of a new activity (Mayston 2014).

With its worldwide application, the name of the treatment approach changed into Neuro Developmental Treatment (NDT). Moreover, its application became very heterogeneous. NDT varies nowadays from treatment with more hands-on than the Bobaths intended to goal-oriented guidance with minimal hands-on facilitation. The variants occur within and between countries (Dirks et al. 2011; Akhbari Ziegler et al. 2018; Farjoun et al. 2020). This means that studies evaluating the effect of NDT without specifying the contents of NDT assess the effect of a black box. This is presumably a major reason why available studies did not demonstrate a beneficial effect of NDT, as approaches with ample hands-on intervention blur a potentially beneficial effect of the more goal-oriented approaches with minimal hands-on (Blauw-Hospers et al. 2011). Understandably, recent guidelines recommend that NDT as it is currently mostly practised should not be used in older children with CP (Novak et al. 2020).

The application of NDT in early intervention deserves special attention. The application of NDT in babies was largely developed by Elsbeth Köng and Mary Quinton and later described in detail by Lois Bly (1999). Treatment uses the typical sequence of motor milestones as an agenda for goal-setting, but following this sequence is not an obligation. Facilitation by hands-on techniques is a key element in treatment, as is amply illustrated in Bly's book (1999). The hands-on techniques aim at aligning the baby's body during the movement and to provide the infant with guided typical sensorimotor experiences until the baby's own activity takes over. The idea is that hands-on facilitation enables the infant to move. The facilitation techniques are performed in various situations: on the adult's body, on a ball, a bolster or on the floor. NDT regards parents as partners in the baby treatment team. The parents receive instructions how to continue the treatment at home (Bly 1999).

Research suggests that the effect of NDT in early intervention for infants with low to moderate risk of developmental motor disorders may differ from that in infants at high risk. The former group consists especially of infants born preterm without a having acquired a significant lesion of the brain. Systematic reviews revealed that NDT is not effective in promoting developmental outcome in these infants (Blauw-Hospers and Hadders-Algra 2005; Spittle et al. 2015). The study of Blauw-Hospers et al. (2011) even indicated that NDT with much hands-on facilitation was associated with less favourable functional mobility at the age of 18 months.

In children at very high risk of CP (i.e. infants with a significant lesion of the brain), such as periventricular leukomalacia or cortical infarction, the effect of NDT may be different. Two systematic reviews indicated that NDT as performed in the 1980s and 1990s was not associated with a better developmental outcome (Morgan et al. 2016a; Hadders-Algra et al. 2017). However, as suggested by Hadders-Algra et al. (2017), it is conceivable that goal-oriented NDT with minimal hands-on facilitation may be a proper intervention strategy. This suggestion is supported by the results of recent trials on early intervention in infants at very high risk of CP: the intervention that used a combination of goal-directed activities and minimal hands-on support was associated with a better infant motor development (Morgan et al. 2015, 2016b), whereas the intervention with similar goal-directed activities without hands-on support was not associated with an improved motor outcome (Hielkema et al. 2020a).

CURRENT FORMS OF EARLY INTERVENTION

Evidence is accumulating that the effect of early intervention of infants at low to moderate risk of developmental motor disorders differs from that of infants at very high risk. Therefore, the various forms of intervention are discussed for these two groups separately. Very high risk refers to infants with a significant lesion of the brain, such as periventricular leukomalacia, cortical infarction, or periventricular-intraventricular haemorrhages complicated by posthaemorrhagic ventricular dilation or parenchymal haemorrhagic infarction. Importantly, not all infants with an early lesion of the brain will be diagnosed with CP (see Chapters 2 and 3).

Early Intervention in Infants at Low to Moderate Risk of Developmental Motor Disorders

Early intervention in infants at low to moderate risk of developmental motor disorders especially refers to early intervention in medically fragile infants that started their postnatal life in the neonatal intensive care unit (see Chapter 13). Examples are the majority of infants born preterm or with neonatal hypoxic-ischaemic encephalopathy or a complex congenital heart disease, who – despite their challenging neonatal start – did not acquire a significant lesion of the brain.

A wealth of programmes has been developed to support these infants and their families (Puthussery et al. 2018). In general, these programmes start when the infant is still in the hospital, after which they continue during the first months after discharge. The programmes aim to enhance parent–infant inter-action, to reduce parental anxiety and depression, and to promote infant development. They consist of (1) parent education, including teaching and sensitization to the infant's cues; (2) parent support (e.g. guidance and encouragement); and (3) support of infant development. Not all programmes are equally effective, but the components aiming at parental support and education are generally associated with a reduction of maternal stress, anxiety, and depression, and a better maternal sensitivity and responsiveness to the infant (Benzies et al. 2013; Puthussery et al. 2018).

The Cochrane review of Spittle et al. (2015) demonstrated that the early intervention programmes have a significant beneficial effect on the infant's cognitive development. The effect can be demonstrated up to and including preschool age, but no evidence is available that the effect extends to school age. The interventions that were most successful in improving the infant's cognitive outcome especially supported parent–infant interaction and infant development.

Spittle's review also revealed that the early intervention programmes had substantially less effect on the child's motor outcome. Early intervention was only associated with a minor effect on motor devel-opment in infancy; it had no effect on later motor development. As was true for cognitive development, the interventional components that contributed most to the minor aggregate effect on motor outcome were support of parent–infant interaction and infant development.

The *Infant Behavioral Assessment and Intervention Program (IBAIP)* was the only intervention pro-gramme reported in the review, that was able to achieve a significant effect on the infant's motor development. The other programs had an insignificant effect on motor development but contributed to the aggregate effect. IBAIP consists of one intervention session shortly before discharge and six to eight sessions at home until the infant has reached the age of 6 months corrected age. IBAIP aims to enhance the infant's social and environmental interactions without causing distress in the infant and – therewith – in the caregivers. IBAIP uses a combination of support and education of the caregiver and instructions on infant development. On the basis of shared behavioural observations, the therapist aims to sensitize caregivers to the infant's way to handle environmental information, and to assist caregivers how to adjust the daily environment to the infant's needs. Moreover, caregivers are taught how they may offer co-regulatory support during their interaction with the infant, for instance by bringing the infant's hands to the midline or to the infant's mouth (Koldewijn et al. 2009, 2010). The IBAIP resulted in better improvements in motor outcome up to and including the age of 2 years than standard care of very preterm infants. The latter implied that typical physiotherapeutic intervention was only provided when the paediatrician had recommended it (Koldewijn et al. 2010). Follow-up studies at the ages of 3.5 and 5.5 years demonstrated that the effect was not sustained after the age of 2 years – at least, not when Bonferroni correction for multiple testing was applied (Verkerk et al. 2011; Van Hus et al. 2013; see also Spittle et al. 2015). The IBAIP also affected cognitive outcome, an effect that was expressed at 5.5 years in a lower prevalence of children with a performance intelligence quotient below 85 (Van Hus et al. 2013). In addition, mothers of infants who had received IBAIP reported more happiness and less distractibility in their infants than mothers of infants who had received standard care (Meijssen et al. 2011). Yet, IBAIP had a mixed effect on the mothers. When the infant was 6 months, IBAIP was associated with higher maternal sensitivity (Meijssen et al. 2010). But when the infant was 1–2 years, IBAIP mothers reported more often feelings of social isolation (Meijssen et al. 2011). The latter may be attributed to IBAIP's aim to increase parental availability and responsibility. This may have resulted in a parental feeling that care-taking activities should be performed only by the parents and not by other persons. Consequently, parents would have less time available for social activities (Meijssen et al. 2011).

After the publication of Spittle's Cochrane review, studies evaluating the effect of two other intervention programmes reported significant beneficial effects of the intervention on motor development of infants at low to moderate risk of developmental disorders (Sgandurra et al. 2016, 2017; Akhbari Ziegler et al. 2020). As both programmes, the family centred program Coping with and Caring for infants with special needs (COPCA) and CareToy, have been designed for infants with special needs in general, and in particular for infants at very high risk for developmental disorders, the programmes will be discussed in the following section.

In conclusion: the current state of the art is that early intervention in infants at low to moderately increased risk of developmental disorders and their families profit from early intervention. Parental support and education are associated with better maternal well-being; support of parent–infant interaction and infant development are associated with better cognitive development. Evidence is emerging that programmes that combine support and education of caregivers and infant stimulation may also promote the infant's motor development. The effects of these programmes on family well-being are less clear.

Early Intervention in Infants with or at Very High Risk of Developmental Motor Disorders

Early Intervention Programmes

During the last two decades, five early intervention programmes have been developed for infants with or at very high risk of developmental motor disorders. The programmes aim at optimizing not only mobility (i.e. gross and fine motor skills) but also the child's achievements in the domains of learning and applying knowledge and communication. Four programmes have been evaluated in groups of very high risk infants – they will be discussed below. The fifth programme is the CareToy intervention; it will be described here.

CareToy is a technological and modular system for home intervention for young infants at low to very high risk of developmental disorders that aims to provide by means of tele-rehabilitation a personalized intervention. It has been developed by an international European research group. The system looks like a playpen and consists of four modules: (1) a gym module including a variety of sensorized toys, interactive walls with sound and lights, a belt wall with a sensorized pillow, an arch with lights, and four cameras; (2) a vision module (i.e. a screen wall with a large monitor); (3) a mat module including a sensorized mat and three wearable sensors; and (4) a tele-rehabilitation module allowing communication with the health care centre (Sgandurra et al. 2014). CareToy aims to improve motor, perceptual, and cognitive outcome by provision of the enriched environment of the CareToy system, and to help caregivers in stimulating their infant's development. CareToy professionals design – via telecommunication – series of individual goal-directed activities, so-called scenarios, to be performed in the CareToy environment. The activities focus on postural control, upper limb activities and visual attention and orientation in three positions (supine, prone, and sitting). The caregivers are trained how to playfully perform these activities with the infant in the CareToy system. It is recommended that CareToy training is performed 30–45 minutes per day in bouts of 2–10 minutes (Sgandurra et al. 2014).

CareToy has been evaluated in groups of young low-risk very preterm infants, first in a pilot study, next in a randomized controlled study (RCT; Sgandurra et al. 2016, 2017). The studies compared CareToy intervention with standard care of very preterm infants that generally did not include home-based intervention. Both studies indicated that provision of 4 weeks of CareToy intervention was associated with better motor outcome and better visual acuity than standard care. The effects on motor outcome consisted of better motor skills and an increase of the movement repertoire. CareToy intervention was also associated with a reduction in maternal but not paternal distress. The reduction in maternal stress was correlated with the time during which the mother had performed play activities with the infant in the CareToy system (Sgandurra et al. 2019). This suggests that CareToy could be used in early intervention of low-risk very preterm infants. Nonetheless, the study also indicated that the intervention does not work for all families: more than half of the families that were eligible for the CareToy RCT declined to participate (Sgandurra et al. 2017), a proportion that is much higher than those reported in the studies on the intervention programmes described below. CareToy is currently tested in a RCT of infants at very high risk of CP. To this end, the system has been modified; it now also includes a set of soft and coloured modules with different shapes that can be attached to a mat by Velcro straps. The modules aim at offering postural and perceptive stimuli (Sgandurra et al. 2018).

BABY-CONSTRAINT-INDUCED MOVEMENT THERAPY

Constrained-induced movement therapy (CIMT) is a recognized intervention in children with unilateral spastic CP (Novak et al. 2020). Basically, CIMT consists of the combination of a restraint of the less affected upper limb with intensive training of the most affected upper limb (Eliasson et al. 2014b). The recent Cochrane review of Hoare et al. (2019) reported that CIMT results in better bimanual abilities and better unimanual abilities of the most affected limb when compared to low dosage standard therapy. However, this difference disappears when CIMT is compared to standard therapy focusing on bimanual activities that is equally intensive as CIMT.

Baby-CIMT is the adaptation of CIMT for infants with signs that may indicate the development of unilateral CP, that is, a clear asymmetry in hand function. It has been developed by Ann-Christin Eliasson (Eliasson et al. 2014a). Baby-CIMT is a home-based intervention. It consists of restraining the infant's less affected upper limb for a period of 30 minutes per day. This can be achieved by simple means, such as a sock, a mitt, or a bag clip at the end of a long-sleeved sweater. During the period of restraint, upper limb activities are trained by the presentation of a variety of attractive toys, therewith creating an enriched environment. The caregivers are in charge of the baby-CIMT intervention; they also take care that the infant is optimally seated during the training. The task of the therapist is to train and coach the caregivers. The latter includes advice, such as to be patient, to provide the infant with positive feedback, and to sit in front of the infant during the activities in order to facilitate communication with the infant. The therapist also supports caregivers' sense of self-efficacy and problem-solving capacities.

Three studies have shed light on the effectiveness of baby-CIMT. A retrospective study suggested that baby-CIMT could be useful in promoting the use of the most affected hand in bimanual activities (Nordstrand et al. 2015). A following RCT indicated that baby-CIMT and the control intervention of baby massage had an equal effect on hand function of infants who had presented with clear asymmetrical hand function. However, when the analysis was restricted to the children who were diagnosed with unilateral CP, baby-CIMT was associated with better use of the most affected hand in bimanual activities (Eliasson et al. 2018). A second RCT, performed in infants with unilateral CP (Chamudot et al. 2018), demonstrated that the effectiveness of baby-CIMT in promoting hand function was similar to that of equally intensive bimanual therapy – just as in older children.

Baby-CIMT and intensive bimanual therapy may also be used in infants with neonatal brachial plexus palsy (Frade et al. 2019). Yet, the effects of these interventions have not been studied systematically.

GOALS – ACTIVITY – MOTOR ENRICHMENT INTERVENTION

The Goals – Activity – Motor Enrichment (GAME) intervention has been developed by Cathy Morgan and colleagues. It is an intervention designed for infants with or at high risk of a developmental disorder (Morgan et al. 2014). It is based on three theoretical assumptions: (1) goal-oriented intervention enhances motivation to practice activities; (2) intensive practice is crucial for learning new activities; (3) environmental enrichment is associated with better developmental outcome. GAME is a home-based intervention consisting of three components: goal-oriented intensive motor training, parent education, and strategies to enrich the infant's motor learning environment. The goals of the motor training are the result of shared decision making. The therapist has an important role in assisting the caregivers to set realistic goals. Parents are taught and coached how the goals can be reached by intensive practice. The practice consists of performing activities that are appropriate for the infant's level of functional development and the tasks are scaffolded in such way that the infant is always able to actively complete part of the task. Minimal manual assistance is provided, that is, hands-on support is given when the infant learns a new task for reasons of safety or 'to give the infant an "idea" of the movement' (Morgan et al. 2015). When the infant has mastered a task, variability of practice is introduced. The environmental enrichment consists of informing caregivers about the use of varied toys and typical baby equipment during the tasks. In addition, the interventionist discusses with caregivers the importance of reading books with the infant, reducing the amount of screen-time, sleep hygiene, and – when needed – options for feeding interventions.

GAME has been evaluated in two RCTs in infants at very high risk of CP, one being a pilot study (Morgan et al. 2015, 2016b). Both studies compared the effect of GAME with that of typical infant physiotherapy as currently practised in Australia. The latter implies a mix of clinic-based appointments and home visits. In the pilot study (Morgan et al. 2015) intervention was provided for 12 weeks. GAME interventionists visited families once a week for 60–90 minutes. The families in the control group received three times less professional intervention. Also, a large difference was found in the hours that the families in both groups practised: 140 versus 54 hours. The latter implies that the GAME families practised more than 1.5 hours per day. The study showed that the infants of the GAME intervention group immediately after the intervention had better motor abilities than the control infants. In the other RCT (Morgan et al. 2016b), the interventions were provided for a longer period (GAME: 37 weeks, control intervention: 32 weeks). The GAME intervention had a lower intensity than in the pilot study. This time the therapist paid a fortnightly visit to the family and caregivers practised about 50 minutes per day (control group: 30 minutes). At the age of 1 year the infants of the GAME group had a better motor and cognitive outcome than the infants of the control group. The GAME and control intervention had a similar effect on parental anxiety and depression. In addition, the authors reported that four of the 15 GAME families had dropped out of the study, mainly because they moved to receive more family support. None of the control families dropped out of the study.

SMALL STEP PROGRAM

The Small Step Program (SSP) bears large similarities to the GAME intervention. It has been developed by Ann-Christin Eliasson and colleagues. SSP has been designed for infants of at least 4 months of age with a very high risk of a developmental motor disorder. It aims to promote the infant's abilities in the mobility and communication domains and to support the families (Eliasson et al. 2016). It is a home-based programme providing individualized, goal directed, and intensive intervention focusing on mobility (fine and gross motor abilities) and communication. Like GAME it uses the concept of the enriched environment by designing a variety of tasks with a variety of toys to promote self-produced fine motor and gross motor actions. The tasks are adapted to the infant's developmental level. The caregivers provide the training on a daily basis. Once a week the caregivers are trained and coached by therapists. The training and coaching includes recommendations such as to be patient with the infant, provide positive feedback, avoid forcing the infant to perform an action, and to help and guide the child by means of hands-on support 'when necessary' (Eliasson et al. 2016). SSP does not specify what coaching implies, but the provided information indicates that the programme uses parental training as the main parental approach. SSP pays more explicit attention than GAME to communication. To this end caregivers are made aware of the way the infant communicates verbally and non-verbally and enjoys to be engaged in imitation and conversation.

The provision of 35 weeks of SSP was evaluated in one RCT in infants at very high risk of CP (Holmström et al. 2019). The effect of SSP was compared to that typical infant physiotherapy in Sweden, which consists of having a therapy session in an outpatient setting once every 3–4 weeks including a discussion of the home programme for the coming period. Motor abilities of both intervention groups were similar immediately after the intervention period and at the age of 2 years. Yet, the results also suggested that the infants with the most severe motor impairments at the start of the intervention profited more from SSP than from the control intervention. SSP and standard care had a similar effect on maternal well-being.

COPING AND CARING FOR INFANTS WITH SPECIAL NEEDS – A FAMILY-CENTRED PROGRAMME

The family centred programme COPing and CAring for infants with special needs (COPCA) was developed by Tineke Dirks and Mijna Hadders-Algra. It is a home-based, family relationship-oriented programme that has been designed for infants at low and at very high risk of developmental motor disorders from term age onwards. COPCA aims to empower the family in coping with the situation of having an infant with special needs and to promote the infant's activities and participation. Related to these two aims, COPCA has two components: a family component and an infant neurodevelopmental component (Dirks et al. 2011; Dirks and Hadders-Algra 2011; Akhbari Ziegler et al. 2019). COPCA's starting point is family autonomy. It considers caregivers as the experts of their child's needs and recognizes that caregivers will have to deal for a prolonged time with the situation of having a child with special needs. Therefore COPCA considers it quintessential that caregivers make informed decisions in accordance with their own culture and their own specific parenting style. The consequence of these starting points is that COPCA does not use caregiver training but caregiver coaching. In the literature and in practice, coaching is used in different ways and its definitions are characterized by ambiguity (Akhbari Ziegler and Hadders-Algra 2020). In COPCA the approach and definition of coaching of the International Coaching Federation is used. Coaching is defined as 'an ongoing relationship which focuses on coaches taking action toward the realization of the families' visions, goals, and desires. Coaching uses a process of inquiry and personal discovery to build the family's awareness and responsibility and provides the family with structure, support, and feedback' (Rush and Shelden 2011, p. 3). (Note that I replaced the word 'coachee' in the definition by 'family'.) In COPCA, coaching is used to promote the creative exploration of the competencies of the family and infant, therewith empowering the family to find their own solutions.

The infant component of COPCA is primarily based on the Neuronal Group Selection Theory (see Chapter 3), but it also uses the transactional model of Sameroff (Sameroff 2009). The latter emphasizes the bidirectional and transactional nature of the interaction between caregiver and infant. Based on the theoretical principles COPCA recommends (1) to expose the infant to varied conditions and varied positions (e.g. during carrying, dressing, bathing; and playing); the varied positioning also serves the prevention of contractures and deformities; (2) to playfully challenge the infant with a variety of attractive toys to perform by means of self-produced movements activities that are just at the limit of his capabilities (i.e. activities that sometimes can and sometimes cannot be performed successfully); (3) to explain that in infants with impaired postural abilities activities either should challenge the postural abilities or the manual skills, not both abilities simultaneously; during the manual activities the infant deserves proper postural support (De Graaf-Peters et al. 2006; Hadders-Algra 2013); (4) to perform the activities as often as feasible in the family setting during daily care-giving activities – the family decides and sets the goals; (5) to explain that learning by trial and error is the road to success (i.e. to master a skill); (6) to explain that the movement strategies that the child with special needs selects to achieve functional goals may differ from typical movement strategies and that this is fine as long as it serves functional goals; (7) to explain that infants with special needs may have less exploratory drive and may react differently than typically developing infants (Festante et al. 2019), but that this does not mean that the infant is not interested in being engaged in play and interaction; (8) to experience the joy of playful interaction, that is, the shared exploratory journey of discovering new motor, cognitive, language, and social competencies. Play is an integral ingredient of COPCA (see also Chapter 6). It does not only refer to motor play but it also includes singing or reading a book with the infant, or having shared screen-time with the child. Initially, COPCA did not use hands-on techniques, but on the basis of new knowledge (Hadders-Algra et al. 2017; Hielkema et al. 2020a) COPCA currently includes hands-on techniques. It recommends using it as little as possible and to restrict it to minimal postural support in the initial phases of learning a new motor skill, such as standing up.

In practice, COPCA is implemented in the following way. During the first visit the coach explains the nature of COPCA's coaching and the active role of the family members in the intervention (Akhbari Ziegler and Hadders-Algra 2020). Next, the coach visits the family once a week. The coach listens and observes, while the caregiver is involved in daily routines with the child, including feeding and play. This creates a situation in which caregivers feel free to explore and discuss various alternative strategies. In the discussion – based on a bidirectional dialogue – the coach shares the information of the above described recommendations with the caregivers. The caregiver is free to pick and choose strategies and to try them out; the caregivers determine the goals for the next intervention period. When the parents suggest that the caregivers of the day care centre also need to be included in the coaching, this certainly is an option. In general, the frequency of the visits of the coach can be gradually reduced, as the families – in an own process of trial and error – learn the basic principles of coping and caring of an infant with special needs. A qualitative study indicated that caregivers especially valued COPCA's home-based setting, the support from the coach, and the experience being able to participate as active partners in the intervention and make their own decisions (Akhbari Ziegler et al. 2020).

COPCA has been studied in three RCTs in which its effect was compared to that of typical infant physiotherapy. Each study combined the RCT with a process evaluation based on a quantitative analysis of the contents of video-taped intervention sessions. The latter was done to cope with the large heterogeneity in the contents of physiotherapy sessions and to understand which elements in the intervention are associated with better outcome. One RCT was a small study in very preterm infants with a low to moderately increased risk of developmental motor disorders (Akhbari Ziegler et al. 2020). The effect of COPCA was compared to that of typical infant physiotherapy in Switzerland. Swiss typical therapy is characterized by a relatively frequent application of hands-on facilitation and is mostly organized in clinic-based settings (Akhbari Ziegler et al. 2018). Both interventions were applied for 6 months with one intervention session of equal duration per week. Motor outcome immediately after the end of the intervention was similar in both groups. Yet, at later follow-up at 18 months the infants in the COPCA group had improved significantly more in motor outcome than the control infants; the COPCA infants especially had profited in terms of an increase in motor skills and an increase of the movement repertoire. The process evaluation indicated that coaching during the intervention was associated with better motor outcomes at 18 months, whereas training and the application of hands-on techniques were associated with less favourable motor outcomes. The COPCA and the control group did not differ in cognitive development and family empowerment.

The other two RCTs compared the effect of COPCA with that of typical infant physiotherapy in the Netherlands in infants at very high risk of developmental motor disorders. Dutch typical therapy is mostly provided at home. In the first RCT infants were included on the basis of definitely abnormal movements at 10 weeks corrected age; about a quarter of the infants were later diagnosed with CP (Hielkema et al. 2011; Blauw-Hospers et al. 2011). The randomized intervention was provided from 3 to 6 months corrected age with two intervention sessions per week in the COPCA group and about one session per week in the control group. Motor outcome in both groups was similar, whereas the infants in the COPCA group improved slightly more in cognitive scores between 6 and 18 months than the control infants. The process evaluation indicated that the associations between the contents of the intervention and developmental outcome differed for the children who were diagnosed with CP and those who were not. In children with CP, the intervention elements 'coaching' and 'being challenged to produce self-generated movements' were associated with better motor outcomes at 18 months. In the children without CP, coaching was associated with better functional abilities at 18 months, whereas application of hands-on techniques was associated with less favourable mobility. An additional process evaluation, based on quantification of videos of the daily care-taking activity of bathing, revealed that caregivers in the COPCA group bathed their 6-month-old infants significantly more often in a challenging sitting position than caregivers in the control group. In turn, being bathed in a sitting position at 6 months was associated with better functional mobility at 18 months, suggesting that implementation of COPCA principles in daily care giving activities was associated with better outcome (Dirks et al. 2016). The children of this RCT were reassessed at the age of 8 years (Hamer et al. 2017). Functional outcome of the two intervention groups at 8 years was similar. Yet, process evaluation indicated that the intervention elements 'training' and 'instruction' were associated with less favourable mobility scores at school age.

The other Dutch RCT was performed in infants with a significant lesion of the brain; about 50% of the infants were diagnosed with CP (Hielkema et al. 2020a,b). The intervention was provided for a year with weekly intervention sessions in both groups. At the end of the intervention and at the age of 21 months both groups had similar outcomes in the mobility, learning and applying knowledge and behaviour domains. Yet, in the COPCA group the family's quality of life improved significantly, whereas that in the control group did not. Both groups did not differ in family empowerment scores, but the process evaluation indicated that coaching was associated with better empowerment. Through the process evaluation, the insight emerged that the COPCA approach would benefit from inclusion of minimal hands-on support.

GENERAL CONSIDERATIONS ON EARLY INTERVENTION PROGRAMMES IN INFANTS AT VERY HIGH RISK

What can be learned from the above described intervention programmes and studies? First, that all current programmes recommend that early intervention of infants with or at very high risk of a developmental disorder occurs in the home setting. This includes home visits of the therapist. It is conceivable that in case of a prolonged need of early intervention part of the visits, for example, during the second year, can be replaced by teleconsultation, for instance by sessions using videophones. A point of concern is that health insurances in many countries do not cover the costs associated with professional home visits.

The above described programmes also share other insights (Table 14.1). They agree about the following principles: (1) intervention aims at support of the family and at improving the infant's activities in the domains of mobility, learning and applying knowledge and communication, and at optimizing participation of infant and family; (2) intervention is goal-oriented; (3) a key element of intervention is challenging the infant to try out the activities all by himself, with trial and error; (4) the use of hands-on support is restricted to a minimum and is only applied in the initial stages of learning a new motor skill; (5) intervention profits from an enriched environment, that is, the use of a variety of attractive toys, tasks and infant positions; (6) in infants with clear asymmetries in hand use intervention may include the approaches of CIMT or bimanual training; (7) early integration of assistive devices; (8) a high dosage of intervention is associated with better outcomes.

The principle of high dosage introduces a dilemma (Kruijsen-Terpstra et al. 2014): How much is feasible, that is, how much is compatible with daily family life? The study of Campbell et al. (2012) suggested that families indeed have limits in the amount of intervention tasks that they can cope with. The study evaluated the effect of a 10-month-programme of intensive motor practice and environmental enrichment in very high-risk infants. It revealed that families practised less than scheduled, especially during the final months of the intervention. In this respect, the COPCA approach may offer a solution: the family learns the principles of infant development and implements them in their own way and in their preferred intensity. The studies on COPCA indicated that this does not result in an immediate effect on infant development; the effect emerges in the long run, as families continue to implement the intervention principles, thereby generating a slowly accumulating higher dosage of practice (Blauw-Hospers et al. 2011; Akhabari Ziegler et al. 2020).

The programmes also differ – especially in the role that they attribute to the family (Table 14.1). In CareToy, CIMT, GAME, and SSP the main role of the caregivers is to train the infant. In COPCA, caregivers continue to raise the child according to their own family perspectives; they are not regarded as trainers. The difference in role of the family is associated with differences in who is in charge of decision-making (family and professional versus family), in the role of the professional (being a teacher and a coach vs being a coach) and in the associated educational and communication skills used by the professional (Table 14.1; Akhbari Ziegler et al. 2019; Akhbari Ziegler and Hadders-Algra 2020). Currently, it is not entirely clear which approach is best. Nonetheless, the COPCA trials suggest that coaching is preferred, as coaching was associated with better mobility outcomes, whereas training was associated with less favourable outcomes. Also, the review of Hutchon et al. (2019) concluded that coaching is the preferred approach. Coaching is possible in all families (Rush and Sheldon 2011), but it requires an explanation of the coaching process to the families, as the coaching approach differs from the traditional physiotherapeutic approach. It also requires specific education of the professional, as becoming a coach involves acquiring knowledge of adult learning processes, changing of habits, and attitudes and beliefs (Akhbari Ziegler et al. 2018; Akhbari Ziegler and Hadders-Algra 2020).

The use of assistive devices is mentioned in two of the programmes, SSP and COPCA (Table 14.1). It is getting increasingly evident that assistive devices for lying, sitting, standing, walking, and communication certainly deserve a place in early intervention. The use of assistive devices in early intervention is discussed in Chapter 15.

Whether treadmill training deserves a place in early intervention is less clear. Some evidence is available that treadmill intervention may accelerate the development of independent walking in children with trisomy 21 (Down syndrome). It also may accelerate motor skill attainment in children with CP and general developmental delay (Valentín-Gudiol et al. 2017).

EARLY INTERVENTION IN INFANTS AT VERY HIGH RISK ADDRESSING SPECIFIC SIGNS AND SYMPTOMS

- *Feeding difficulties.* Infants with or at very high risk of developmental motor disorders often have feeding difficulties. These difficulties are associated with impaired growth, aspiration pneumonia, and death (Khamis et al. 2020). The study of Benfer et al. (2017) indicated that at the age of 18–24 months about 80% of children with CP have oropharyngeal dysphagia. After that age, the prevalence gradually declines, especially in children functioning at GMFCS levels I and II. The management of oropharyngeal dysphagia consists of (1) direct interventions, including adaptations of the texture or taste of the fluid or food, (2) indirect interventions, such as exercises to improve oral

Table 14.1 Recently developed programs for infants with or at very high risk of developmental motor disorders

Component of intervention	Baby-CIMT	GAME	Small Step Program	COPCA
Site of				
– professional support	Home	Home	Home	Home
– intervention	Home	Home	Home	Home
Role of family	Training infant	Training infant	Training infant	Family, raising child according to family perspectives
In charge of decision-making	Family and professional	Family and professional	Family and professional	Family
Role of professional	Coach and trainer	Coach and trainer	Coach and trainer	Coach
Skills used by professional	Coaching,* training, and education of caregivers so that they become confident service providers; no details provided	Coaching,* training, and education of caregivers; no details provided	Coaching,* training, and education of caregivers; no details provided	Coaching; listening; observing; giving hints and suggestions; allowing families to cope in their own way with the situation of having a child with special needs
Goals of intervention (in order of priority)	– Optimal child development (mobility; learning and applying knowledge; communication) – Reduction of family stress and anxiety	– Optimal child development (mobility; learning and applying knowledge; communication)	– Optimal child development (mobility; learning and applying knowledge; communication) – Reduction of family stress and anxiety	– Family empowerment, learning to cope with the situation of having a child with special needs – Optimal child development (mobility; learning and applying knowledge; communication)

(Continued on next page)

Table 14.1 Recently developed programs for infants with or at very high risk of developmental motor disorders (Continued)

Component of intervention	Baby-CIMT	GAME	Small Step Program	COPCA
Means to achieve goals	– Application of simple restraint of the least-involved hand (e.g. mitten, sock), 30 min/day, presentation of interesting objects that are appropriate for the infant's developmental abilities, while sitting upright and stable (e.g. in infant chair) – Additional flyer with CIMT information	– Training according to written home program, promoting self-initiated actions by use of meaningful and motivating activities and toys; to explore with trial and error – Encouragement of interaction and language-facilitating communication during daily activities – Integration of CIMT optional	– Training sessions in home environment promoting self-initiated actions by use of meaningful and motivating activities and toys – Encouragement of interaction and language-facilitating communication during daily activities – Integration of CIMT optional	– Playful interaction during daily caregiving activities, accompanied by dialogue between caregiver and child – During the interactions: challenging infant to self-produced movements, to explore with trial and error performance of own body, objects, environment, communication, and social interaction, appropriate for infant's current abilities and context – Integration of CIMT optional
Hands-on	No hands-on during CIMT-sessions	Hands-on when learning new skills for safety and to give the infant an idea of the movement'	Hands-on when learning new skills, to provide postural stability	Only hands-on in infants at very high risk of CP and only to provide postural stability
Assistive devices	No specific assistive devices used	Early introduction of postural equipment and mobility devices	Early introduction of postural equipment and mobility devices	Early introduction of postural equipment and mobility devices

Based on Akhbari Ziegler et al. (2019), Dirks et al. (2011), Dirks and Hadders-Algra (2011), Eliasson et al. (2014a, 2016), Hielkema et al. (2010), Holmström et al. (2019), Morgan et al. (2014, 2015).

*Note that the approaches of training and coaching do not match. The descriptions of the programmes indicate that parental training is the main approach used.

motor function, and (3) compensatory techniques, such as provision of an optimal sitting condition and using adapted utensils (Morgan et al. 2012). The motor learning interventions aim to improve suck–swallow–breathe coordination, the oral skills for bolus formation, and swallowing skills while minimizing safety risks. To this end the interventions use, for instance, biting and chewing practice, and changes in texture, taste, and temperature of food to increase oral awareness. The evidence on the effectiveness of these intervention strategies is very weak (Khamis et al. 2020). In children in whom the feeding difficulties are associated with growth impairment, feeding via gastrostomy tube is recommended as an effective, long-term nutritional intervention. The tube feeding should not be delayed, but should start before the development of malnutrition (Romano et al. 2017).

- *Drooling.* Many children with CP are impaired by drooling, that is, clearly visible spilling of saliva from the month (McInerney et al. 2019). It is estimated that about 40% of children with CP at schoolage have this impairment. The systematic review of McInerney et al. (2019) indicated that in children with CP aged 5 years and older a large variety of behavioural interventions are used to alleviate drooling, including reinforcement, prompting, self-management, extinction, overcorrection, instruction, and fading (i.e. a feedback technique with decreasing promptness of feedback over time; Lancioni et al. 2009). Yet, the evidence that these interventions are successful is low. No systematic studies on drooling interventions in young children are available.
- *Spasticity.* Current early intervention programmes do not focus on impairments such as spasticity; focus is on activities and participation. In older children botulinum toxin is used to reduce spasticity in targeted muscles. This treatment is successful, but limited in time (Basu et al. 2015). Recent studies indicate that caution is warranted as repeated botulinum toxin treatment in children with CP may be associated with impaired muscle growth (Schless et al. 2019). In young children, botulinum toxin, oral baclofen, and NDT are used to manage tone; however, no evidence is available about the effectiveness of these treatments (Ward et al. 2017).
- *Pain.* Children with CP often have pain – a prevalence of about 75% has been reported (Novak et al. 2012). The systematic review of Ostojic and colleagues on pain management in children with CP indicated that the level of evidence of the various interventions is weak (Ostojic et al. 2019). Relatively good evidence is available that intrathecal baclofen in children with spastic or spastic-dyskinetic CP is able to reduce pain. Whether botulinum toxin has the same effect in children with spastic CP is less clear. The review did not specify the ages of the children evaluated in the various interventions, but presumably most of them were older than 2 years of age.
- *Epilepsy.* About a quarter of children with CP have epilepsy (Novak et al. 2012). The epilepsy deserves pharmacological treatment. The details of the antiepileptic treatment are beyond the scope of this chapter.
- *Cerebral visual impairment.* Function in daily life of children with CP may also be impaired by cerebral visual impairment. Its reported prevalence varies from 4% to 11% (Sellier et al. 2020). It occurs especially in children with complex multidisability. Children with this impairment profit from good lighting, optimal contrast and a relatively simple and structured visual environment (Ortibus et al. 2019). The effect of specific interventions in young children with cerebral visual impairment has not been investigated.

STEM CELL INTERVENTIONS: A FUTURE OPTION?

Theoretically, stem cells may have a positive effect on the injured developing brain. This effect is presumably less due to replacement or engrafting but more related to paracrine effects (i.e. the factors secreted by the stem cells facilitating neurogenesis, angiogenesis, and immunomodulation) (Jantzie et al. 2018). However, currently caution for its clinical use is warranted. Two reviews indicated that up until now heterogeneous studies have been performed. The studies suggested that stem cell therapy might be associated with a minor beneficial effect on gross motor function; however, the effect is far from proven (Novak et al. 2016; Eggenberger et al. 2019).

CONCLUDING REMARKS

Early intervention programmes are family centred. The intervention programmes designed for infants who were critically ill in the neonatal period without acquiring a significant lesion of the brain focus on caregiver support and education, support of sensitive and responsive parent–infant interaction, and infant stimulation. These programmes are associated with a reduction in maternal stress, anxiety and depression, and better infant cognitive development. Most programmes have not been associated with a significant effect on infant motor development, but there are exceptions: IBAIP, CareToy, and COPCA have been associated with improved motor outcome.

In early intervention in infants with or at very high risk of developmental motor disorders, two approaches for the family are available: family-centred programmes that focus on the infant and the infant's development (CareToy, CIMT, GAME, SSP) and the family-centred programme COPCA that focusses on the family. The difference in focus results in differences in the roles of the family and the professional, in differences in approaches and communication. COPCA's approach is associated with increased family empowerment.

The programmes for infants with or at very high risk of motor developmental disorders agree that (1) early intervention should not only focus on mobility, but also address learning and applying knowledge and communication; (2) intervention primarily addresses activities, not impairments such as deviant muscle tone or abnormal reflexes; (3) important ingredients of intervention are self-generated movements, challenging the infant with activities at the limit of his abilities, and trial and error; (4) minimal use of hands-on techniques; it is restricted to minimal postural support in the initial phases of learning a new activity by trial and error; (5) in infants with severe impairments, assistive devices are used from early age onwards to provide postural support, to prevent contractures and deformities, and to assist mobility and communication.

Finally, the chapter underscores the notion that research in early intervention is challenging. The challenges are caused by the presence of multiple sources of heterogeneity: diversity in the children studied, for example variations in brain lesion and variations in resilience, diversity in families, for instance in educational level and cultural background, regional diversity in health care available, and diversity in contents, frequency, and duration of the intervention (Hadders-Algra et al. 2017). In addition, the results of the study are often heterogeneous as different outcome measures are used. To deal with the major sources of this challenging heterogeneity the following two strategies may be used: (1) multicentre RCTs, where the multicentre approach allows for larger numbers of children, which increases the likelihood that two intervention groups are comparable in child and family characteristics, and (2) smaller RCTs or studies with case series that accurately document not only child and family characteristics, but also precisely document the contents of the intervention and its implementation in the home situation. The former can be done, for stance, by quantifying video-recordings of intervention sessions (e.g. Blauw-Hospers et al. 2011; Hielkema et al. 2020a,b; Akhbari-Ziegler et al. 2020) and the latter by quantifying video-recordings of home activities (Dirks et al. 2016).

Specific questions that urgently need to be addressed are:

- Which intervention approach benefits families best: training or coaching? Does the effect of the approaches differ for different families? Does it matter whether the effect is evaluated immediately after the intervention or on the long run?

- What is the optimal dosage of intervention (i.e. what is the optimal balance between the proven research adage 'more is better' and the quality of life of the family of the infant with or at high risk of a developmental disorder)?
- Which children may profit from some hands-on techniques and in which situations? What are the key-components of such hands-on techniques?

During the last decades, the scientific community dealing with developmental disorders really provided insight into the do's and don'ts in early intervention. Yet, the goal of knowing 'what intervention is best for which infant and which family' has not been reached. I suggest that the intervention programs and their evaluation use an approach including all aspects of the ICF-CY (see Chapter 1). This means that not only attention is paid to impairments in body structure and function and limitations in activities and participation, but also to the environment. The latter involves family empowerment and the application of assistive devices, such as adaptive seating systems and power mobility. These assistive devices may assist the infant in the discovery of the world and the interaction with other people therewith promoting cognitive and personal development (see the next chapter).

REFERENCES

Adolph KE, Cole WG, Komati M, et al. (2012) How do you learn to walk? Thousands of steps and dozens of falls per day. *Psychol Sci* **23**: 1387–1394. doi: 10.1177/0956797612446346.

Akhbari Ziegler S, von Rhein M, Meichtry A, et al. (2020) The coping with and caring for infants with special needs intervention was associated with improved motor development in preterm infants. *Acta Paediatr*, epub ahead of print. doi: 10.1111/apa.15619.

Akhbari Ziegler S, Hadders-Algra M (2020) Coaching approaches in early intervention and paediatric rehabilitation. *Dev Med Child Neurol* **62**: 569–574. doi: 10.1111/dmcn.14493.

Akhbari Ziegler S, Dirks T, Reinders-Messelink HA, Meichtry A, Hadders-Algra M (2018) Changes in therapist actions during a novel pediatric physical therapy program: success and challenges. *Pediatr Phys Ther* **30**: 223–230. doi: 10.1097/PEP.0000000000000509.

Akhbari Ziegler S, Dirks T, Hadders-Algra M (2019) Coaching in early physical therapy intervention: the COPCA program as an example of translation of theory into practice. *Disabil Rehabil* **41**: 1846–1854. doi: 10.1080/09638288.2018.

Akhbari Ziegler S, Mitteregger E, Hadders-Algra M (2020) Caregivers' experiences with the new family-centred paediatric physiotherapy programme COPCA: a qualitative study. *Child Care Health Dev* **46**: 28–36. doi: 10.1111/cch.12722.

d'Avignon M, Norén L, Arman T (1981) Early physiotherapy ad modum Vojta or Bobath in infants with suspected neuromotor disturbance. *Neuropediatrics* **12**: 232–241.

Ayres AJ (1966) Interrelationships among perceptual-motor functions in children. *Am J Occup Ther* **20**: 68–71.

Basu AP, Pearse J, Kelly S, Wisher V, Kisler J (2015) Early intervention to improve hand function in hemiplegic cerebral palsy. *Front Neurol* **5**: 281. doi: 10.3389/fneur.2014.00281.

Benfer KA, Weir KA, Bell KL, Ware RS, Davies PSW, Boyd RN (2017) Oropharyngeal dysphagia and cerebral palsy. *Pediatrics* **140** pii: e20170731. doi: 10.1542/peds.2017-0731.

Benzies KM, Magill-Evans JE, Hayden KA, Ballantyne M (2013) Key components of early intervention programs for preterm infants and their parents: a systematic review and meta-analysis. *BMC Pregnancy Childbirth* **13** (Suppl 1): S10.

Blanche EI, Chang MC, Gutiérrez J, Gunter JS (2016) Effectiveness of a sensory-enriched early intervention group program for children with developmental disabilities. *Am J Occup Ther* **70**: 7005220010, 1–8. doi: 10.5014/ajot.2016.018481.

Blank R, Barnett AL, Cairney J, et al. (2019) International clinical practice recommendations on the definition, diagnosis, assessment, intervention, and psychosocial aspects of developmental coordination disorder. *Dev Med Child Neurol* **61**: 242–285. doi: 10.1111/dmcn.14132.

Blauw-Hospers CH, Hadders-Algra M (2005) A systematic review of the effects of early intervention on motor development. *Dev Med Child Neurol* **47**: 421–432.

Blauw-Hospers CH, Dirks T, Hulshof LJ, Bos AF, Hadders-Algra M (2011) Pediatric physical therapy in infancy: from nightmare to dream? A two-arm randomized trial. *Phys Ther* **91**: 1323–1338. doi: 10.2522/ptj.20100205.

Bleyenheuft Y, Gordon AM (2013) Precision grip control, sensory impairments and their interactions in children with hemiplegic cerebral palsy: a systematic review. *Res Dev Disabil* **34**: 3014–3028. doi: 10.1016/j.ridd.2013.05.047.

Bly L (1999) *Baby Treatment Based on NDT Principles.* Austin, TX: Pro-ed.

Bobath K (1980) *A Neurophysiological Basis for the Treatment of Cerebral Palsy*, 2nd edn. London: William Heinemann Medical Books.

Bobath K, Bobath B (1950) Spastic paralysis treatment by the use of reflex inhibition. *Br J Phys Med* **13**: 121–127.

Bobath K, Bobath B (1984) The Neuro-Developmental Treatment. In: Scrutton D, editor, *Management of the Motor Disorders of Children with Cerebral Palsy.* Oxford: Blackwell Scientific Publications, pp. 6–18.

Bourke-Taylor H, O'Shea R, Gaebler-Spira D (2007) Conductive education: a functional skills program for children with cerebral palsy. *Phys Occup Ther Pediatr* **27**: 45–62.

Bos AF, van Asperen RM, de Leeuw DM, Prechtl HF (1997) The influence of septicaemia on spontaneous motility in preterm infants. *Early Hum Dev* **50**: 61–70.

Bremner JD (2013) Post-traumatic stress disorder (PTSD). In: Ochsner KN, Kosslyn S, editors, *The Oxford Handbook of Cognitive Neuroscience. Volume 2. The Cutting Edges.* Oxford: Oxford Handbooks Online. doi: 10.1093/oxfordhb/9780199988709.013.0027.

Buntinx WHE (2013) Understanding disability: a strengths-based Approach. In: Wehmeyer ML, editor, *The Oxford Handbook of Positive Psychology and Disability.* Oxford: Oxford Handbooks On-line, doi: 10.1093/oxfordhb/9780195398786.013.013.0002.

Butler C, Darrah J (2001) Effects of neurodevelopmental treatment (NDT) for cerebral palsy: an AACPDM evidence report. *Dev Med Child Neurol* **43**: 778–790.

Campbell SK, Gaebler-Spira D, Zawacki L, et al. (2012) Effects on motor development of kicking and stepping exercise in preterm infants with periventricular brain injury: a pilot study. *J Pediatr Rehabil Med* **5**: 15–27. doi: 10.3233/PRM-2011-0185.

Chamudot R, Parush S, Rigbi A, Horovitz R, Gross-Tsur V (2018) Effectiveness of modified constraint-induced movement therapy compared with bimanual therapy home programs for infants with hemiplegia: a randomized controlled trial. *Am J Occup Ther* **72**: 7206205010p1-7206205010p9. doi: 10.5014/ajot.2018.025981.

De Graaf-Peters VB, De Groot-Hornstra AH, Dirks T, Hadders-Algra M (2006) Specific postural support promotes variation in motor behaviour of infants with minor neurological dysfunction. *Dev Med Child Neurol* **48**: 966–972.

Dirks T, Hadders-Algra M (2011) The role of the family in intervention of infants at high risk of cerebral palsy: a systematic analysis. *Dev Med Child Neurol* **53** (Suppl 4): 62–67. doi: 10.1111/j.1469-8749.2011.04067.x.

Dirks T, Blauw-Hospers CH, Hulshof LJ, Hadders-Algra M (2011) Differences between the family-centered 'COPCA' program and traditional infant physical therapy based on neurodevelopmental treatment principles *Phys Ther* **91**: 1303–1322. doi: 10.2522/ptj.20100207.

Dirks T, Hielkema T, Hamer EG, Reinders-Messelink HA, Hadders-Algra M (2016) Infant positioning in daily life may mediate associations between physiotherapy and child development – video-analysis of an early intervention RCT. *Res Dev Disabil* **53–54**: 147–157. doi: 10.1016/j.ridd.2016.02.006.

Edelman GM (1989) *Neural Darwinism. The Theory of Neuronal Group Selection.* Oxford: Oxford University Press.

Eggenberger S, Boucard C, Schoeberlein A, et al. (2019) Stem cell treatment and cerebral palsy: systematic review and meta-analysis. *World J Stem Cells* **11**: 891–903. doi: 10.4252/wjsc.v11.i10.891.

Eliasson AC, Holmström L, Aarne P, et al. (2016) Efficacy of the small step program in a randomized controlled trial for infants below age 12 months with clinical signs of CP: a study protocol. *BMC Pediatr.* **16**: 175. doi: 10.1186/s12887-016-0711-x.

Eliasson A-C, Krumlinde-Sundholm L, Gordon AM, et al. (2014b) Guidelines for future research in constraint-induced movement therapy for children with unilateral cerebral palsy: an expert consensus. *Dev Med Child Neurol* **56**: 125–137. doi: 10.1111/dmcn.12273.

Eliasson AC, Nordstrand L, Ek L, et al. (2018) The effectiveness of baby-CIMT in infants younger than 12 months with clinical signs of unilateral cerebral palsy: an explorative study with randomized design. *Res Dev Disabil* **72**: 191–201. doi: 10.1016/j.ridd.2017.11.006.

Eliasson AC, Sjöstrand L, Ek L, Krumlinde-Sundholm L, Tedroff K (2014a) Efficacy of baby-CIMT: study protocol for a randomized controlled trial on infants below age 12 months, with clinical signs of unilateral CP. *BMC Pediatr* **14**: 141. doi: 10.1186/1471-2431-14-141.

Farjoun N, Mayston M, Florencio LL, Fernández-De-Las-Peñas C, Palacios-Ceña D (2020) Essence of the Bobath concept in the treatment of children with cerebral palsy. A qualitative study of the experience of Spanish therapists. *Physiother Theory Pract,* epub ahead of print. doi: 10.1080/09593985.2020.1725943.

Festante F, Antonelli C, Chorna O, Corsi G, Guzzetta A (2019) Parent-infant interaction during the first year of life in infants at high risk for cerebral palsy: a systematic review of the literature. *Neural Plast* **2019**: 5759694. doi: 10.1155/2019/5759694.

Frade F, Gómez-Salgado J, Jacobsohn L, Florindo-Silva F (2019) Rehabilitation of neonatal brachial plexus palsy: integrative literature review. *J Clin Med* **8**: E980. doi: 10.3390/jcm8070980.

Gordon AM (2011) To constrain or not to constrain, and other stories of intensive upper extremity training for children with unilateral cerebral palsy. *Dev Med Child Neurol* **53** (Suppl 4): 56–61. doi: 10.1111/j.1469-8749.2011.04066.x.

Gorter JW, Ketelaar M, Rosenbaum P, Helders PJ, Palisano R. (2009) Use of the GMFCS in infants with CP: the need for reclassification at 2 years or older. *Dev Med Child Neurol* **51**: 46–52. doi: 10.1111/j.1469-8749.2008.03117.x.

Granild-Jensen JB, Rackauskaite G, Flachs EM, Uldall P (2015) Predictors for early diagnosis of cerebral palsy from national registry data. *Dev Med Child Neurol* **57**: 931–935. doi: 10.1111/dmcn.12760.

Guttmann K, Flibotte J, DeMauro SB (2018) Parental perspective on diagnosis and prognosis of neonatal intensive care unit graduates with cerebral palsy. *J Pediatr* **203**: 156–162. doi: 10.1016/j.jpeds.2018.07.089.

Guttmann K, Flibotte J, DeMauro SB, Seitz H (2020) A mixed methods analysis of parental perspectives on diagnosis and prognosis of neonatal intensive care graduates with cerebral palsy. *J Child Neurol* **35**: 336–343. doi: 10.1177/0883073820901412.

Hadders-Algra M (2007) Putative neural substrate of normal and abnormal general movements. *Neurosci Biobehav Rev* **31**: 1181–1190.

Hadders-Algra M (2013) Typical and atypical development of reaching and postural control in infancy. *Dev Med Child Neurol* **55** (Suppl 4): 5–8. doi: 10.1111/dmcn.12298.

Hadders-Algra M (2018a) Early human motor development: from variation to the ability to vary and adapt. *Neurosci Biobehav Rev* **90**: 411–427. doi: 10.1016/j.neubiorev.2018.05.009.

Hadders-Algra M (2018b) Neural substrate and clinical significance of general movements: an update. *Dev Med Child Neurol* **60**: 39–46. doi: 10.1111/dmcn.13540.

Hadders-Algra M, Boxum AG, Hielkema T, Hamer EG (2017) Effect of early intervention in infants at very high risk of cerebral palsy: a systematic review. *Dev Med Child Neurol* **59**: 246–258. doi: 10.1111/dmcn.13331.

Hamer EG, Hielkema T, Bos AF, et al. (2017) Effect of early intervention on functional outcome at school age: follow-up and process evaluation of a randomized controlled trial in infants at risk. *Early Hum Dev* **106–107**: 67–74. doi: 10.1016/j.earlhumdev.2017.02.002.

Hamer EG, La Bastide-Van Gemert S, Boxum AG, et al. (2018) The tonic response to the infant knee jerk as an early sign of cerebral palsy. *Early Hum Dev* **119**: 38–44. doi: 10.1016/j.earlhumdev.2018.03.001.

Hari M, Tillemans T (1984) Conductive education. In: Scrutton D, editor, *Management of the Motor Disorders of Children with Cerebral Palsy.* Oxford: Blackwell Scientific Publications, pp. 19–35.

Heineman KR, Bos AF, Hadders-Algra M (2008) The Infant Motor Profile: a standardized and qualitative method to assess motor behaviour in infancy. *Dev Med Child Neurol* **50**: 275–282. doi: 10.1111/j.1469-8749.2008.02035.x.

Hielkema T, Blauw-Hospers CH, Dirks T, Drijver-Messelink M, Bos AF, Hadders-Algra M (2011) Does physiotherapeutic intervention affect motor outcome in high-risk infants? An approach combining a randomized controlled trial and process evaluation. *Dev Med Child Neurol* **53**: e8–15. doi: 10.1111/j.1469-8749.2010.03876.x

Hielkema T, Hamer EG, Reinders-Messelink HA, et al. (2010) LEARN2MOVE 0–2 years: effects of a new intervention program in infants at very high risk for cerebral palsy; a randomized controlled trial. *BMC Pediatr* **10**: 76. doi: 10.1186/1471-2431-10-76.

Hielkema T, Boxum AG, Hamer EG, et al. (2020b) LEARN2MOVE 0–2 years, a randomized early intervention trial for infants at very high risk of cerebral palsy: family outcome and infant's functional outcome. *Disabil Rehabil* **42**: 3762–3770. doi: 10.1080/09638288.2019.1610509.

Hielkema T, Hamer EG, Boxum AG, et al. (2020a) LEARN2MOVE 0–2 years, a randomized early intervention trial for infants at very high risk of cerebral palsy: neuromotor, cognitive, and behavioural outcome. *Disabil Rehabil* **42**: 3752–3761. doi: 10.1080/09638288.2019.1610508.

Hielkema T, Toonen RF, Hooijsma SJ, et al. (2018) Changes in the content of pediatric physical therapy for infants: a quantitative, observational study. *Phys Occup Ther Pediatr* **38**: 457–488. doi: 10.1080/01942638.2017.1405863.

Hoare BJ, Wallen MA, Thorley MN, Jackman ML, Carey LM, Imms C (2019) Constraint-induced movement therapy in children with unilateral cerebral palsy. *Cochrane Database Syst Rev* **4**: CD004149. doi: 10.1002/14651858.CD004149.pub3.

Holmström L, Eliasson AC, Almeida R, et al. (2019) Efficacy of the small step program in a randomized controlled trial for infants under 12 months old at risk of cerebral palsy (CP) and other neurological disorders. *J Clin Med* **8** pii: E1016. doi: 10.3390/jcm8071016.

Howle JM (2002) *Neurodevelopment Treatment Approach: Theoretical Foundations and Principles of Clinical Practice.* Laguna Beach, CA: Neuro-Developmental Treatment Association.

Hubner LM, Feldman HM, Huffman LC (2016) Parent-reported shared decision making: autism spectrum disorder and other neurodevelopmental disorders. *J Dev Behav Pediatr* **37**: 20–32. doi: 10.1097/DBP.0000000000000242.

Hutchon B, Gibbs D, Harniess P, et al. (2019) Early intervention programmes for infants at high risk of atypical neurodevelopmental outcome. *Dev Med Child Neurol* **61**: 1362–1367. doi: 10.1111/dmcn.14187.

Jantzie LL, Scafidi J, Robinson S (2018) Stem cells and cell-based therapies for cerebral palsy: a call for rigor. *Pediatr Res* **83**: 345–355. doi: 10.1038/pr.2017.233.

Jung MW, Landenberger M, Jung T, Lindenthal T, Philippi H (2017) Vojta therapy and neurodevelopmental treatment in children with infantile postural asymmetry: a randomised controlled trial. *J Phys Ther Sci* **29**: 301–306. doi: 10.1589/jpts.29.301.

Kanda T, Pidcock FS, Hayakawa K, Yamori Y, Shikata Y (2004) Motor outcome differences between two groups of children with spastic diplegia who received different intensities of early onset physiotherapy followed for 5 years. *Brain Dev* **26**: 118–126.

Khamis A, Novak I, Morgan C, et al. (2020) Motor learning feeding interventions for infants at risk of cerebral palsy: a systematic review. *Dysphagia* **35**: 1–17. doi: 10.1007/s00455-019-10016-x.

King G, Chiarello L (2014) Family-centered care for children with cerebral palsy: conceptual and practical considerations to advance care and practice. *J Child Neurol* **29**: 1046–1054. doi: 10.1177/0883073814533009.

King S, Teplicky R, King G, Rosenbaum P (2004) Family-centered service for children with cerebral palsy and their families: a review of the literature. *Semin Pediatr Neurol* **11**: 78–86.

Kolb B, Harker A, Gibb R (2017) Principles of plasticity in the developing brain. *Dev Med Child Neurol* **59**: 1218–1223. doi: 10.1111/dmcn.13546.

Koldewijn K, Vvan Wassenaer A, Wolf MJ, et al. (2010) A neurobehavioral intervention and assessment program in very low birth weight infants: outcome at 24 months. *J Pediatr* **156**: 359–365. doi: 10.1016/j.jpeds.2009.09.009.

Koldewijn K, Wolf MJ, Van Wassenaer A, et al. (2009) The Infant Behavioral Assessment and Intervention Program for very low birth weight infants at 6 months corrected age. *J Pediatr* **154**: 33–38.e2. doi: 10.1016/j.jpeds.2008.07.039.

Köng E (1966) Very early treatment of cerebral palsy. *Dev Med Child Neurol* **8**: 198–202.

Kruijsen-Terpstra AJ, Ketelaar M, Boeije H, et al. (2014) Parents' experiences with physical and occupational therapy for their young child with cerebral palsy: a mixed studies review. *Child Care Health Dev* **40**: 787–796. doi: 10.1111/cch.12097.

Lach LM, Rosenbaum P, Bailey S, Bogossian A, MacCulloch R (2014) Parenting a child with cerebral palsy: family and social issues. In: Dan B, Mayston M, Paneth N, Rosenbloom L, editors, *Cerebral palsy: Science and Clinical Practice.* London: Mac Keith Press, pp. 27–41.

Lancioni GE, Singh NN, O'Reilly MF, et al. (2009) Technology-assisted programs to promote mouth drying and reduce the effects of drooling with two persons with developmental disabilities. *J Dev Phys Disabil* **21**: 555–564. doi: 10.1007/s10882-009-9153-9.

Lecuona E, Van Jaarsveld A, Raubenheimer J, Van Heerden R (2017) Sensory integration intervention and the development of the premature infant: a controlled trial. *S Afr Med J* **107**: 976–982. doi: 10.7196/SAMJ.2017. v107i11.12393.

Marvin RS, Pianta R C (1996) Mothers' reactions to their child's diagnosis: relations with security of attachment. *J Clin Child Psychol* **25**: 436–445.

Mayston M (2004) Physiotherapy management in cerebral palsy: an update on treatment approaches. In: Scrutton D, Damiano D, Mayston M, editors, *Management of the Motor Disorders of Children with Cerebral Palsy*, 2nd edn. London: Mac Keith Press, pp. 147–160.

Mayston M (2008) Bobath concept: Bobath@50: mid-life crisis – what of the future? *Physiother Res Int* **13**: 131–136. doi: 10.1002/pri.413.

Mayston M (2014) Intervention planning, implementation and evaluation. In: Dan B, Mayston M, Paneth N, Rosenbloom L, editors, *Cerebral Palsy: Science and Clinical Practice*. London: Mac Keith Press, pp. 329–360.

Mayston M (2016) Bobath and NeuroDevelopmental Therapy: What is the future? *Dev Med Child Neurol* **58**: 994. doi: 10.1111/dmcn.13221.

McInerney MS, Reddihough DS, Carding PN, Swanton R, Walton CM, Imms C (2019) Behavioural interventions to treat drooling in children with neurodisability: a systematic review. *Dev Med Child Neurol* **61**: 39–48. doi: 10.1111/dmcn.14048.

Meijssen D, Wolf MJ, Koldewijn K, et al. (2010) The effect of the Infant Behavioral Assessment and Intervention Program on mother-infant interaction after very preterm birth. *J Child Psychol Psychiatry* **51**: 1287–1295. doi: 10.1111/j.1469-7610.2010.02237.x.

Meijssen DE, Wolf MJ, Koldewijn K, Van Wassenaer AG, Kok JH, van Baar AL (2011) Parenting stress in mothers after very preterm birth and the effect of the Infant Behavioral Assessment and Intervention Program. *Child Care Health Dev* **37**: 195–202. doi: 10.1111/j.1365-2214.2010.01119.x.

Morgan AT, Dodrill P, Ward EC (2012) Interventions for oropharyngeal dysphagia in children with neurological impairment. *Cochrane Database Syst Rev* **10**: CD009456. doi: 10.1002/14651858.CD009456.pub2.

Morgan C, Darrah J, Gordon AM, et al. (2016a) Effectiveness of motor interventions in infants with cerebral palsy: systematic review. *Dev Med Child Neurol* **58**: 900–909. doi: 10.1111/dmcn.13105.

Morgan C, Novak I, Dale RC, Guzzetta A, Badawi N (2014) GAME (Goals – Activity – Motor Enrichment): protocol of a single blind randomized controlled trial of motor training, parent education and environmental enrichment for infants at high risk of cerebral palsy. *BMC Neurol* **14**: 203. doi: 10.1186/s12883-014-0203-2.

Morgan C, Novak I, Dale RC, Badawi N (2015) Optimising motor learning in infants at high risk of cerebral palsy: a pilot study. *BMC Pediatr* **15**: 30. doi: 10.1186/s12887-015-0347-2.

Morgan C, Novak I, Dale RC, Guzzetta A, Badawi N (2016b) Single blind randomised controlled trial of GAME (Goals – Activity – Motor Enrichment) in infants at high risk of cerebral palsy. *Res Dev Disabil* **55**: 256–267. doi: 10.1016/j.ridd.2016.04.005.

Myrhaug HT, Odgaard-Jensen J, Østensjø S, Vøllestad NK, Jahnsen R (2018) Effect of a conductive education course in young children with cerebral palsy: a randomized controlled trial. *Dev Neurorehabil* **21**: 481–489. doi: 10.1080/17518423.2017.1360961.

Myrhaug HT, Odgaard-Jensen J, Jahnsen R (2019) The long-term effects of conductive education courses in young children with cerebral palsy: a randomized controlled trial. *Dev Neurorehabil* **22**: 111–119. doi: 10.1080/17518423.2018.1460771.

Nordstrand L, Holmefur M, Kits A, Eliasson AC (2015) Improvements in bimanual hand function after baby-CIMT in two-year old children with unilateral cerebral palsy: a retrospective study. *Res Dev Disabil* **41–42**: 86–93. doi: 10.1016/j.ridd.2015.05.003.

Novak I, Hines M, Goldsmith S, Barclay R (2012) Clinical prognostic messages from a systematic review on cerebral palsy. *Pediatrics* **130**: e1285–312. doi: 10.1542/peds.2012-0924.

Novak I, Morgan C, Adde L, et al. (2017) Early, accurate diagnosis and early intervention in cerebral palsy: advances in diagnosis and treatment. *JAMA Pediatr* **171**: 897–907. doi: 10.1001/jamapediatrics.2017.1689.

Novak I, Morgan C, McNamara L, Te Velde A (2019) Best practice guidelines for communicating to parents the diagnosis of disability. *Early Hum Dev* **139**: 104841. doi: 10.1016/j.earlhumdev.2019.104841.

Novak I, Morgan C, Fahey M, et al. (2020) State of the evidence traffic lights 2019: systematic review of interventions for preventing and treating children with cerebral palsy. *Curr Neurol Neurosci Rep* **20**: 3. doi: 10.1007/s11910-020-1022-z.

Novak I, Walker K, Hunt RW, Wallace EM, Fahey M, Badawi N (2016) Concise review: stem cell interventions for people with cerebral palsy: systematic review with meta-analysis. *Stem Cells Transl Med* **5**: 1014–1025. doi: 10.5966/sctm.2015-0372.

Odding E, Roebroeck ME, Stam HJ (2006) The epidemiology of cerebral palsy: incidence, impairments and risk factors. *Disabil Rehabil* **28**: 183–191.

Ortibus E, Fazzi E, Dale N (2019) Cerebral visual impairment and clinical assessment: the European perspective. *Semin Pediatr Neurol* **31**: 15–24. doi: 10.1016/j.spen.2019.05.004.

Ostojic K, Paget SP, Morrow AM (2019) Management of pain in children and adolescents with cerebral palsy: a systematic review. *Dev Med Child Neurol* **61**: 315–321. doi: 10.1111/dmcn.14088.

Peiper A (1963) *Cerebral Function in Infancy and Childhood*, 3rd edn. New York: Consultants.

Pekçetin S, Akı E, Üstünyurt Z, Kayıhan H (2016) The efficiency of sensory integration interventions in preterm infants. *Percept Mot Skills* **123**: 411–423. doi: 10.1177/0031512516662895.

Petö A (1955) Konductive Mozgásterápia mint guópedagógia. *Gyópedagógia* 1: 15–21.

Prechtl HFR (1990) Qualitative changes of spontaneous movements in fetus and preterm infant are a marker of neurological dysfunction. *Early Hum Dev* **23**: 151–158.

Puthussery S, Chutiyami M, Tseng PC, Kilby L, Kapadia J (2018) Effectiveness of early intervention programs for parents of preterm infants: a meta-review of systematic reviews. *BMC Pediatr* **18**: 223. doi: 10.1186/s12887-018-1205-9.

Reddihough DS, King J, Coleman G, Catanese T (1998) Efficacy of programmes based on conductive education for young children with cerebral palsy. *Dev Med Child Neurol* **40**: 763–770.

Rentinck IC, Ketelaar M, Jongmans MJ, Gorter JW (2007) Parents of children with cerebral palsy: a review of factors related to the process of adaptation. *Child Care Health Dev* **33**: 161–169.

Romano C, van Wynckel M, Hulst J, et al. (2017) European Society for Paediatric Gastroenterology, Hepatology and Nutrition guidelines for the evaluation and treatment of gastrointestinal and nutritional complication in children with neurological impairment. *J Pediatr Gastroenterol Nutr* **65**: 242–264. doi: 10.1097/MPG.0000000000001646.

Rosenbaum P (2011) Family and quality of life: key elements in intervention in children with cerebral palsy. *Dev Med Child Neurol* **53** (Suppl 4): 68–70. doi: 10.1111/j.1469-8749.2011.04068.x.

Rush DD, Sheldon ML (2011) *The Early Childhood Coaching Handbook*. Baltimore, MD: Paul H. Brookes Publ.

Sameroff AJ (2009) *The Transactional Model of Development: How Children and Contexts Shape Each Other*. Washington, DC: American Psychological Association.

Schless SH, Cenni F, Bar-On L, et al. (2019) Medial gastrocnemius volume and echo-intensity after botulinum neurotoxin A interventions in children with spastic cerebral palsy. *Dev Med Child Neurol* **61**: 783–790. doi: 10.1111/dmcn.14056.

Sellier E, McIntyre S, Smithers-Sheedy H, Platt MJ; SCPE and ACPR Groups (2020) European and Australian Cerebral Palsy Surveillance Networks working together for collaborative research. *Neuropediatrics* **51**: 105–112. doi: 10.1055/s-0039-3402003.

Sgandurra G, Bartalena L, Cecchi F, et al. (2016) A pilot study on early home-based intervention through an intelligent baby gym (CareToy) in preterm infants. *Res Dev Disabil* **53–54**: 32–42. doi: 10.1016/j.ridd.2016.01.013.

Sgandurra G, Bartalena L, Cioni G, et al. (2014) Home-based, early intervention with mechatronic toys for preterm infants at risk of neurodevelopmental disorders (CARETOY): a RCT protocol. *BMC Pediatr* **14**: 268. doi: 10.1186/1471-2431-14-268.

Sgandurra G, Beani E, Giampietri M, Rizzi R, Cioni G; Care-Toy-R Consortium (2018) Early intervention at home in infants with congenital brain lesion with CareToy revised: a RCT protocol. *BMC Pediatr* **18**: 295. doi: 10.1186/s12887-018-1264-y.

Sgandurra G, Beani E, Inguaggiato E, Lorentzen J, Nielsen JB, Cioni G (2019) Effects on parental stress of early home-based CareToy intervention in low-risk preterm infants. *Neural Plast* 7517351. doi: 10.1155/2019/7517351.

Sgandurra G, Lorentzen J, Inguaggiato E, et al. (2017) A randomized clinical trial in preterm infants on the effects of a home-based early intervention with the CareToy System' *PLoS One* **12**: e0173521. doi: 10.1371/journal. pone.0173521.

Shafer RL, Newell KM, Lewis MH, Bodfish JW (2017) A cohesive framework for motor stereotypy in typical and atypical development: the role of sensorimotor integration. *Front Integr Neurosci* **11**: 19. doi: 10.3389/ fnint.2017.00019.

Smith BA, Trujillo-Priego IA, Lane CJ, Finley JM, Horak FB (2015) Daily quantity of infants leg movement: wearable sensor algorithm and relationship to walking onset. *Sensors (Basel)* **15**: 19006-19020. doi: 10.3390/ s150819006.

Smithers-Sheedy H, Badawi N, Blair E, et al. (2014) What constitutes cerebral palsy in the twenty-first century? *Dev Med Child Neurol* **56**: 323–328. doi: 10.1111/dmcn.12262.

Spittle A, Orton J, Anderson PJ, Boyd R, Doyle LW (2015) Early developmental intervention programmes provided post hospital discharge to prevent motor and cognitive impairment in preterm infants. *Cochrane Database Syst Rev* CD005495. doi: 10.1002/14651858.CD005495.pub4.

Stewart SL, Applequist K (2019) Diverse families in early intervention: professionals' views of early intervention. *J Res Childh Educ* **33**: 242–256. doi: 10.1080/02568543.2019.1577777.

Trujillo-Priego IA, Lane CJ, Vanderbilt DL, et al. (2017) Development of a wearable sensor algorithm to detect the quantity an kinematic characteristics of infant arm movement bouts produced across a full day in the natural environment. *Technologies (Basel)* **5**, pii: 39. doi: 10.3390/technologies5030039.

Valentín-Gudiol M, Mattern-Baxter K, Girabent-Farrés M, Bagur-Calafat C, Hadders-Algra M, Angulo-Barroso RM (2017) Treadmill interventions in children under six years of age at risk of neuromotor delay. *Cochrane Database Syst Rev* **7**: CD009242. doi: 10.1002/14651858.CD009242.pub3.

Van Balen LC, Boxum AG, Dijkstra LJ, et al. (2018) Are postural adjustments during reaching related to walking development in typically developing infants and infants at risk of cerebral palsy? *Infant Behav Dev* **50**: 107–115. doi: 10.1016/j.infbeh.2017.12.004.

Van Hus JW, Jeukens-Visser M, Koldewijn K, et al. (2013) Sustained developmental effects of the infant behavioral assessment and intervention program in very low birth weight infants at 5.5 years corrected age. *J Pediatr* **162**: 1112–1119. doi: 10.1016/j.jpeds.2012.11.078.

Verkerk G, Jeukens-Visser M, Koldewijn K, et al. (2011) Infant behavioral assessment and intervention program in very low birth weight infants improves independency in mobility at preschool age. *J Pediatr* **159**: 933–938.e1. doi: 10.1016/j.jpeds.2011.05.035.

Vojta V (1968) Reflexkriechen und seine Bedeutung für krankengymnastische Frühbehandlung. *Z Kinderheilkd* **104**: 319–330.

Vojta V (1976) *Die cerebralen Bewegungsstörungen im Säuglingsalter. Frühdiagnose und Frühtherapie*, 2nd edn. Stuttgart: Ferdinand Enke Verlag.

Vojta V (1984) The basic elements of treatment according to Vojta. In: Scrutton D, editor, *Management of the Motor Disorders of Children with Cerebral Palsy*. Oxford: Blackwell Scientific Publications, pp. 75–85.

Ward R, Reynolds JE, Bear N, Elliott C, Valentine J (2017) What is the evidence for managing tone in young children with, or at risk of developing, cerebral palsy: a systematic review. *Disabil Rehabil* **39**: 619–630. doi: 10.3109/09638288.2016.1153162.

White R (1984) Sensory-integrative therapy for the cerebral-palsied child. In: Scrutton D, editor, *Management of the Motor Disorders of Children with Cerebral Palsy*. Oxford: Blackwell Scientific Publications, pp. 86–95.

Wilson PH, Smits-Engelsman B, Caeyenberghs K, et al. (2017) Cognitive and neuroimaging findings in developmental coordination disorder: new insights from a systematic review of recent research. *Dev Med Child Neurol* **59**: 1117–1129. doi: 10.1111/dmcn.13530.

World Health Organization (2001) *International Classification of Functioning, Disability and Health (ICF)*. Geneva: World Health Organization.

World Health Organization (2007) *International Classification of Functioning, Disability and Health, Children and Youth Version (ICF-CY)*. Geneva: World Health Organization.

Zanon MA, Porfírio GJM, Riera R, Martimbianco ALC (2018). Neurodevelopmental treatment approaches for children with cerebral palsy. *Cochrane Database Syst Rev* CD011937. doi: 10.1002/14651858.CD011937.pub.

Environmental Adaptations

Gunilla Thunberg, Roslyn Livingstone, Margret Buchholz, and Debra Field

SUMMARY POINTS

- While outcomes supporting use of environmental adaptations are mainly positive, evidence of effectiveness is weak to moderate and methodological quality is low to moderate.
- As evidence is limited, we recommend the use of valid, reliable outcome measures to evaluate effectiveness of environmental adaptations (postural management, mobility, and communication) for individual children.
- The combination of expert consensus and currently available research suggests the following:
  - Adding support to promote symmetry and increase comfort should be considered for all young children who remain in asymmetrical or frog-leg lying positions from the first few months of life.
  - Early upright positioning promotes visual-motor development, interaction with objects, and may facilitate overall development and inclusion.
  - Supported standing should be introduced starting between 9 and 12 months for children who are not pulling to stand.
  - Gait trainers or walkers may be introduced around 12 months to assist with development of independent stepping for children who are unable to walk without support.
  - Power mobility interventions (switch-adapted ride-on toys as well as powered wheelchairs) can promote developmental change, enhance social relationships and child engagement, and should be considered for young children with limited mobility starting from 9 to 12 months.
  - There is strong evidence that early communication intervention should include parent support and should primarily include guidance in the use of responsive communication strategies. Augmentative and alternative communication (AAC) should be introduced as soon as communication difficulties are identified or expected due to diagnosis.
  - AAC interventions facilitate communication and give the non-speaking child access to language when oral speech is insufficient. AAC does not hinder speech development. Direct intervention for young children with communication impairments is more effective when implemented within play and daily routines, and based on the child's interests.
  - Children with more severe motor impairment may use alternative access methods including eye-gaze technology.
  - Assessment and implementation of assistive technology is a complex process that should involve a professional team and the child's supportive network.

According to the World Health Organization's International Classification of Functioning, Disability and Health Children and Youth version (ICF-CY), environmental factors are defined as 'the physical, social and attitudinal environment in which people live and conduct their lives' (World Health Organization 2007). The paradigm shift from a medical to ICF-CY's broader biopsychosocial model of disability requires special attention to environmental factors. This is certainly true for young children with disabilities whose development depends on persons in their immediate environment and who require toys and other products that are accessible and adapted to their developmental level.

Environmental adaptations include assistive devices used by an individual in daily life for personal mobility and communication (World Health Organization 2007). Use of these devices may be influenced by accessibility in the child's physical environment at home or in the community. Use may also be influenced by the knowledge and attitudes of those around the child, including parents (who are especially important for young children), siblings, extended family, friends, others in their social and cultural communities, as well as health care and early childhood professionals. It is important to remember that environmental adaptations are a right of the child with disabilities, as stated in the United Nations Convention on the Rights of Persons with Disabilities (United Nations GA 2006). We live in a technological era, which means that new and exciting options for children with motor and communication challenges may be available in the near future.

This chapter describes the current evidence supporting the efficacy and effectiveness of different environmental adaptations with young children at risk for, or diagnosed with developmental motor disorders, such as cerebral palsy (CP). The first section describes the use of postural management or positioning equipment in lying, sitting, and standing positions. The second section describes mobility interventions including supported walking, manual wheeled mobility, and power mobility. The third section introduces communication support and the use of augmentative and alternative communication (AAC) strategies, including eye-gaze technology.

Environmental adaptations using positioning, mobility, and communication strategies provide opportunities for children to learn about their own bodies, the properties of objects and the people around them, which in turn guides further action – perception – action interaction (Huang 2018). A State of the Evidence systematic review of intervention effectiveness (Novak et al. 2020) identified a significant body of lower-quality evidence supporting use of environmental adaptations interventions for children with CP. Therefore, we start our chapter with a caveat. Research into environmental adaptations has mainly been conducted with children over 2 years of age. In this chapter, we drew evidence wherever possible from research involving children under 6 years of age and we extrapolated the findings to the age-group addressed in this book. Nonetheless, the majority of our descriptions have been derived from research including older children. In addition, some communication intervention research also included children with minimal motor disabilities.

POSTURAL MANAGEMENT

Children with CP may adopt unstable and asymmetrical body positions because of altered muscle tone, strength imbalance, stereotyped or involuntary movements. These atypical positions reduce function and may lead to pain and postural deformity. Postural management is the use of equipment and strategies to support posture and function in lying, sitting, and standing. Common goals are to promote body alignment and stability, communication, cognitive development, prevent deformity, enhance functional abilities, and optimize participation in daily life. These interventions are particularly relevant for children classified at Gross Motor Function Classification System (GMFCS) levels III, IV, and V (Gericke 2006).

Lying

Expert consensus recommends use of night-time or sleep positioning systems from as soon after birth as possible for GMFCS IV-V (Gericke 2006). A systematic review on the effectiveness of sleep positioning systems, including all available study designs, found low-quality evidence supporting improvements in sleep quality, hip stability, and quality of life (Humphreys et al. 2019). Yet, the review also noted that the two randomized trials found no difference in sleep quality or pain among children who used and who did not use sleep positioning systems. The same research group conducted a Delphi consensus of 43 clinicians experienced in postural management. Their unpublished study supported use of sleep positioning systems to promote hip stability and postural alignment or body symmetry, increase comfort, reduce pain, and improve sleep quality in children functioning at GMFCS IV-V and possibly GMFCS III. Both the systematic review and consensus recommend professional support to help families implement support systems in lying with attention to potential safety risks such as pressure management, respiratory status, and reflux or vomiting.

Sitting

Expert consensus (Gericke 2006) recommends positioning in upright sitting from 6 months for children functioning at GMFCS IV-V and promoting active sitting for children functioning at GMFCS III. Ryan's (2012) overview of five systematic reviews of adaptive seating interventions for children with CP (from birth to 19 years) found inconclusive evidence because of differences in participant characteristics, seating interventions and outcome measures. A more recent review examining adaptive seating for those classified as GMFCS IV and V, noted that none of the nine studies reviewed reported significant adverse effects (Angsupaisal et al. 2015). Novak et al. (2020) suggested there is weak positive evidence supporting the use of adaptive seating to improve postural support, hand function, pulmonary function, and pressure management, and they advocated for continued measurement of individual outcomes. Based on evidence and clinical experience, we suggest that children functioning at GMFCS IV-V should be supported in reclined sitting starting at 3 months and progress towards supported upright sitting by 6 months. Examples of supportive seating are shown in Figure 15.1. The importance of upright positioning to facilitate visual abilities, hand use, and object exploration for advancement of cognition, language, and social interaction was highlighted in a perspective article by Lobo et al. (2013).

Standing

Clinical practice recommends the introduction of supported standing and weight-bearing for children functioning at GMFCS III-V from 9 months of age, when children typically begin pulling to stand. Examples of supported standing are shown in Figure 15.2. Novak et al. (2020) concluded that strong evidence supports the impact of weight-bearing on bone mineral density for children functioning at GMFCS III (weak positive for GMFCS IV-V) and that weak positive evidence supports impact of postural management on hip stability. An earlier synthesis of stretching interventions suggested that there is insufficient evidence to either support or refute the use of supported standing equipment to maintain range of motion and prevent contractures (Craig et al. 2016). Although clinical practice promotes neutral to abducted hip positioning, there is debate in the literature about specific hip angles and positions as well as dosage. Expert opinion along with weak research evidence supports a positive influence on bowel function, range of motion, activity, and participation outcomes. Surveys, qualitative studies, and expert opinion are generally supportive of introducing supported standing from 9 to 12 months of age.

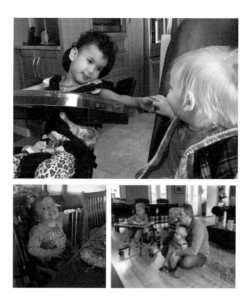

Figure 15.1   Supportive seating promotes child participation in a variety of functional activities. Top: Specialized seating on a high–low indoor base with a tray promotes social engagement and communication. Bottom left: supportive seat (with lateral trunk and pelvic supports), attached to a dining chair, develops independent eating and participation in family meals. Bottom right: an activity chair (with tray for added postural support) promotes play and inclusion in family life. Published with permission of the parents.

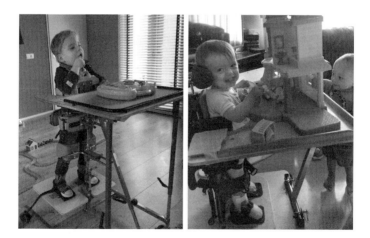

Figure 15.2   Supported standing promotes early upright orientation and weight-bearing to enhance and maintain body function and structures as well as promote activity and participation. Left: a prone to upright standing frame. Right: a supine to upright standing frame. Published with permission of the parents.

MOBILITY

In young children who are typically developing, independent mobility increases exploration enhancing cognitive, motor, social, and perceptual development. For children whose mobility is limited in early childhood, alternative means of mobility can promote overall development and minimize secondary impairments. Given that neuroplasticity is greatest in the first 2 years of life, providing opportunity to enhance young children's development by augmenting mobility is important during this sensitive time period. There is a reciprocal, and reinforcing relationship between self-initiated independent mobility and young children's development, engagement, and participation in daily life.

Walkers and Gait Trainers

Expert opinion supports introduction of walkers or gait trainers for young children with CP around 12 months. For children functioning at GMFCS II and III, gait trainers may allow earlier independent walking and exploration of the environment (Fig. 15.3), and may be replaced with hand-held walkers, crutches, or unaided walking at older ages. Walkers are defined as frames with two or four casters that may be used with the frame in front (anterior), or behind (posterior) the body to provide hand-held support for children who are unable to walk independently. Walkers are most often used by very young children classified as GMFCS II prior to independent walking and by school-aged children classified as GMFCS III. Gait trainers are more supportive walkers for children who require additional trunk or pelvic support (GMFCS IV-V), and have a seat for body-weight support (Paleg and Livingstone 2015).

One systematic review evaluated anterior versus posterior walkers for children with CP (Poole 2018); fewer than 16 children under 6 years of age were included. No firm conclusions could be drawn as evidence level and quality was very low. Nonetheless, the review suggested that posterior

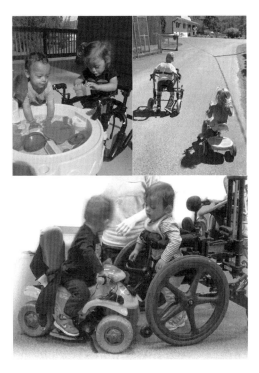

Figure 15.3   Gait trainers promote active movement and fitness. Top left: a posterior orientation gait trainer with a sling seat, used for play in standing. Top right: an anterior orientation gait trainer with a dynamic seat used for active stepping and play outdoors. Bottom: a switch adapted ride-on toy and a hands-free dynamic gait trainer promote active play and interaction. Published with permission of the parents.

walkers may positively influence posture, stability, and speed of walking and tend to be preferred by children and parents. The one systematic review available on gait trainer interventions reported mainly activity level outcomes (increased number of steps or walking distance) and only one included study reported increased participation (Paleg and Livingstone 2015). Novak et al. (2020) concluded that mobility training (using gait trainers) may assist children classified as GMFCS IV-V to take more steps. Gait trainers may be an important means of facilitating upright positioning, active exploration, and physical fitness.

Manual Mobility

Little research has explored the use of manual mobility equipment in very young children with CP (Fig. 15.4). Novak et al. (2020) concluded that adaptive equipment (including manual mobility devices) decreased the burden of care for parents. Small manual wheeled mobility devices that are low to the ground and promote bimanual self-propulsion are popular for young children, but research has yet to explore impact on development. A cross-sectional analysis of 2328 children with CP aged 1–11 years found that very few were independent using manual wheelchairs, especially outdoors, regardless of GMFCS level or hand function (Rodby-Bousquet et al. 2016). The literature suggests that manual wheelchairs or buggies/strollers are ineffective in promoting independent mobility in young children with CP although such passive transport devices may help ease caregiving.

Power Mobility

Power mobility interventions include ride-on toys (Fig. 15.3), specialty mobility devices and child-sized wheelchairs that are electrically powered and operated by joysticks, switches, or other specialized controls (Fig. 15.4). A systematic review found strongest evidence supporting a positive impact on mobility,

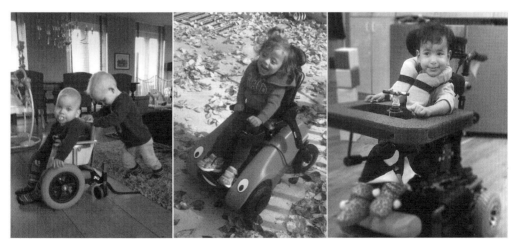

Figure 15.4 Wheeled mobility promotes independent exploration and participation. Left: a toddler sized manual wheelchair may be useful in indoor settings. Centre: a child-sized power mobility device enables independent play and exploration outdoors. Right: a child-sized power wheelchair with supportive seating and adaptations encourages independent mobility experience for a child classified as GMFCS V. Published with permission of the parents.

overall development, and independence; however, most research was descriptive rather than experimental (Livingstone and Field 2014). The common fear that power mobility use at an early age will negatively impact motor development was not supported. A positive impact on play skills was quantified in one group study, although qualitative literature provides the most evidence supporting impact on children's participation in daily life (Livingstone and Field 2015). These two complementary reviews, taken together, included 107 children under 6 years with the diagnosis of CP.

Few studies have included children with CP under the age of 2 years, with most case studies reporting on children of at least 3 or 4 years. Nonetheless, a short-term power mobility training intervention to increase use and awareness of the more affected arm and hand was published for an 11-month-old at risk for CP. Children with disabilities under 12 months have not been shown to independently steer a power mobility device, although they may be able to activate a single switch to initiate movement through space and explore their environment. Successful use of a joystick for steering has been reported between 18 and 24 months for children without brain involvement (Livingstone and Paleg 2014).

A more recent scoping review of modified ride-on toy car interventions (James et al. 2019) identified 13 case studies and one non-randomized two-group comparison design reporting a positive impact on young children's social-emotional development and mobility. Seven children 2 years or younger with CP were included in an intervention that was feasible and appropriate. The ride-on toy cars were all accessed by a single-switch and most children used the switch to stop and go, while adults steered. This appeared to provide meaningful mobility, but whether it is effective for independence and exploration depends on the child's profile and other environmental factors.

Research and expert opinion supports introduction of power mobility, starting around 12 months for children who will never walk, children who are predicted to have inefficient mobility and also children who will not achieve independent autonomous mobility during the first few years (Livingstone and Paleg 2014). In contrast to manual mobility devices, power mobility devices are more likely to promote independence (Rodby-Bousquet et al. 2016) and should be considered starting at very young ages.

COMMUNICATION SUPPORT AND AUGMENTATIVE AND ALTERNATIVE COMMUNICATION

Challenges in Early Communication Development

Typical development of communication, characterized by mutual exchanges between the child and their communication partners, may become problematic when the child has a disability (Simeonsson et al. 2012). Parents of children with disabilities may have difficulties detecting and interpreting their child's communication attempts, and they may become more directive and less responsive in their communication with the child (Pennington et al. 2004). For instance, studies including children with CP have shown that parents – not children – initiate most conversational topics, ask closed questions (requiring yes/no responses) and ask for information that is already known (Pennington et al. 2004). Breakdowns in the early interactions between the child with a disability and their parent may in the long run restrict social participation and the child's development of important social, cognitive, and communicative skills. Research has also shown that the interaction imbalance is further impacted in children with severe expressive problems, such as dysarthria or anarthria (Geytenbeek et al. 2015; Smith and Hustad 2015).

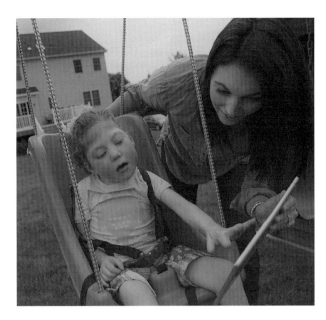

Figure 15.5 AAC in everyday life. The communication device as a shared resource for interaction between the young child and the parent in daily and motivating activities. The mother has just pointed to the tablet commenting on the swinging and now the child wants to take her turn. Published with permission of the parents and by courtesy of Tobii Dynavox.

Early Communication Intervention

A comprehensive review of 155 intervention studies with preschool-aged children with different communication disabilities, concluded that early communication intervention should include: (1) guidance and instruction to parents in responsive communication strategies; (2) training of communication skills within natural environments and through play (Fig. 15.5); and (3) introduction of multimodal AAC as early as possible, modelled by parents and other important communication partners (Eberhart et al. 2017). The majority of studies included instructions and support to the parents during group sessions or individual visits, typically at home. More recent studies often included the use of video coaching, where parents had the opportunity to watch themselves implementing the communication strategies with their child and receive feedback from the therapist and/or other parents (Eberhart et al. 2017).

Augmentative and Alternative Communication Strategies

AAC comprises different strategies and modes of communication, such as body language, tangible objects, manual signs, graphic symbols, or speech-generating devices (Fig. 15.6). Sometimes, parents worry that AAC introduction may hinder the development of speech. The research points in the opposite direction: meta-analyses and other studies show that AAC intervention should be started as soon as communication difficulties are observed or suspected. AAC facilitates communication and language development and also stimulates speech production (Branson and Demchak 2009; Romski et al. 2010). There are no age-limits or prerequisites that need to be met before AAC is introduced. This is important for all children with motor impairments, especially when there is a gap between comprehension of spoken language (receptive) and communication output (expressive) (Geytenbeek et al. 2015). AAC

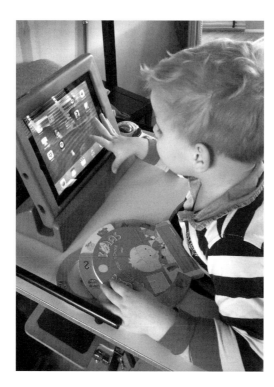

Figure 15.6 Use of a speech-generation device during play. The boy has access to communication opportunities (in this case using a speech-generating device) during toy play. Published with permission of the parents.

intervention may also be effective in decreasing challenging behaviours related to communication difficulties. Potential for success is increased when the social network around a child is supported to increase communication opportunities, uses responsive strategies, and incorporates AAC into natural daily interactions (Eberhart et al. 2017).

No mode of AAC has been shown to be better than any other for young children with motor challenges; multimodal AAC is recommended, although manual signing may be less useful (Clarke and Price 2012). Transparent naturalistic graphic symbols are most easily learned, and the combination of auditory and visual feedback seems to be effective (Eberhart et al. 2017). Recent research suggests that using photos and videos of meaningful activities and people, paired with spoken messages (referred to as hot spots), may be highly motivating for the young child and quickly learned (Light et al. 2019). For children unable to directly touch the talking display due to motor difficulties, alternative access methods may be an option. Introduction of such applications, integrated in play and meaningful activities should be complemented with generic or core vocabulary to promote communication and language use in different environments. AAC incorporating early literacy learning has been shown to be successful and is important for social participation (Light et al. 2019). Most importantly AAC strategies and devices should be used and modelled (i.e. aided language input) by the child's communication partners to promote learning and spontaneous symbol use (Eberhart et al. 2017; Light et al. 2019).

In spite of the fact that as many as 85% of 2-year-old children with CP have significant speech and language impairments (Smith and Hustad 2015), most research has included few participants with motor disorders. Since children with CP may experience a range of medical problems during the first years, and parents are often focused on gross motor development, communication impairments may not be so obvious at this young age (Smith and Hustad 2015). Professionals should guide parents to communication intervention and AAC implementation much earlier and more frequently, given the pivotal function of communication and language in the child's cognitive, social, and literacy development. Intervention should preferably be started during the first year and/or as soon as communication difficulties are identified.

Access to Communication Technology and Eye-Gaze Technologies

Digital technology today is typically operated with touch screens (for both assistive devices and off-the-shelf products) (Light and Drager 2007). These devices are often intuitive, adaptable, and work well for many users. Although children who have more severe motor impairments may not be able to use touch screens effectively, alternative access methods for communication technology, toys or computers may enhance play and increase self-determination and social participation (Light and Drager 2007), for example, by eye-gaze technology (Fig. 15.7).

Assistive Technology Assessment

A thorough trans-disciplinary assessment (including occupational therapists and speech and language therapists) is recommended for determining most appropriate assistive technologies and access methods for the child (Holmqvist and Buchholz 2011). Assessing children with disabilities that affect their communication, motor, and cognitive skills is complex; the ultimate goal is to determine how the child can communicate and perform activities independently. Positioning is crucial and should be the first step in the assessment to evaluate optimal motor function for accessing different assistive technologies. A thorough motor assessment is carried out, often in several positions (e.g. sitting, standing, lying). When evaluating assistive technology solutions, it is important to consider cognition, vision, hearing, etc, as well as the perspective of the child and the family. Actually trying out and comparing different technology solutions is critical. This may involve comparing software solutions, application settings and different physical devices (Holmqvist and Buchholz 2011).

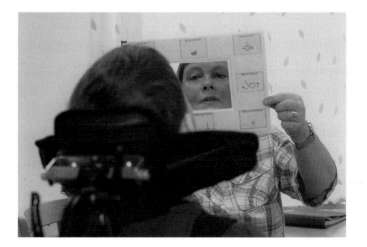

Figure 15.7 Use of an eye-gaze manoeuvred communication book. Child communicates by using eye pointing on an eye-gaze enabled communication book. The therapist can easily see which symbols the child is looking at. Published with permission of the parents.

Assistive Technology Devices

Trackballs, joysticks, and adapted keyboards are commonly used to enable computer access for children with motor difficulties (Higginbotham et al. 2007). If the child has limited hand function, other body parts can be used. For example, a head-operated mouse translates movements from the child's head into proportional mouse pointer movements, and switches combined with scanning software can be used with any body part (Higginbotham et al. 2007). For children who have very limited voluntary motor function eye-gaze technology can be useful (Borgestig et al. 2017). Eye movements are translated into mouse pointer movements using an eye-tracker camera and associated software. These systems can be used with communication software on a tablet computer (Holmqvist and Buchholz 2011) or be integrated into a speech-generating device (Borgestig et al. 2017). During an assessment for eye-gaze control technologies, there are specific considerations regarding the child's vision and gaze, as well as unique technology characteristics that need to be taken into account (Holmqvist and Buchholz 2011). When introducing eye-gaze enabled speech-generating devices (Fig. 15.8), there is a need for close collaboration among child, family, and professionals as well as extensive technical and AAC implementation support, especially in the initial stages (Holmqvist et al. 2018).

Use of Eye-Gaze Technology

There are few studies on eye-gaze control technology, as it is fairly new. In a systematic review on the effectiveness of this technology for communication, only two studies met inclusion criteria (Karlsson et al. 2018). The introduction of an eye-gaze enabled speech-generating device allowed children to express themselves and perform activities independently, achieving their communication and activity goals (Borgestig et al. 2017; Holmqvist et al. 2018). The appropriate age of introduction for eye-gaze technologies is yet unknown. In a case report, a 9-month-old Swedish child with a high spinal cord injury was introduced to an eye-gaze enabled speech-generating device (Hemmingsson et al. 2018) and was followed until 36 months of age. At this young age, the child could use eye-gaze control

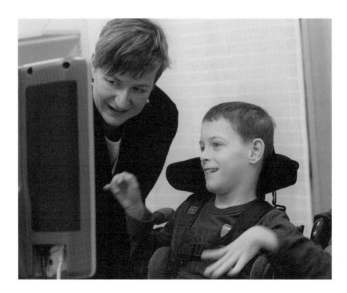

Figure 15.8   Introduction of eye-gaze control technology. Published with permission of the parents.

technology in progressively more complex play activities, choice-making, and social interaction with his parents.

Assessing and Introducing Assistive Technologies for Environmental Adaptations

When carrying out an assessment and introducing assistive technologies, professionals need to have good knowledge of the child's preferred activities, the technology options and the child's environment (Holmqvist and Buchholz 2011). The integration of assistive technologies into the child's everyday life requires extensive training and ongoing support. It is important that family members are provided with the necessary knowledge and skills to support the child (Holmqvist et al. 2018).

CONCLUDING REMARKS

Systematic reviews supporting interventions for children with motor impairments identify the need for research focusing on all environmental adaptations. Strong conclusions cannot be drawn from the current evidence and further research with longer-term follow-up is needed. Desired outcomes should be monitored for individual children using valid and responsive outcome measures.

REFERENCES

Angsupaisal M, Maathuis CGB, Hadders-Algra M (2015) Adaptive seating systems in children with severe cerebral palsy across International Classification of Functioning, Disability and Health for Children and Youth version domains: a systematic review. *Dev Med Child Neurol* **57**: 919–930. doi: 10.1111/dmcn.12762.

Borgestig M, Rytterström P, Hemmingsson H (2017) Gaze-based assistive technology in daily activities in children with severe physical impairments – an intervention study. *Dev Neurorehabil* **20**: 129–141. doi: 10.3109/17518423.2015.1132281.

Branson D, Demchak M (2009) The use of augmentative and alternative communication methods with infants and toddlers with disabilities: a research review. *Augment Altern Commun* **25**: 274–286. doi: 10.3109/07434610903384529.

Clarke M, Price K (2012) Augmentative and alternative communication for children with cerebral palsy. *Paediatr Child Health* **22**: 367–371. doi: 10.1016/j.paed.2012.03.002.

Craig J, Hilderman C, Wilson G, Misovic R (2016) Effectiveness of stretch interventions for children with neuromuscular disabilities: evidence-based recommendations. *Pediatr Phys Ther* **28**: 262–275. doi: 10.1097/PEP.0000000000000269.

Eberhart B, Forsberg J, Nilsson L, et al. (2017) Tidiga kommunikations- och språkinsatser till förskolebarn [Early communication intervention for pre-school aged children]. Report published by the Swedish National Society for Habilitation Services.

Gericke T (2006) Postural management for children with cerebral palsy: consensus statement. *Dev Med Child Neurol* **48**: 244. doi: 10.1017/S0012162206000685.

Geytenbeek JJM, Vermeulen RJ, Becher JG, Oostrom KJ (2015). Comprehension of spoken language in non-speaking children with severe cerebral palsy: an explorative study on associations with motor type and disabilities. *Dev Med Child Neurol* **57**: 294–300. doi: 10.1111/dmcn.12619.

Huang H-H (2018) Perspectives on early power mobility training, motivation, and social participation in young children with motor disabilities. *Front Psychol* **8**: 1–8. doi: 10.3389/fpsyg.2017.02330.

Humphreys G, King T, Jex J, Rogers M, Blake S, Thompson-Coon J (2019) Sleep positioning systems for children and adults with a neurodisability: a systematic review. *Brit J Occup Ther* **82**: 5–14. doi: 10.1177/0308022618778254.

Hemmingsson H, Ahlsten G, Wandin H, Rytterström P, Borgestig M (2018) Eye-gaze control technology as early intervention for a non-verbal young child with high spinal cord injury: A case report. *Technol* **6**: 12. doi: 10.3390/technologies6010012.

Higginbotham DJ, Shane H, Russell S, Caves K (2007) Access to AAC: present, past, and future. *Augment Altern Commun* **23**: 243–257. doi: 781353683 [pii]10.1080/07434610701571058.

Holmqvist E, Buchholz M (2011) A model for gaze control assessments and evaluation. In Majaranta P, Aoki H, Donegan M et al. editors, *Gaze Interaction and Applications of Eye Tracking: Advances in Assistive Technologies.* Hershey, PA. IGI Global pp. 36–47. doi: 10.4018/978-1-61350-098-9.ch005.

Holmqvist E, Thunberg G, Peny Dahlstrand M (2018) Gaze-controlled communication technology for children with severe multiple disabilities: Parents and professionals' perception of gains, obstacles, and prerequisites. *Assist Technol* **30**: 201–208. doi: 10.1080/10400435.2017.1307882.

James D, Pfaff J, Jeffries LM (2019) Modified ride-on cars as early mobility for children with mobility limitations: a scoping review. *Phys Occup Ther Pediatr* **39**: 525–542. doi: 10.1080/01942638.2018.1547808.

Karlsson P, Allsop A, Dee-Price BJ, Wallen M (2018) Eye-gaze control technology for children, adolescents and adults with cerebral palsy with significant physical disability: Findings from a systematic review. *Dev Neurorehabil* **21**: 497–505. doi: 10.1080/17518423.2017.1362057. https://www.spinalinjury101.org/details/levels-of-injury.

Light J, Drager K (2007) AAC technologies for young children with complex communication needs: state of the science and future research directions. *AAC: Augmentative and Alternative Communication*. doi: 10.1080/07434610701553635.

Light J, McNaughton D, Caron J (2019) New and emerging AAC technology supports for children with complex communication needs and their communication partners: State of the science and future research directions. *Augment Altern Commun* **35**: 26–41. doi: 0.1080/07434618.2018.1557251.

Livingstone R, Field D (2014) Systematic review of power mobility outcomes for infants, children and adolescents with mobility limitations. *Clin Rehabil* **28**: 954–964. doi: 10.1177/0269215514531262.

Livingstone R, Field D (2015) The child and family experience of power mobility: a qualitative synthesis. *Dev Med Child Neurol* **57**: 317–327. doi: 10.1111/dmcn.12633.

Livingstone R, Paleg G (2014) Practice considerations for the introduction and use of power mobility for children. *Dev Med Child Neurol* **56**: 210–221. doi: 10.1111/dmcn.12245.

Lobo MA, Harbourne RT, Dusing SC, McCoy SW (2013) Grounding early intervention: physical therapy cannot just be about motor skills anymore, *Phys Ther* **93**: 94–103. doi: 10.2522/ptj.20120158.

Novak I, Morgan C, Fahey M, et al. (2020) State of the evidence traffic lights 2019: Systematic review of interventions for preventing and treating children with cerebral palsy. *Curr Neurol Neurosci Rep* **20**: 1–21. doi: 10.1007/s11910-020-1022-z.

Paleg G, Livingstone R (2015) Outcomes of gait trainer use in home and school settings for children with motor impairments: A systematic review. *Clin Rehabil* **28**: 1077–1091. doi: 10.1177/0269215514565947.

Pennington L, Goldbart J, Marshall J (2004) Interaction training for conversational partners of children with cerebral palsy: a systematic review. *Int J Lang Commun Dis* **39**: 151–170.

Poole M, Simkiss D, Rose A (2018) Anterior or posterior walkers for children with cerebral palsy? A systematic review. *Dis Rehabil: Assist Technol* **13**: 422–433. doi: 10.1080/17483107.2017.1385101.

Rodby-Bousquet E, Paleg G, Casey J, Wizert A, Livingstone R (2016) Physical risk factors influencing wheeled mobility in children with cerebral palsy: a cross-sectional study. *BMC Pediatr* **16**: 165. doi: 10.1186/s12887-016-0707-6.

Romski MA, Sevcik RA, Adamson LB, et al. (2010) Randomized comparison of augmented and nonaugmented language interventions for toddlers with developmental delays and their parents. *J Speech, Lang Hear Res* **53**: 350–364. doi: 10.1044/1092-4388(2009/08-0156).

Ryan SE (2012) An overview of systematic reviews of adaptive seating interventions for children with cerebral palsy: Where do we go from here? *Disabil Rehabil: Assist Technol* **7**: 104–111. doi: 10.3109/17483107.2011.595044.

Simeonsson RJ, Bjorck-Akesson E, Lollar DJ (2012) Communication, disability, and the ICF-CY. *Augment Altern Commun* **28**: 3–10. doi: 10.3109/07434618.2011.653829.

Smith AL, Hustad KC (2015) AAC and early intervention for children with cerebral palsy: Parent perceptions and child risk factors. *Augment Altern Commun* **31**: 336–350. doi: 10.3109/07434618.2015.1084373.

United Nations GA (2006) *Convention on the Rights of Persons with Disabilities and Optional Protocol.* https://www.refworld.org/docid/4680cd212.html [accessed 18 March 2020].

World Health Organization (2007) *International Classification of Functioning, Disability and Health – Children and Youth.* Geneva, WHO.

RECOMMENDED READING

Majaranta P, Aoki H, Donegan M, et al. (2011) *Gaze Interaction and Applications of Eye Tracking: Advances in Assistive Technologies.* Hershey, PA: IGI Global.

Concluding Remarks

Mijna Hadders-Algra

This book provides an overview on early detection and early intervention in developmental motor disorders, in particular cerebral palsy (CP) and developmental coordination disorder (DCD). These disorders are characterized by limitations in mobility, that is, limitations in changing and maintaining body position, moving around and walking, and carrying, moving, and handling objects. The disorders originate from an altered organization of the brain that starts in the prenatal, perinatal, or neonatal period. Generally, the altered organization of the brain is not limited to the networks involved in mobility. Neural networks do not function in isolation but in continuously changing coalitions of circuitries that are shared and reused (Anderson 2016). As a result infants with or at risk of developmental motor disorders frequently exhibit comorbidity in the form of, for example, limitations in learning and communication, behavioural disorders, or epilepsy.

EARLY DETECTION: A CHALLENGE

The early origin of developmental motor disorders offers an opportunity to start intervention at young age (i.e. during a period when the brain is characterized by high neuroplasticity) (see Chapter 3). Yet, it is not easy to detect at an early age all children that later in life are diagnosed with a developmental motor disorder (Chapters 2 and 3). The early detection of these children largely depends on their early medical history. Basically, two groups of infants can be distinguished: (1) infants, who postnatally needed advanced medical care, for instance, admission to a neonatal intensive care unit (NICU); and (2) infants with an uneventful neonatal period.

In the first group, infants having a very high risk of a developmental motor disorder can be detected relatively reliably, especially when using neonatal magnetic resonance imaging of the brain and general movement assessment at 3 months of age (Novak et al. 2017; see Chapters 2 and 10). (Recall all ages mentioned in the book are corrected ages unless specified otherwise.) Fortunately, the large majority of infants have an uneventful prenatal, perinatal, and neonatal period. In these children the risk of being diagnosed with a developmental motor disorder is much lower than that in the infants who start postnatal life in the NICU. Yet, children with an uneventful early medical history constitute a substantial proportion of the children diagnosed with CP or DCD. To detect developmental motor disorders in low-risk infants, we need to combine careful history taking that pays specific attention to the infant's developmental history and clinical instruments, such as standardized neurological examinations, general movements assessment (GMA), and specific motor tests, including the Alberta Infant Motor Scale and the Infant Motor Profile (see Chapters 10 and 11). The assessments, except for GMA, can also be used to monitor developmental progress throughout infancy in infants at risk of or with a developmental motor disorder. Other tests, such as cognitive and sensory tests, can be used to document the infant's strengths and limitations in these domains (see Chapter 4). The use of standardized assessments is strongly recommended (see Chapter 9).

FAMILY-CENTRED EARLY INTERVENTION

The difficulty of diagnosing developmental motor disorders early in life does not preclude early intervention. Early intervention is meant for all infants at risk of a developmental disorder. It is always family centred (see Chapter 12), even though opinions differ about what this means for the practical implementation of early intervention (see Chapter 14). In medically fragile newborn infants, intervention in the NICU consists of family-centred developmental care or rather family integrated care. The latter means that parents are encouraged to provide all care for their fragile infant, except for the most advanced medical care, while being coached by health professionals (see Chapter 13).

For infants who are cared for at home, basically two (overlapping) groups of intervention programmes are available. The first group consists of programmes for infants who were critically ill in the neonatal period without having acquired a significant brain lesion (i.e. infants who are at low to moderate risk of developmental motor disorders). Early intervention programs designed for these infants focus on support and education of the caregivers, support of sensitive and responsive parent–infant interaction, and infant stimulation. The programs are associated with improved infant cognitive development and better maternal well-being. But only three of the many programmes available have been associated with improved infant motor development (IBAIP, CareToy, and COPCA; see Chapter 14).

The second group of programmes are programmes designed for infants at very high risk of a developmental disorder. The programmes have a family and an infant development component. Components of the latter are: (1) they do not only address mobility, but also learning and applying knowledge and communication; (2) they primarily addresses activities, not impairments such as deviant muscle tone or abnormal reflexes; (3) they stress the importance of self-generated movements, trial and error, and challenging the infant to perform actions at the limit of his abilities; (4) they restrict hands-on techniques to minimal postural support in the initial phases of learning a new activity by trial and error; and (5) they support the use of assistive devices in infants with severe impairments. The programmes agree that dosage of intervention matters (i.e. more practice is associated with better achievements). Yet, it is gradually acknowledged that more practice, more diagnostics, and more intervention also have their drawbacks. Intensive practice and intensive monitoring may have a negative impact on the well-being of family and child (see Chapter 14 and Textbox 16.1).

Early intervention of infants with or at high risk of developmental disorders preferably is performed at home, including home visits of the health professional. The intervention takes into account that families of infants with or at very high risk of developmental motor disorders deal with prolonged periods of stress and uncertainty. This is true for the period before disclosure of the diagnosis and the period thereafter.

Currently, two family approaches are available: one advocating a combination of training and coaching, and the other applying only coaching. Nonetheless, it should be realized that the term coaching is used heterogeneously in early intervention. It is often used for parent education that uses a combination of training, instruction, and teaching. Yet, the concepts of training, instruction and teaching are incompatible with coaching as they are based on different attitudes and tune into different goals. Therefore, it is recommended to reserve the term coaching for relationship-directed family-centred interventions and to label intervention forms that primarily use training, instruction

Health professionals in early intervention commit themselves whole heartedly to achieve optimal well-being and participation of infants and families. However, the commitment and activities of health professionals may also have side-effects. Jan Grue (2018, Fig. 16.1) grippingly recounted the side-effects in his autobiographic book. He is a writer and professor at the department of special needs education of the University of Oslo. He has a congenital muscular dystrophy. He describes how the frequent visits to medical doctors and therapists for diagnostics, monitoring and intervention induced in himself the feeling of being 'a case', a creature characterized by impairments. Only when he reached adult age, when he got a partner and a son, did he realize that he has a life just as anyone else and that his life is just as much worth as that of others. His book invites us to reflect about the right quantity of well-meant care. It should be realized that every encounter in a health care context unintentionally changes the receiver of care – child or adult – in a 'medical case'. Each intervention session carries the implicit message that 'something is wrong'.

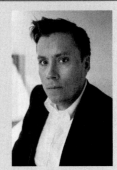

Figure 16.1   Jan Grue.

and teaching as parent training. Recent studies indicate that coaching in relationship-directed family interventions is associated with better family well-being and infant motor outcome (see Chapter 14).

FUTURE PERSPECTIVES IN EARLY DETECTION AND EARLY INTERVENTION

Most likely, technologies of antenatal and postnatal neuroimaging will increasingly improve over the years, allowing for more accurate prediction of developmental outcome in infants with a complicated prenatal, perinatal, and neonatal history. It is also likely that in the next decade low-cost automated GMA will become available. Automated GMA certainly will help the detection of infants at very high risk among the infants who were critically ill in the neonatal period. The value of automated GMA in the general population is less clear (Bouwstra et al. 2010). As is true for any screening instrument, the psychological burden of its false negatives and false positives need to be critically evaluated (Kaplan 2012).

In early intervention, we presumably will use increasingly often telecommunication technology – we improved our internet communication skills rapidly during the COVID-19 pandemic of 2020. We need to determine which professional attitude suits families and infants best: the attitude that uses parent training or the one that uses parent coaching. It could be that the best choice is the family's choice. Other areas that deserve further investigation are the effect of assistive devices on the infant's activities and participation and the effect of hands-on techniques (how, when, how little) on developmental outcome of infants with or at very high risk of a motor disorder.

Early detection and early intervention in developmental motor disorders will remain an area that is challenged by distress and uncertainty – this is inherent to the nature of the developing nervous system and its responses to adversities. Nevertheless, families, infants and professionals will get increasingly better in coping with this situation, resulting in optimal well-being and participation of infant and family.

REFERENCES

Anderson ML (2016) Neural reuse in the organization and development of the brain. *Dev Med Child Neurol* **58** (Suppl 4): 3–6. doi: 10.1111/dmcn.13039.

Bouwstra H, Dijk-Stigter GR, Grooten HM, et al. (2010) Predictive value of definitely abnormal general movements in the general population. *Dev Med Child Neurol* **52**: 456–461. doi: 10.1111/j.1469-8749.2009.03529.x.

Grue J (2018) *Jeg lever et liv som ligner deres*. Oslo: Gyldendal Norsk Forlag.

Kaplan RM (2012) Uncertainty, variability, and resource allocation in the health care decision process. In: Friedman HS, editor, *The Oxford Handbook of Health Psychology*. Oxford: Oxford: Oxford Handbooks On-line. doi: 10.1093/oxfordhb/9780195342819.013.0005.

Novak I, Morgan C, Adde L, et al. (2017) Early, accurate diagnosis and early intervention in cerebral palsy: advances in diagnosis and treatment. *JAMA Pediatr* **171**: 897–907. doi: 10.1001/jamapediatrics.2017.1689.

Index

NOTE: *b* = boxed section; *f* = figure; *t* = table.

Other titles from Mac Keith Press www.mackeith.co.uk

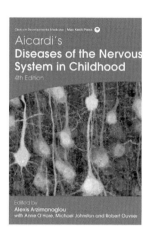

Aicardi's Diseases of the Nervous System in Childhood, 4th Edition
Alexis Arzimanoglou, Anne O'Hare, Michael V Johnston and Robert Ouvrier (Editors)

Clinics in Developmental Medicine
2018 ▪ 1524pp ▪ hardback ▪ 978-1-909962-80-4

This fourth edition retains the patient-focussed, clinical approach of its predecessors. The international team of editors and contributors has honoured the request of the late Jean Aicardi, that his book remain 'resolutely clinical', which distinguishes *Diseases of the Nervous System in Childhood* from other texts in the field. New edition completely updated and revised and now in full colour.

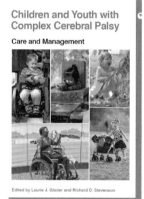

Children and Youth with Complex Cerebral Palsy: Care and Management
Laurie J. Glader and Richard D. Stevenson (Editors)

A Practical Guide from Mac Keith Press
2019 ▪ 404pp ▪ softback ▪ 978-1-909962-98-9

This is the first practical guide to explore management of the many medical comorbidities that children with complex CP face, including orthopaedics, mobility needs, cognition and sensory impairment, difficult behaviours, respiratory complications and nutrition, amongst others. Uniquely, contributors include children and parents, providing applied wisdom for family-centred care. Clinical Care Tools are provided to help guide clinicians and include a Medical Review Supplement, Equipment and Services Checklist and an ICF-Based Care: Goals and Management Form.

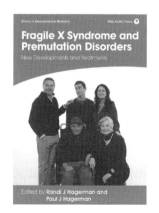

Fragile X Syndrome and Premutation Disorders: New Developments and Treatments
Randi J Hagerman and Paul J Hagerman (Editors)

Clinics in Developmental Medicine
2020 ▪ 192pp ▪ hardback ▪ 978-1-911612-37-7

Fragile X syndrome results from a gene mutation on the X-chromosome, which leads to various intellectual and developmental disabilities. *Fragile X Syndrome and Premutation Disorders* offers clinicians and families a multidisciplinary approach in order to provide the best possible care for patients with Fragile X. Unique features of the book include what to do when an infant or toddler is first diagnosed, the impact on the family and an international perspective on how different cultures perceive the syndrome.

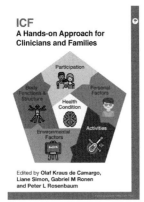

ICF: A Hands-on Approach for Clinicians and Families
Olaf Kraus de Camargo, Liane Simon, Gabriel M. Ronen and Peter L. Rosenbaum (Editors)

A practical guide from Mac Keith Press
2019 ▪ 192pp ▪ softback ▪ 978-1-911612-04-9

This accessible handbook introduces the World Health Organisation's International Classification of Functioning, Disability and Health (ICF) to professionals working with children with disabilities and their families. It contains an overview of the elements of the ICF but focusses on practical applications, including how the ICF framework can be used with children, families and carers to formulate health and management goals.

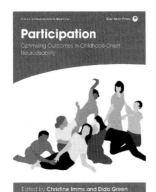

Participation: Optimising Outcomes in Childhood-Onset Neurodisability
Christine Imms and Dido Green (Editors)

Clinics in Developmental Medicine
2020 ▪ 288pp ▪ hardback ▪ 978-1-911612-17-9

This unique book focuses on enabling children and young people with neurodisability to participate in the varied life situations that form their personal, familial and cultural worlds. Chapters provide diverse examples of evidence-based practices and are enriched by scenarios and vignettes to engage and challenge the reader to consider how participation in meaningful activities might be optimised for individuals and their families. The book's practical examples aim to facilitate knowledge transfer, clinical application and service planning for the future.

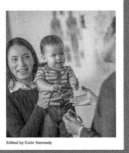

Principles and Practice of Child Neurology in Infancy, 2nd Edition
Colin Kennedy (Editor)

A Practical Guide from Mac Keith Press
2021 ▪ 552pp ▪ softback ▪ 978-1-911612-00-1

Management of neurological disorders presenting in infancy poses many challenges for clinicians. Using a symptom-based approach, and covering a wide range of scenarios, the latest edition of this comprehensive practical guide provides authoritative advice from distinguished experts. It now includes revised coverage of disease prevention, clinical assessment, and promotion of neurodevelopment.

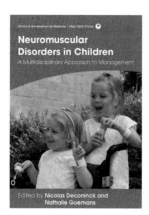

Neuromuscular Disorders in Children: A Multidisciplinary Approach to Management
Nicolas Deconinck and Nathalie Goemans (Editors)

Clinics in Developmental Medicine
2019 ▪ 468pp ▪ hardback ▪ 978-1-911612-09-4

Neuromuscular Disorders in Children: A Multidisciplinary Approach to Management critically reviews current evidence of management approaches in the field of neuromuscular disorders (NMDs) in children. Uniquely, the book focusses on assessment as the cornerstone of management and highlights the importance of a multidisciplinary approach.

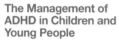
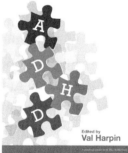

The Management of ADHD in Children and Young People
Val Harpin (Editor)

A Practical Guide from Mac Keith Press
2017 ▪ 292pp ▪ softback ▪ 978-1-909962-72-9

This book is an accessible and practical guide on all aspects of assessment of children and young people with Attention Deficit Hyperactivity Disorder (ADHD) and how they can be managed successfully. The multi-professional team of authors discusses referral, assessment and diagnosis, psychological management, pharmacological management, and co-existing conditions, as well as ADHD in the school setting. New research on girls with ADHD is also featured. Case scenarios are included that bring these topics to life.

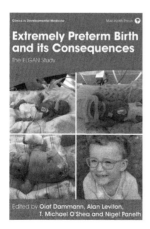

Extremely Preterm Birth and its Consequences: The ELGAN Study
Olaf Dammann, Alan Leviton, Thomas Michael O'Shea and Nigel Paneth (Editors)

Clinics in Developmental Medicine
2020 ▪ 256pp ▪ hardback ▪ 978-1-911488-96-5

The ELGAN (Extremely Low Gestational Age Newborns) Study was the largest and most comprehensive multicentre study ever completed for this population of babies born before 28 weeks' gestation. The authors' presentation and exploration of the results of the research will help clinicians to prevent adverse health outcomes and promote positive health for these children.

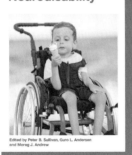

Nutrition and Neurodisability
Peter B. Sullivan, Guro L. Andersen and Morag J. Andrew (Editors)

A Practical Guide from Mac Keith Press
2020 ▪ 208pp ▪ softback ▪ 978-1-911612-26-1

Feeding difficulties are common in children with neurodisability and disorders of the central nervous system can affect the movements required for safe and efficient eating and drinking. This practical guide provides strategies for managing the range of nutritional problems faced by children with neurodevelopmental disability. The easily accessible information on aetiology, assessment and management is informed by a succinct review of current evidence and guidelines to inform best practice.

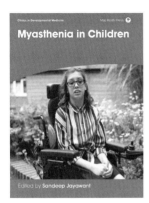

Myasthenia in Children
Sandeep Jayawant (Editor)

Clinics in Developmental Medicine
2019 ▪ 144pp ▪ hardback ▪ 978-1-911612-30-8

Myasthenia is a rare, but underdiagnosed and sometimes life-threatening disorder in children. There are no guidelines for diagnosing and managing these children, especially those with congenital myasthenia, a more recently recognised genetic condition, but there have been significant developments in identification and treatment of myasthenia in recent years. This book will help clinicians and families of children with this rare condition direct management effectively.

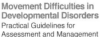
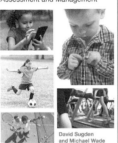

Movement Difficulties in Developmental Disorders
David Sugden and Michael Wade (Authors)

A Practical Guide from Mac Keith Press
2019 ▪ 240pp ▪ softback ▪ 978-1-909962-95-8

This book presents the latest evidence-based approaches to assessing and managing movement disorders in children. Uniquely, children with developmental coordination disorder (DCD) and children with movement difficulties as a co-occurring secondary characteristic of another development disorder, including ADHD, ASD, and Dyslexia, are discussed. It will prove a valuable guide for anybody working with children with movement difficulties, including clinicians, teachers and parents.